Tarascon General Surgery Pocketbook

From the publishers of the *Tarascon Pocket Pharmacopoeia*®

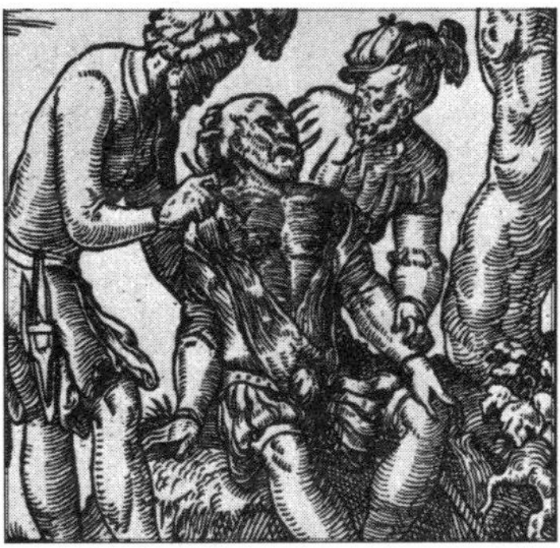

James A. Chambers, MD, MPH
Lt Col, USAF, MC, SFS
Staff Surgeon
San Antonio Military Health System
San Antonio, TX

JONES & BAR
LEARNING

World Headquarters
Jones & Bartlett Learning
5 Wall Street
Burlington, MA 01803
978-443-5000
info@jblearning.com
www.jblearning.com

Jones & Bartlett Learning books and products are available through most bookstores and online booksellers. To contact Jones & Bartlett Learning directly, call 800-832-0034, fax 978-443-8000, or visit our website, www.jblearning.com.

Substantial discounts on bulk quantities of Jones & Bartlett Learning publications are available to corporations, professional associations, and other qualified organizations. For details and specific discount information, contact the special sales department at Jones & Bartlett Learning via the above contact information or send an email to specialsales@jblearning.com.

Production Credits

Executive Publisher: Christopher Davis
Senior Acquisitions Editor: Nancy Anastasi Duffy
Associate Editor: Laura Burns
Production Assistant: Leia Poritz
Marketing Manager: Rebecca Rockel
Manufacturing and Inventory Control Supervisor: Amy Bacus
Composition: Exemplarr Worldwide Ltd.
Cover Design: Kristin E. Parker
Cover Image: © Courtesy of The National Library of Medicine
Printing and Binding: Malloy, Inc.
Cover Printing: Malloy, Inc.

ISBN: 978-1-4496-2862-8

6048

Printed in the United States of America
16 15 14 13 12 10 9 8 7 6 5 4 3 2 1

DEDICATION

Dedicated to Sylvia, Neil, Brette, and my parents. Your love and patience have made everything possible.

Thank you to Drs. Robert McClelland and Gary Purdue for your encouragement and example.

CONTENTS

EDITORIAL BOARD

Affiliations are given for information purposes only, and no affiliation sponsorship is claimed. James A. Chambers, MD, MPH authored this book in his private capacity. The views expressed in this book do not necessarily represent the views of either the United States Air Force or the United States Government.

A NOTE FROM THE AUTHOR

Tarascon General Surgery Pocketbook is intended as a quick reference for the practice of general surgery. It represents a compilation of facts and techniques that I have found useful and are referenced where thought to be particularly important. If you find an error or wish to make a suggestion, please let us know (email: editor@tarascon.com).

CHAPTER 1

FLUIDS, ELECTROLYTES, METABOLISM, AND NUTRITION

I. FLUIDS

A. **24 h:** 100 mL/kg for 1st 10 kg (1000 mL), 50 mL/kg for 2nd 10 kg (500 mL), 20 mL/kg thereafter.

B. **Per h:** 4 mL/kg for 1st 10 kg (40 mL), 2 mL/kg for 2nd 10 kg (20 mL), 1 mL/kg thereafter.

C. **Body fluids and IVF composition:**

TABLE 1.1. Body Fluid Volume and Composition

Source	Vol/24h	Osm	Na^+	Cl^-	K^+	Bicarb
Saliva	1000	Hypo	30–80	70	20	30
Stomach	1000–2000	Hypo	60–80	100	15	0
Pancreas	1000	Iso	140	60–90	5–10	40–100
Bile	1000	Iso	140	100	5–10	40
Small Bowel	2000–3000*	Iso	140	100	20	25–50
Large Bowel	200–1500	Hypo	75	30	30	0
Sweat	200–1000	Hypo	20–70	40–60	5–10	0

*Ileostomy initially puts out up to 1–2 L/d, gradually slows to 500–800 cc/d.

TABLE 1.2. Crystalloid Composition

Crystalloid	Kcal / L	Osm	Na^+	Cl^-	K^+	Ca^{++}	Mg^{++}	Lactate
NS (0.9%)	0	Iso	154	154	0	0	0	0
D5W	170	Hypo	0	0	0	0	0	0
LR	9	Iso	130	109	4	1.5	0	28
Plasmalyte	21	Iso	140	98	5	0	3	*
D5 ½ NS	170	Hypo	77	77	0	0	0	0
D5 ⅓ NS	170	Iso			0	0	0	0
D5 ¼ NS	170	Iso	38	38	0	0	0	0
3% NS	0	Hyper	513	513	0	0	0	0

*Plasmalyte uses 27 mEq of acetate and 23 mEq of gluconate as buffers instead of lactate. One advantage of Plasmalyte over RL is its lack of calcium, which makes RL incompatible w/ blood infusions.

TABLE 1.3. Appropriate Replacement Fluids

Maintenance	D5 1/2 NS w/ 20 KCl
Traumatic hypovolemia	LR
Stomach	D5 1/2 NS w/ 20 KCl
Emesis/ NGT	LR
Biliary	D5 LR w/ 25 mEq/L HCO_3 (1/2 amp/L)
Pancreatic	D5 LR w/ 50 mEq/L HCO_3 (1 amp/L)
Diarrhea, secretory	D5 LR w/ 15 mEq/L HCO_3

*Note: for pediatric pts, maintenance fluid of D5 1/4 NS w/ 20 KCl is appropriate for up to age 5.

D. Body fluid composition/rate:

1. *Total body water* (TBW): overall average, 55% body wt is water.
   a. 35% is intracellular, 20% extracellular, 16% interstitial, 4% intravascular.
2. *GI fluids*:
   a. Hypotonic from mouth to upper esophagus and in colon at low rates
   b. Isotonic from stomach through small intestines and in colon at massive rates
   c. *Acid*: stomach—2/3 of Na^+ replaced by H^+, full amount of Cl^-, little HCO_3^-
   d. *Alkaline*: lower GI, w/ full Na^+, part of the Cl^- replaced by HCO_3^- (80–90 Cl^-, 30–50 HCO_3^-)

II. ELECTROLYTES

A. Sodium: normal is 140 (135–145).

1. *Plasma osmolality* = $(2 \times Na^+)$ + (Glucose/18) + (Bun/2.8).
2. *Hypernatremia* can result from loss of hypotonic fluids or gain of hypertonic fluids.
   a. Therapy depends on extracellular fluid status.
      i. *Sx of possible metabolic encephalopathy*: altered MS, generalized seizures, and focal neuro deficits.
   b. If pt does not have invasive monitors, consider:
      i. *Recent loss of wt?* (suggests decreased ECV if no edema)
      ii. *Peripheral edema?* (suggests increased ECV if adequate proteinemia)
      iii. *Spot sodium < 10 mEq/L?* (suggests decreased ECV)
   c. *Low ECV* (most common): from loss of hypotonic fluids. Total Na^+ is *decreased* (lost sodium but even more free water), must replace quickly; follow by replacing the free water deficit more slowly.
      i. Crystalloid of choice is isotonic saline, *not* hypotonic.
      ii. Once hypovolemia is corrected, replace the free water deficit:
         - Calculate *normal TBW*.
            - *For hypernatremia*: male TBW → lean body kg × 0.5; female TBW → lean body kg × 0.4. (When not in this circumstance, males are 60% and females 50%.)
         - Calculate *current TBW*: normal TBW × (140/current P_{Na}).
         - Calculate *TBW deficit* (L): normal TBW – current TBW.
         - Calculate *replacement volume* (L): TBW deficit × (1/1 – X). (*Note*: X = Na^+ in replacement fluid / 154.)
      iii. *Replace volume*: free water deficit should be replaced over 48–72 h.
   d. *Normal ECV*: from net loss of free water, usu. when hypotonic fluid is replaced w/ isotonic saline 1:1. Slowly replace the free water deficit.
      i. Can also occur w/ diabetes insipidus (DI), w/ dilute urine but hypertonic plasma; confirmed if complete fluid restriction does not increase urine osm > 30 mOsm/L w/in hours. Vasopressin (5 U IV) can differentiate between the 2 types.
         - *Central DI* (secondary to closed head injury, meningitis, hypoxic encephalopathy): urine osm often < 200; vasopressin increases by 50+% urine osmolality very quickly.

- *Nephrogenic DI* (secondary to hypokalemia, aminoglycosides, amphotericin, iodinated contrast, or polyuric ATN): urine osm usu. 200–500, unaffected by vasopressin.

ii. *Tx for DI*: replace free water only. Calculate TBW deficit, replace over 2–3 d to reduce risk of cerebral edema. If central DI, then generally need to give 5–10 U aqueous vasopressin SC every 6–8 h (monitor Na^+ carefully).

e. *High ECV*: from gain of hypertonic fluids. Seen w/ excessive use of hypertonic saline, sodium bicarbonate, or PO salt. May need furosemide and replace w/ fluids relatively hypotonic to the urine (usu. ~ 75 mEq/L of Na^+ in urine from furosemide diuresis).

3. *Hyponatremia*: therapy depends on volume status, urine sodium, and if sx present. In general, pts w/ low urine sodiums are easier to manage as body trying to retain sodium. Major risk is potentially irreversible encephalopathy from cerebral edema.

a. *Pseudohyponatremia*:

i. Not an issue if using ion-specific electrodes (encountered w/ older, flame emission spectrophotometry).

ii. *Hypertriglyceridemia*: mEq/L decrease in plasma sodium = plasma triglycerides (g/L) × 0.002.

iii. *Hyperproteinemia*: mEq/L decrease in plasma sodium = plasma protein – 8 (g/dL) × 0.025.

b. True hyponatremia is, like hypernatremia, classified by ECV status.

i. *Low ECV (hypovolemic)*: from fluid losses that are insufficiently replaced by fluids that are hypotonic relative to the lost fluids. A spot urine sodium may be useful:

TABLE 1.4. Interpretation of Spot Urine Sodium in Hypovolemia

Urine Sodium	Site of Sodium Loss
> 20 mEq/L	Renal (diuretics, adrenal insufficiency)
< 20 mEq/L	Extrarenal (diarrhea, vomiting)

- Infuse hypertonic (3%) saline if symptomatic, and normal saline if asymptomatic.

ii. *Normal ECV (isovolemic)*: from gain of up to 5 L of excess water that is not clinically apparent. Spot urine sodium and urine osmolality can be helpful:

TABLE 1.5. Interpretation of Spot Urine Sodium and Osmolality

U Na^+	U Osm	Etiology
> 20	> 100	SIADH (plasma tonicity usu. < 290 also)
< 10	< 100	Water intoxication

- Combine furosemide diuresis w/ infusion of hypertonic saline if symptomatic, or w/ normal saline if asymptomatic.

iii. *High ECV (hypervolemic)*: gain water > gain Na^+. Spot urine sodium can be helpful, although diuretics can confuse the situation.

TABLE 1.6. Interpretation of Spot Urine Sodium in Hypervolemia

U Na^+	Etiology
< 20	Extrarenal (cardiac failure, cirrhosis)
> 20	Renal failure

- Start furosemide diuresis if asymptomatic; combine w/ judicious use of hypertonic saline if sx.

c. Major concern w/ rapid correction is central pontine myelinolysis. To avoid, in plasma Na^+ should NOT > 0.5 mEq/L/h and final plasma Na^+ should not > 130 mEq/L.

i. *Calculate sodium deficit in mEq*: normal TBW × (130 – current PNa).

- TBW men = 0.6 × lean body wt kg . . . TBW women = 0.5 × kg.
  - *Calculate replacement volume* based on [Na^+] in replacement fluid.

- *Calculate infusion time in hours*: (130 – current PNa) / 0.5 mEq/H.
- *Calculate infusion rate*: (replacement vol)/(infusion time).

d. Rarely, profound alkalemia (i.e., pH > 7.5) may need to be initially lowered relatively rapidly w/ 0.1 N HCl through a central vein.
   i. Hydrogen deficit (mEq) = 0.3 × wt (kg) × (measured bicarb – desired bicarb).
      - An appropriate goal for initial desired bicarb is 35.
      - Rate of hydrogen replacement = 0.2 mEq/kg/h.
      - Using 0.1 N hydrochloric acid (H^+ = 100 mEq/h):
         - Volume (L) = hydrogen deficit/100.
         - Infusion rate (L/h) = 0.2 × wt (kg)/100.

B. Potassium: normal is 4 (3.5–4.5).

1. *Hypokalemia*
   a. *Etiology*: K^+ ⟶ inside cell w/ alkalosis, insulin/anabolism, adrenergic state (can occur w/ beta agonist inhalers), and hypothermia. Most diuretics, steroids, hyperaldosteronism ⟶ renal loss of K^+.
   b. *Presentation*: ileus, asthenia. *EKG*: ↑ digitalis effect, flat/inverted T waves, QT prolongation, ST segment depression. Nephrotoxic if chronic.
   c. *Tx*:
      i. Keep above 4 in critically ill pts. Give as KCl (20, 40, 60 mEq) or KPhos (15, 30, 45 mmol).
      ii. Usu. keep administration < 10 mmol/h, although 2× this rate is tolerated.
      iii. Only 2% of body K^+ is extracellular and deficit of 200–400 mmol ↓ serum [K^+] by only 1 mmol/L. After initial 1 mmol ↓, higher total losses (200–400 mmol) required to ↓ K^+. Only 100–200 mmol ↑ in total K^+ required to ↑ normal [K^+] by 1 mmol/L increments.
      iv. *Acidosis*: if prolonged, body will lose lots of K in urine. Watch for hypokalemia if rapidly correct prolonged acidosis.
      v. *Alkalosis*: although little plasma K^+, kidney must trade to retain Na^+ (harder to retain HCO_3^- to balance or trade H^+ in alkalosis, so K^+ is used instead), ⟶ urinary loss. Eventually, when K^+ gets too low, kidneys will revert to trading H^+ again, resulting in *paradoxical aciduria* (strong sign of total K^+ depletion).
         - *Note*: difficult to reverse alkalosis w/out first correcting K^+ deficit, as kidneys continue to trade H^+ to retain Na^+ (or resorb HCO_3^- to balance) if not enough K^+ to do the job.
         - *Note*: impossible to correct K^+ deficit w/ KCl alone if Mg^{++} is deficient. First replace the Mg^{++} (important to replace Mg^{++} for hypocalcemic pts as well).
2. *Hyperkalemia*
   a. K^+ released w/ acidosis, starvation/catabolism, and cell death.
   b. Manifests as paralysis, loss of deep tendon reflexes. *EKG*: peaked T waves (esp. in precordial leads), ↑ PR interval +/– widened QRS. Arrhythmias, ultimately VFib. Increases action of digitalis (tx w/ 2 g IV $MgSO_4^-$ NOT Ca^{++}, +/– digitalis Ab).
   c. *Tx*:
      i. *Ca^{++} chloride*, 500–1000 mg IVP (5–10 cc of 10% solution).
         - Protects heart from dysrhythmias.
         - Effects in 1–3 min, lasting 30–60 min.
      ii. 1 ampule D_{50} (50 cc) + 10 U regular *insulin* IVP.
         - Effects in 30 min, lasting 4–6 h.
      iii. Nebulized *albuterol*, 10–20 mg nebulized over 15 min.
         - Effects in 15 min, lasting 15–90 min.
      iv. *$NaHCO_3$* 1 mEq/kg IVP.
         - Effects in 5–10 min, lasting 1–2 h.
      v. Consider *furosemide*, 40–80 mg IVP.
      vi. Consider *Kayexalate*, 20–50 g PO in (50 cc) or PR (retention enema) in (200 cc) 20% sorbitol.
         - Effects in 1–2 h, lasting 4–6 h.
      vii. If above fails, consult for *dialysis*.

C. Cl^-: normal is 100 (99–109).

1. *Hyperchloremia*
   a. W/ inpts, usu. due to excess IV NS → non-gap metabolic *acidosis*. *Tx*: change IVF (i.e., Na^+ acetate).
2. *Hypochloremia*
   a. May be from excess GI losses (i.e., gastric outlet obstruction) or volume contraction. Freq. assoc. w/ *alkalosis*. Spot urine Cl^- may help determine if alkalosis will be chloride-responsive.
      i. *Chloride-responsive alkalosis* (most common w/ inpts): ↓ U Cl^- (< 15 mEq/L), usu. from gastric losses, diuretics, intravascular volume ↓, or metabolic compensation for respiratory acidosis. *Note*: diuretic usage can sometimes result in chloride-responsive alkalosis w/ a high U Cl^-. Tx w/ IV NS:
         - Chloride deficit (mEq) = 0.3 × wt (kg) × (100 – plasma [Cl^-])
         - Volume of NS (0.9% saline) to administer = chloride deficit/154
      ii. *Chloride-resistant alkalosis*: ↑ U Cl^- (> 25 mEq/L), usu. from K^+ depletion a/o excess mineralocorticoid activity; assoc. w/ volume expansion. Pts usu. euchloremic.

D. Calcium (*total* 8.0–10.2 mg/dL or 2.2–2.5 mmol/L; *ionized* 2.5–5.0 mg/dL or 0.8–1.6 mmol/L).

1. ~ 50% bound to plasma proteins (80% is albumin). Ionized fraction is physiologically active. Hypoproteinemia decreases total Ca^{++}, but does not affect the ionized fraction.
2. *Hypocalcemia* (50–65% of ICU admissions)
   a. *Etiology*: alkalosis, blood transfusions, cardiopulmonary bypass, drugs (aminoglycosides, cimetidine, heparin, theophylline), fat embolism, magnesium depletion, pancreatitis, renal insufficiency, sepsis.
      i. Corrected serum Ca^{++} mg/dL = serum Ca^{++} mg/dL (0.8 × [4.0 – albumin g/dL]).
   b. *Clinical effects*
      i. *Neuromuscular excitability*: hyperreflexia, seizures, tetany. Chvostek sign is nonspecific (25% in normal adults), Trousseau sign insensitive (30% false-negative).
   c. *Cardiovascular*
      i. Hypotension, decreased CO, ventricular ectopy (ionized Ca < 0.65 mmol/L assoc. w/ VTach and refractory hypotension).
   d. *Tx*:
      i. IV Ca^{++} only indicated for symptomatic hypocalcemia or ionized level < 0.65 mmol/L.
      ii. 10% Ca^{++} chloride or 10% Ca^{++} gluconate. Ca^{++} chloride has 3× the elemental Ca^{++} (27 mg/mL vs 9 mg/mL), but is also much more osmolar (2000 vs 680 mOsm/L).
      iii. Because of high osmolarity, give either form through central vein if possible; if not, use Ca^{++} gluconate through peripheral vein.
      iv. Bolus 200 g elemental Ca^{++} (in 100 mL NS over 10 min); as levels will fall again after 30 min, f/u w/ an infusion of 1–2 mg/kg/h elemental Ca^{++} for at least 6 h.
      v. Maintain w/ dosage of 2–4 g/d in adults orally w/ calcium carbonate or calcium gluconate tabs.
      vi. Treat any assoc. Mg^{++} depletion as well as hypomagnesemia that impairs PTH release and end-organ responsiveness.
3. *Hypercalcemia*
   a. 90% from malignancy or hyperparathyroidism. Occ. from prolonged immobility, thyrotoxicosis, or drugs (lithium, thiazide diuretics).
   b. Clinical effects (usu. if serum Ca^{++} > 12 mg/dL or ionized Ca > 3.0 mmol/L).
      i. *Gastrointestinal*: N/V, constipation, ileus, pancreatitis.
      ii. *Cardiovascular*: hypovolemia, hypotension, shortened QT interval.
      iii. *Renal*: polyuria, urolithiasis.
      iv. *Neuro*: confusion, depressed consciousness, coma.
   c. *Tx*: (if symptomatic or serum Ca^{++} > 14 mg/dL or ionized Ca > 3.5 mmol/L).
      i. *Saline infusion*: first step as hypercalcemia leads to an osmotic diuresis.
      ii. *Furosemide*: give w/ saline as 40–80 mg IV q 2 h to achieve 100–200 mL/min, which MUST be replaced w/ NS.

iii. *Calcitonin*: most effective for cases of bone resorption (i.e., from cancer). Use salmon calcitonin, 4 U/kg SQ or IM q 12 h. Effects w/in a few hours, but are mild (0.5 mmol/L).

iv. *Hydrocortisone*: most useful for multiple myeloma or renal failure, esp. if given w/ calcitonin. Usu. 200 mg IV daily in 2–3 divided doses.

v. *Bisphosphonates*: more potent than calcitonin, but delayed onset. Pamidronate is agent of choice, given as 90-mg IV infusion over 24 h; peak effect in 4–5 d; can also be repeated in 4–5 d.

vi. *Plicamycin*: more potent than calcitonin, but delayed onset. 25 mcg/kg IV over 4 h, can be repeated in 24–48 h. Less often used than bisphosphonates because of side effects (i.e., bone marrow suppression).

vii. *Dialysis*: for pts w/ renal failure.

E. Magnesium

1. *Range*:
   a. *Total* (1.4–2.0 mEq/L or 0.7–1.0 mmol/L).
   b. *Ionized* (0.8–1.1 mEq/L or 0.4–0.6 mmol/L).
   c. *Urinary* (5–15 mEq/24 h or 2.5–7.4 mmol/24 h).
2. Helps maintain cell gradient and calcium movement in smooth muscle. < 1% in the plasma (50% in bone)—can have total body depletion w/ normal plasma levels. In these cases, urine Mg^{++} will be abnormally low, however. 55% is in the ionized, active form; most assays only report total Mg^{++}, though.
3. *Hypomagnesemia*: up to 65% ICU pts.
   a. Caused by furosemide (most common), aminoglycosides, amphotericin, digitalis, cisplatin, cyclosporine, secretory diarrhea, chronic alcoholism, diabetes mellitus, acute MI.
   b. *Findings*: *hypokalemia* (40%; often need to fix Mg^{++} before K^+ can be fixed), *hypophosphatemia* (30%; often *causes* Mg^{++} depletion), *hyponatremia* (27%), *hypocalcemia* (22%; again may need to fix Mg^{++} before Ca^{++}), *thiamin deficiency*.
      i. *Cardiac*: ischemia, arrhythmias, digitalis toxicity. Mg^{++} infusion can often stop digitalis toxicity and refractory arrhythmias even in absence of hypomagnesemia.
      ii. *Neurologic*: altered mentation, generalized seizures, tremors, and hyperreflexia. Reactive CNS syndrome presents w/ ataxia, slurred speech, metabolic acidosis, excessive salivation, diffuse muscle spasms, seizures, and obtundation.
   c. *Tx*: if sx (+) or severe deficiency, IV route preferred. If renal insufficiency, reduce doses by $^1/_2$, monitor.
      i. *Mild*, asymptomatic cases.
         - Assume deficit of 1–2 mEq/kg.
         - Assume 50% replacement lost in urine; need to replace twice the deficit.
         - Replace 1 mEq/kg the 1st 24 h, then 0.5 mEq/kg/d and over the next 3–5 d.
         - If serum Mg^{++} > 1 mEq/L, can use oral Mg^{++}.
      ii. *Moderate* cases (serum Mg^{++} < 1, or other electrolyte problems).
         - Add 6 g $MgSO_4$ (48 mEq Mg^{++}) to 250–500 mL of NS, infused over 3 h.
         - Follow w/ 5 g $MgSO_4$ (40 mEq Mg^{++}) in 250–500 mL NS, infused over 6 h.
         - Continue w/ 5 g $MgSO_4$ every 12 h by continuous infusion for the next 5 d.
      iii. *Life-threatening* cases (seizures or serious arrhythmias).
         - Infuse 2 g $MgSO_4$ (16 mEq Mg^{++}) IV over 2 min.
         - Follow w/ 5 g $MgSO_4$ (40 mEq Mg^{++}) in 250–500 NS infused over 6 h.
         - Continue w/ 5 g $MgSO_4$ every 12 h by continuous infusion for the next 5 d.
      iv. *Parenteral*: each gram of $MgSO_4$ has 8 mEq (4 mmol) of elemental Mg^{++}. Dilute w/ NS, not LR.
         - $MgSO_4$ 20%, 200 mg/mL (1.6 mEq/L).
         - $MgSO_4$ 10%, 100 mg/mL (0.8 mEq/L).
4. *Hypermagnesemia*
   a. Rare in absence of renal impairment (creatinine clearance < 30); massive hemolysis ↑ risk.
      i. DKA, adrenal insufficiency, hyperparathyroidism, Li^+ excess can also ↑ levels.

b. *Manifestation*: clinically, antagonize calcium's effects. Serum $Mg^{++} > 4$ mEq/L may cause hyporeflexia; > 5.0 prolongs AV conduction; > 10 → complete heart block; > 13 → cardiac arrest.

c. *Tx*:

i. Severe → hemodialysis.

ii. Calcium gluconate, 1 g IV over 2–3 min for temporary control of cardiac effects.

iii. If renal function is not impaired, aggressive IVF w/ furosemide can be useful.

F. **Phosphorus** (2.5 mg/dL or 0.8 mmol/L to 5.0 mg/dL or 1.6 mmol/L)

1. Inorganic state is predominantly intracellular; utilized in glycolysis and high-energy molecule formation.

2. *Hyperphosphatemia*

a. *Etiology*: usu. from renal insufficiency or massive cell necrosis (crush injury, tumor lysis, etc.). Less often from DKA.

b. *Manifestation*: may deposit calcium-phosphate complexes in soft tissue a/o calciphylaxis, typically when product of calcium and phosphorus levels exceeds 60–70.

c. *Tx*:

i. *Severe* → consider hemodialysis.

ii. *Mild/moderate*: aluminum-containing compounds (i.e., antacids, carafate, etc.), or, if pt is hypocalcific, calcium acetate tablets (PhosLo), given as 2 tablets 3 times per day (each tablet is 667 mg w/ 8.45 mg calcium).

3. *Hypophosphatemia*

a. *Etiology*:

i. Intracellular shift (usual cause), ↑ renal excretion, or ↓ gut absorption.

ii. *Glucose loading "refeeding syndrome"*: glucose transported w/ P into cells, clinically significant in malnourished pts starting parenteral or enteral feeds; effect starts 1st d, begins to plateau after 7–10 d. Also seen w/ respiratory alkalosis, which raises intracellular pH, stimulating glycolysis.

iii. Al-containing substances (sucralfate, Amphogel) bind inorganic P, preventing upper GI absorption.

iv. Hyperglycemia-induced osmotic diuresis → excessive renal losses of P, aggravated w/ insulin as it drives glucose (and thus phosphorus) into cells.

v. Beta agonists (i.e., bronchodilators) can also increase intracellular movement of P, though rarely significantly. Sepsis is assoc. w/ hypophosphatemia; mechanism not established.

b. *Manifestation*:

i. *Severe depletion can*:

- ↓ myocardial contractility.
- ↓ RBC deformability (leading to hemolytic anemia).
- ↓ 2,3-DPG (shifts oxyhemoglobin dissociation curve left; ↓ O_2 off-loading to tissues).
- ↓ glycolytic pathway and production of ATP.

c. *Tx*:

i. *IV replacement* if < 1.0 mg/dL or 0.3 mmol/L, or if cardiac dysfunction, respiratory failure, generalized weakness, or impaired tissue oxygenation.

ii. *Oral replacement*: Neutra-Phos or K-Phos, 1200–1500 mg PO_4 q d. Higher doses may cause diarrhea.

III. METABOLISM

A. **Glycolysis:** 1 mole glucose → 2 moles ATP + 2 moles lactic acid

B. **Lactic acid** (via pyruvate kinate) → pyruvate (via Krebs cycle)

C. **Krebs cycle:**

1. 2 moles of pyruvate (from 1 glucose → 2 lactate → 2 pyruvate) yields acetyl CoA that enters TCA cycle NADH + $FADH_2$ (water, CO_2, electrons, etc.).
2. NADH + $FADH_2$ enter electron transport chain → ATP.
3. Total yield of *1 mole glucose → 36 mole ATP*.

D. **Gluconeogenesis occurs via 2 pathways:**
   1. *Lactic acid* in muscles transported to liver, then via Cori cycle, is converted to pyruvate then → → *glucose*.
   2. Amino acids (*alanine* is predominant substrate for gluconeogenesis; alanine and phenylalanine actually increase during stress/starvation).
   3. Lipids do not participate in gluconeogenesis. Acetyl-CoA (breakdown product of lipids) unable to be converted to pyruvate.

E. **Tissue and fuel consumption**
   1. In absence of stress/starvation, tissues utilize glucose for energy.
   2. During stress/starvation, fat/ketones become primary source of energy.
   3. *Obligate glucose consumers*: RBC, WBC, adrenal medulla, peripheral nerves.
   4. *Facultative glucose consumer*: brain (usu. uses glucose, but can adapt to use ketones during starvation).
   5. No pt should go w/out nutrition > 7 d. Gut is preferred route to avoid immunologic, metabolic, and infectious complications.
   6. Feeding after prolonged starvation may result in "refeeding syndrome" w/ intacellular hunger for K^+, Mg^{++}, and PO_4^{---} resulting in low serum levels of these molecules. Gradual reintroduction of feeds may prevent this complication.

F. **Cori cycle:**
   1. *Gluconeogenesis*: liver > kidneys—function of Cori cycle is restore glucose from pyruvate.
   2. Converts pyruvate to oxaloacetate in mitochondrium. Oxaloacetate (→ malate [to cytosol] → oxaloacetate [cytosol]) → PEP → → glucose.
      a. Requires amino acids for majority.
      b. During starvation (oxaloacetate level is low, shunted to gluconeogenesis) acetyl-CoA is shunted from TCA cycle to form ketones (i.e., for brain).
      c. Fatty acid-derived acetyl-CoA cannot be converted back to pyruvate . . . not able to contribute to gluconeogenesis.
      d. Fatty acids fuel for heart, liver, skeletal muscle, can be oxidized in mitochondria (transport of acetyl-CoA via carnitine).
      e. Glutamine important for transport of nitrogen between organs.
      f. Alanine most important for gluconeogenesis, transported to liver and converted to pyruvate → → → glucose.

G. **Urea cycle:**
   1. Amine group that is discarded from alanine is eliminated, joins alpha ketoglutarate, which can go to TCA → ammonia.

IV. NUTRITION

A. **Calories**
   1. *Generally*: 30 kcal/kg/d. Most need about 2000–2500 kcal/d.
   2. *Alternately*, can use Harris-Benedict equation to determine basal metabolic rate:
      a. *Male* = 66 + (13.7 × wt in kg) + (5 × ht in cm) – (6.8 × age in yr).
      b. *Female* = 65.5 + (9.6 × wt in kg) + (1.7 × ht in cm) – (4.7 × age in yr).
   3. *Add*: 10% for head injury, 30% for polytrauma, 75% for sepsis, 150% for extensive burns.
   4. Calculate above kcals from carbohydrate or fats (up to 30% of total); do not include protein calories in this total.

B. **Protein:** in general need 0.66–1.2 g/kg/d minimum.
   1. 1 g protein = 4 kcal. However, plan for caloric needs to come from sugar or fat, as proteins use up some energy in metabolism.
   2. Protein is 16% nitrogen (or, conversely, 1 g N_2 = 6.25 g protein).
      a. Most pts need about 150 g nonprotein kcal per g nitrogen (150:1).
      b. Pts in renal failure may need a ratio of 400:1, while severely stressed pts may need up to 80:1.

3. Calculate nitrogen balance to determine if adequate protein needs are being met: + value means anabolic; – value means catabolic. N balance = ($N_{in} - N_{out}$) = ([prot/6.25] – [24 h urine N = 4 g]).
4. *Deficiency*
   a. *Syndromic*:
      i. Marasmus = pure caloric deficiency. Assoc. w/ normal WBC, transferrin, and albumin.
      ii. Kwarsiorkor = protein-calorie malnutrition, assoc. w/ depressed WBC, transferrin, and albumin.
   b. *Albumin*: goal < 3.5—single best prognostic nutritional marker. Half-life 21 d.
      i. < 3.0 = 23.7% 30 d mortality.
      ii. < 2.5 = 43% mortality.
      iii. < 2.1 = 62 % mortality.
   c. *Transferrin*: half-life 9 d. < 200 abnormal. Influenced by body iron levels.
   d. *Prealbumin*: half-life 3 d. < 15 abnormal.
   e. *Lymphocyte count* < 1500 mm^3.
   f. *Hypersensitivity skin test*: presence or absence of anergy has not consistently been shown to be useful as a preoperative marker.

C. Fats

1. 1 g fat = 9 kcal.
2. May be given as 2–5% daily calories (safflower or soybean oil) or ~ 40 g of emulsion weekly.
3. Infuse no faster than 0.1 g/kg/h to avoid hepatic dysfunction.
4. Avoid lipid emulsion if serum triglycerides exceed 400 mg/dL. Levels > 800 mg/dL may induce pancreatitis. Excess lipid infusion may also worsen ALI/ARDS.

D. Carbohydrates

1. Usu. 1 g carbohydrates = 4 kcal, but parenteral dextrose is 3.4 kcal.

E. Vitamin and mineral deficiency

1. *Vitamins*
   a. *Water soluble*
      i. *B_1 (thiamin)*:
         - "Beriberi" usu. from alcoholism (ethanol inhibits movement of thiamin from enterocyte into portal circulation) in United States; sx (anorexia, paresthesias, irritability, a/o muscle cramps) may be precipitated by beginning pts w/ marginal levels on IV dextrose solutions.
            - *"Wet" form*: cardiovascular sx (peripheral vasodilation, high-output heart failure, dyspnea, peripheral/pulmonary edema).
            - *"Dry" form*: nervous sx (paresthesias, hyporeflexia, pain, Wernicke-Korsakoff syndrome: nystagmus/ophthalmoplegia, ataxia, confusion, amnesia, etc.).
         - *Tx*: 100 mg thiamin daily.
      ii. *B_2 (riboflavin)*: angular stomatitis, glossitis, cheilosis, asthenia, anemia.
      iii. *Niacin (nicotinic acid)*: pellagra (dermatitis—dry, hyperpigmented, scaly; diarrhea; dementia) may develop after initial sx of anorexia, asthenia, and glossitis.
      iv. *B_6 (pyridoxine)*:
         - Assoc. w/ INH, penicillamine, OCPs, and alcoholism.
         - *Sx*: glossitis, sore mouth, cheilosis, asthenia, peripheral neuropathy, microcytic anemia.
      v. *B_{12} (cyanocobalamin)*:
         - Seen after gastric or ileal resection. Require parenteral B_{12}. Pernicious vs microcytic anemia if gastric resection, as stomach and duodenum have crucial role in iron absorption.
      vi. *C (ascorbic acid)*:
         - Poverty, cancer, smoking, CRF risk factors for clinically significant deficiency (scurvy).

- Early sx include fatigue and asthenia, but may progress to anemia a/o bleeding manifest as petechiae/purpura, hemarthroses, bleeding gums. Late cases demonstrate edema, neuropathy, and intracerebral hemorrhage.

b. *Fat soluble*

i. *A*: 5000 μg/d recommended.
- *Early*: night blindness, dry conjunctive (xerosis), white conjunctival patches (Bitot's spots).
- *Late*: keratomalacia, endophthalmitis, blindness.

ii. *D*: osteomalacia, rickets.
- *Tx orally w/ 50,000 U/wk × 8 wk*: IV replacement risks paradoxically include osteomalacia, although standard TPN dose of 200 U tolerated well.

iii. *E*: areflexia, gait disturbances, diminished proprioception/vibration sense, ophthalmoplegia.

iv. *K*: prolongation of PT commonly seen. Addressed w/ 10 mg vitamin K per wk.

v. *Essential fatty acids* (deficiency uncommon in obese pts): dry, flaky skin, red papules, alopecia.

2. *Minerals*

a. *Iron*: microcytic anemia.

i. Initiallly iron and ferritin ↓ and transferrin level ↑; later microcytic, hypochromic anemia as well.

ii. Usual daily dose is 15 mg PO or 1–2 mg parenterally.
- Replacement during active infection or inflammatory state may contribute to immunosuppression or facilitate bacterial proliferation.

b. *Copper*: microcytic anemia.

c. *Zinc*:

i. Catabolism, diarrhea/malabsorption increases risk; serum levels may be normal in the face of significant depletion.

ii. Rash, cutaneous anergy, *altered taste/smell*, impaired wound healing, hyperpigmentation of skin creases, neuritis, poor night vision, photophobia, etc., all reported.

iii. 6 mg/d given if normal GI function; up to 20 mg/d required if malabsorption/diarrhea.

d. *Calcium*: see section IID. above.

e. *Magnesium*: see section IIE. above.

f. *Selenium*: deficiency rare. Proximal muscle weakness, cardiomyopathy, hypopigmentation, and RBC macrocytosis possible.

g. *Chromium*: refractory hyperglycemia. Up to 150 mcg/d may be required for deficient pts.

F. RQ ratio: reflects amount of carbon dioxide produced per unit of oxygen consumed. 1 = carb; 0.7 = fat; 0.85 = protein.

G. Effects of starvation:

1. *Early (1st wk)*: up to 300 g of protein lost from skeletal muscle; hepatic glycogenolysis also provides a relatively small amount of glucose for energy (exhausted within 24 h). Fat conversion to free fatty acids and ketones represents the largest amount of available energy stores.
2. *Late (> 1 wk)*: proteolysis diminishes as lipolysis assumes even greater role for energy provision.

H. Enteral feeds:

1. Tube feed ordering and complications.

a. *Ordering*: begin w/ isotonic TF if possible at 20 cc/h, advance by 25 cc/h q 8 h until reach goal rate. Elevate HOB 30° or have 30° reverse Trendelenburg.

i. *NGT/Dobhoff*: check gastric residual q 4 h.

ii. *Nasojejunal tube*: place NGT to LCWS.

iii. If gastric residual > 500 cc, hold TF, refeed residual volume, and recheck residual volume in 2 h.
- If second volume < 500 cc, then resume TF at prior rate.
- If second volume > 500 cc, then hold TF and investigate further (i.e., AXR).

b. *Diarrhea*: ensure no laxatives in orders and minimize sorbitol (i.e., in elixirs), check for *C. difficile,* consider rectal tube, Imodium (i.e., 10 cc q 6 h).

TABLE 1.7. Enteral Feeds

Nutrients/L	Replete	Subdue	Boost Plus	Magnacal Renal	Choice DM	Isocal HN
Comments	Milk	Milk	Milk	Milk	Milk/soy	Milk/soy
Kcal/cc	1.00	1.00	1.52	2.0	1.06	1.06
Osmolality	300	330	720	570	300	270
Prot g/L	62.4	50	59	75	45	44
Fat g/L	34	34	58	101	51	45
Carbs g/L	113	130	200	200	119	124
Nonprot Kcal/N ratio	75:1	100:1	139:1	144:1	125:1	125:1
Water g/L	845	840	780	710	850	850

c. *Constipation*: minimize narcotic usage, consider AXR and rectal exam as well as bisacodyl (10 mg PR q d), senna (2 tabs per NGT 2 times per day), or Milk of Magnesia (30 cc per NGT q d).

d. *Refeeding syndrome*: watch for decrease in serum potassium and phosphorus.

2. Where and how is water/food digested and absorbed?

a. *Water*: small bowel absorbs 10–12 L/d, leaving ~ 500 cc to be absorbed in colon.

b. *Sodium*: primarily absorbed via active transcellular mechanisms (i.e., N^+-K^+ ATPase pump) in proximal small bowel. Passive absorption less significant.

c. *Carbohydrates*: salivary amylase begins digestion, which finishes in small bowel (pancreatic amylase, etc.) w/ absorption of 3 specific hexoses along brush border (glucose—Na^+ dependent and Na^+ independent; galactose—Na^+ dependent; and fructose—facilitated transport).

d. *Proteins*: digestion begun in stomach (pepsin), finished in small bowel by peptidases (require activation of pancreatic trypsinogen to trypsin by enterokinase from brush border). Direct absorption of both amino acids and oligopeptides possible through wide variety of uptake mechanisms.

e. *Fats*:

i. Triglycerides (glycerol w/ 3 fatty acid chains) constitute bulk of dietary fat.

ii. Digestion begins in stomach (acid hydrolysis, gastric lipase), but absorption extremely limited.

iii. Emulsification in duodenum w/ bile salts and phospholipids facilitates exposure to pancreatic lipase, which is responsible for brush border membrane absorption.

- *Micelles* contain free fatty acids, monoglycerides, and cholesterol in small spheres w/ hydrophobic core; interior contents absorbed at brush border into enterocytes, leaving bile salts in gut lumen.
- Alternately, short-chain and medium-chain fatty acids cross brush border directly by simple diffusion. Long-chain fatty acids require specific uptake mechanism.

iv. Inside enterocyte, fatty acids re-esterified back into triglycerides. These new triglycerides combine w/ apoprotein, cholesterol, and phospolipid to form *chylomicron* (fat-soluble vitamins included).

- Chylomicrons absorbed into lacteals, ultimately draining into thoracic duct and systemic venous system.
- Medium-chain and polyunsaturated fatty acids absorbed directly into portal circulation.

f. *Vitamins*:

i. *Water soluble*:

- *Vitamin C*: absorbed in small bowel via Na^+-dependent active transport mechanism.
- *Vitamin B_{12}*: absorption potentially inhibited at several steps.

- Bound to R protein in stomach; requires hydrolysis by pancreatic enzymes in duodenum.
- Intrinsic factor (from gastric parietal cells) protects from enzymatic destruction and serves as cofactor for absorption in terminal ileum.

ii. *Other water soluble* (thiamine, riboflavin, biotin, pantothenic acid): absorbed via Na^+-dependent mechanisms in small bowel.

iii. *Fat soluble* (A [retinol], D, E [tocopherols], K): absorbed in small bowel via passive diffusion; enter lymph in chylomicrons.

- *Vitamin D*:
  - D_3 *(cholecalciferol)*: results from UV-mediated activation of 7-dehydrocholesterol in skin and subsequently undergoes up to 2 hydroxylations:
    - *Liver* (first): to 25-hydroxycholecalciferol.
    - *Kidney* (second): to 1,25-dihydroxycholecalciferol.
  - D_2 *(ergocalciferol)*: most common form in foods.
- *Vitamin K*:
  - K_1 *(phytomenadione)*:
    - Obtained from dietary sources:
      - *High concentration*: alfalfa, spinach, Brussels sprouts, kale, broccoli, lettuce, soybeans, cabbage, beef liver, wheat bran, parsley.
      - *Medium concentration*: bacon, wheat germ, cheese, butter, avocado, pork liver.
    - Absorbed in small bowel via carrier-dependent, bile salt-facilitated process.
  - K_2 *(prenyl menaquinones)*: elaborated by colonic bacteria, passively absorbed.

g. *Minerals*

i. *Calcium*: absorbed predominantly via active transport in duodenum, also through passive diffusion in rest of small intestine. Vitamin D enhances primarily the latter.

ii *Magnesium*: absorbed mostly in the ileum through passive diffusion and carrier-mediated processes.

iii. *Iron*: primarily absorbed through divalent cation transporter in proximal duodenum (has affinity for broad range of divalent cations). In the gut, ferric (Fe^{+++}) iron must be reduced to ferrous (Fe^{++}) form by ferrireductase or ascorbic acid (vitamin C) for absorption.

I. TPN

1. *Indications*: enterocutaneous fistula, short gut syndrome, pancreatitis (although some advocate jejunal feeds), severe ARF, preoperative preparation of pts w/ > 15% wt loss (replete for 5–7 d [Detky AS, et al., *Ann Intern Med.* 1987;107:195; Buzby GP, *N Engl J Med.* 1991;325:525-32.]). Consider starting in adults if no anticipated enteral feeds w/in 1 wk, or in pediatrics w/in 3 d.
2. *Four step process to order* (many different ways to approach this):
   a. Determine amount of protein needed and volume.
   b. Determine amount of kcal from dextrose in volume.
   c. Make up what's lacking in kcals w/ lipids (10% solution = 1 kcal/cc).
   d. Choose electrolytes, other additives.
      i. *Note*: several studies suggest it is better to underfeed than overfeed in terms of kcals. Some studies also suggest fats may not be appropriate in critically ill pts.
3. *Protein* (0.8–1.4 g/kg/d in most people, often 1.5 g/kg/d in ICU pts though).
   a. 5% solution = 5 g/100 cc solution = 50 g/L.
4. *Dextrose* (70% solution in commercial products).
   a. 5% solution = 50 g/L = 170 kcal/L.
   b. 10% solution = 100 g/L = 340 kcal/L.
   c. 70% solution = 700 g/L = 2380 kcal/L.

5. *Fat*
   a. Provides supplemental calories w/ low RQ ratio and essential fatty acids.
   b. 10% solution = 1 kcal/mL; 20% solution = 2 kcal/mL.
   c. Limit to no more than 30% of total kcals.
6. *Electrolytes, other*
   a. Acute deficits should be added as IVPB.
   b. K^+, Na^+ offered w/ Cl^-, acetate as anions. To correct metacidosis, use acetate; to correct metalkalosis, choose Cl^-.
   c. *Daily requirements*:
      i. Na^+, K^+, Cl^- all are 1–2 mEq/kg/d.
      ii. Ca^{++} is 0.2–0.3 mEq/kg/d.
      iii. Mg^{++} is 0.25–0.35 mEq/kg/d.
      iv. Phosphate is 7–9 mmol/1000 kcal/d.
7. If available as total nutrient admixture ("3-in-1" solution), then lipid will already be added. In this case, determine how many kcals come from fat, then make up difference w/ dextrose. Alternatively, in some hospitals, 20% ft emulsions are given as a 250 mL dose 2–3 per wk.

J. **Nutrition adjuncts**

1. *Arginine*: semi-essential amino acid, may augment immune function and release of insulin and growth hormone. Precursor to nitric oxide, which has multiple effects, including vasodilatation and macrophage-mediated immune function.
2. *Glutamine*: primary fuel of small bowel (colon principally fueled by short-chain fatty acid butyrate). Levels fall rapidly during times of stress (i.e., trauma, bone marrow transplantation, etc.). However, specific repletion of glutamine has not demonstrated consistent benefit in literature, and may actually help support tumor cell populations that preferentially metabolize glutamine.
3. *Nucleic acid precursors* (purines, pyramidines): thought by some to be conditionally essential like arginine, but paucity of data for benefit from specific supplementation.
4. *Omega-3 fatty acids*: anti-inflammatory effect w/ beneficial clinical effects reported in myriad of conditions (osteoarthritis, postpartum depression, postcardiac arrhythmias). Cirrhotic pts in particular appear to immunologically benefit from augmentation of omega-3 fatty acids EPA and DHA.

CHAPTER 2

HEMATOLOGY

I. BLOOD COMPONENT THERAPY

A. General:

1. Transfusion indicated if continued hemodynamic instability after 2000 cc bolus or class III, IV shock.
2. In general, H/H (7/21) tolerated by healthy adults, elderly may be optimized at 10/30.
3. For stable pt, platelets of 20–40 K generally adequate, but in trauma pt w/ platelet dysfunction (secondary to hypothermia, massive [> 12 U blood] transfusion, excessive crystalloid dilutional coagulopathy, etc.), consider maintaining > 100 K.
4. In general don't give FFP unless correct hypothermia, acidosis first.

B. Components/products:

1. *Whole blood*: rarely given.
2. *PRBCs*: 300 cc. Each unit should increase Hgb and Hct by 1 and 3, respectively. Children often transfused in 10 cc/kg volumes. Stored in sodium citrate, which binds to and depletes calcium, and is converted to bicarb, potentially leading to alkalosis. "Washed" indicates additional removal of most leukocytes, platelets, and plasma.
3. *Platelets*: 50 cc. 6–10 U given at a time. Each unit should raise plt count 5000–10,000.
   a. *Absolute contraindication*: TTP.
   b. *Relative contraindications* (controversial): HIT, Glanzmann's thrombasthenia (consider giving NovoSeven, DIC).
4. *Fresh frozen plasma*: 250 cc. Adequate source of coagulation proteins, esp. II, V, VII, IX, XI. Do not go by PT/PTT for transfusion unless hypothermia, acidosis corrected.
5. *Cryoprecipitate*: contains factor VIII, von Willebrand factor, and fibrinogen. Not used much in trauma, but useful for von Willebrand's dz, hemophilia A, hypofibrinogenemia, factor XIII deficiency, DIC.
6. *Prothrombin complex concentrate* (PCC):
   a. Contains (vitamin K-dependent) factors II, VII, IX, X—useful for reversing warfarin, but unlike FFP, can be given more quickly (smaller volume and no need to thaw), and works more quickly—INR potentially corrects w/in 10 min; more expensive than FFP as well.
   b. Requires reconstitution. Dosing typically 8.8–50 IU/kg; lower dose typically sufficient for initial INR < 5. IV vitamin K should be co-administered to begin process of autogenous synthesis of factors.
7. *Recombinant factor VIIa* (NovoSeven): introduced in the United States in 1999.
   a. *FDA-approved indications*: hemophilia A or B w/ inhibitors to FVIII or FIX; tx of bleeding w/ FVII deficiency; prevention of bleeding in surgical procedures for both inhibitor pts and FVII-deficient pts.
   b. Widely reported for other uses include polytrauma pts as part of massive transfusion protocol and Glanzmann's thromasthenia. Dose of 2.4 mg assoc. w/ fewer thrombotic complications than 4.8 mg.

C. Caveats and complications of transfusion

1. Product incompatibility. Do not run RBCs w/ hypotonic (i.e., D5W) or calcium-containing IVF (i.e., LR) as will cause hemolysis or clumping, respectively.
2. *Immunologic*
   a. *Acute hemolytic reaction*: 1 per 12,000–25,000; from ABO incompatibility. Presents w/ fever, chills, hemoglobinuria, possibly hypotension and ARF. Laboratory c/w hemolysis (haptoglobin < 50, increased indirect bilirubin). Tx supportive, directed at preventing ATN w/ IVF, alkalinization of urine, +/– diuretics.
   b. *Delayed hemolytic reaction*: up to 2 wk posttransfusion; tx (F, C, anemia, hyperbilirubinemia); supportive care.

c. *Acute febrile nonhemolytic allergic reaction*: most common transfusion reaction—generally resulting from antibody response to leukocytes; tx w/ cessation of transfusion, antipyretics, and administration of leukocyte-poor products in future.

d. *Immunosuppression*: assoc. w/ nosocomial infections and increased levels of inflammatory cytokines.

e. *Transfusion-related acute lung injury* (TRALI): P:F ratio < 300 and bilateral infiltrates on CXR.

   i. 1:1500 transfusions, #1 cause of transfusion-related deaths; implicated products often to mulitiparous female donor.

   ii. Onset classically w/in 6 h of receiving product, esp. plasma. Clinically, P:F ratio < 300, hypotension, leukopenia, and bilateral infiltrates on CXR.

   iii. Supportive tx, no proven role for steroids.

f. *Posttransfusion purpura*:

   i. Typically manifests w/ thrombocytopenia 5–10 d after transfusion containing platelets.

   ii. Majority of pts are multiparous women, previously exposed to human platelet specific antigen.

   iii. Dx confirmed w/ immunologic testing.

   iv. *Tx*: high dose IVIG (2 g/kg) in divided doses over 2–5 d.

3. *Transmission of infectious agents*

   a. *Virus*:

      i. CMV most common (decreased risk if leukocyte reduced).

      ii. HIV, hepatitis C 1 per 2–2.6 million.

      iii. Hepatitis B 1 per 60,000.

   b. *Bacterial*: risk ~ 1 per 40,000 (some report 1 per 2000 plt transfusions).

   c. *Protozoan*: *Babesia microti*, *Trypanosoma cruzi* rarely reported.

4. *Metabolic and other complications*

   a. *Hyperkalemia*: a risk esp. in older units (limit 35 d w/out additives), if infused > 150 cc/min in face of oliguria/renal failure. See Chapter 1 for tx.

   b. *Hypocalcemia*: from citrate binding. Increased risk if > 1 U/5 min or if poor liver function (doesn't clear citrate). Tx w/ calcium gluconate for every 100 cc of citrated blood.

   c. *Hypothermia*: results in platelet dysfunction, respiratory and cardiac depression, leftward shift on oxygen dissociation curve, other deleterious effects.

   d. *pH derangements*: although older units of blood may in themselves be acidemic (as low as pH 6.7), large transfusions may result in alkalosis from citrate → bicarb. Increased systemic pH decreases ability to release O_2 (increased O_2 affinity) and decreases inotropy.

   e. *Tissue hypoxia*: in addition to alkalosis, oxygen off-loading may be compromised in older units of blood due to decreased levels of 2,3-DPG.

II. HEMOSTASIS

A. Steps in hemostasis:

1. Injury to vessel wall.
2. Primary vasoconstriction.
3. Primary hemostasis (formation of platelet plug).

   a. Independent of coagulation cascade.

   b. Adhesion of platelets to subendothelial collagen mediated by von Willebrand factor (found in plasma, platelets, subendothelial tissue) via glycoprotein Ia/IIa receptor, activating platelets.

   c. Activated platelets convert arachidonic acid to thromboxane A_2 via cyclo-oxygenase (NSAIDs inhibit this step), causing platelet aggregation and vasoconstriction. Platelets also release ADP from alpha granules, augmenting platelet aggregation.

   d. Activated platelets then bind to fibrinogen via glycoprotein IIa-IIIb complex.

4. Secondary hemostasis (stabilization of clot).

   a. *Extrinsic pathway*:

      i. Begins w/ activation of factor VII by tissue factor in exposed endothelium.

b. *Intrinsic pathway*:
   i. Begins w/ activation of factor XII (Hageman factor), high-molecular weight kinogen (HMWK), and prekallikrein (PK), which in turn activate factor XI that activates factor IX.
c. *Common pathway*:
   i. Both intrinsic and extrinsic pathways culminate in activation of factor X, which converts prothrombin to thrombin.
   ii. Thrombin converts fibrinogen to fibrin, which crosslink, reinforcing the platelet plug.

5. Clot dissolution, prevention of future thromboses.
   a. Platelet aggregation naturally inhibited by endothelial elaboration of nitric oxide (NO) and prostacyclin (PG_{12}).
   b. Naturally occurring heparin potentiates antithrombin III (AT III, also known simply as antithrombin), which inhibits thrombin generation.
   c. Protein C inhibits activation of factors VIII and V, potentiated by thrombomodulin (TM).
   d. Tissue plasminogen activator (tPA) is elaborated by endothelium, transforming plasminogen to plasmin, which affects fibrinolysis.

B. Assays for hemostasis

1. *Protime (PT)*
   a. Measures extrinsic (FVII) and common (FX, FV, FII) pathways.
   b. *Prolonged w/*:
      i. Isolated factor deficiency, vitamin K deficiency, hepatic insufficiency.
      ii. Vitamin K deficiency (biliary obstruction, Coumadin).
      iii. Vitamin K-dependent factors = II, VII, IX, X.
      iv. Hepatic insufficiency.
         - All factors (except VIII) and fibrinogen synthesized exclusively by liver.
2. *PTT*
   a. Measures intrinsic (PK, HMWK, FXII, FXI, FIX, FVIII) and common (FX, FV, FII) pathways.
   b. *Prolonged w/*:
      i. *Isolated factor deficiency*:
         - PK, HMWK deficiency actually *pro-thrombotic*.
         - VIII = hemophilia A, vWF; IX = hemophilia B.
      ii. *Heparin usage*: cofactor w/ antithrombin to inactivate II, X, IX, XI, XII.
      iii. *"Lupus anticoagulant*:*"* Ab that binds to phospholipids; not just in lupus pts, usu. *pro-thrombotic*.
      iv. *Hepatic insufficiency*:
         - 1:1 dilution w/ normal (control) plasma can be performed if unsure of etiology. If corrects, then factor deficiency; if persistent, then antibody is present (usu. VIII, IX, or X; can also be lupus anticoagulant).
3. *TT*
   a. Measures amount of time needed for thrombin to convert fibrinogen to fibrin.
   b. Indirect test for adequate fibrinogen level.
   c. Could bypass by ordering fibrinogen level.
   d. *Note*: fibrinogen deficiency can manifest w/ platelet dysfunction *and* PT/PTT prolongation.

C. Specific disorders of hemostasis (hypocoagulable state)

1. *von Willebrand dz*
   a. Most common hereditary bleeding diathesis.
   b. Deficiency or dysfunction of von Willebrand factor (functions in platelet adherence and carrier for factor VIII).
   c. Manifests as primarily a platelet dysfunction problem (mild operative bleeding d/o, epistaxis, etc.), but as vWF is a carrier for FXIII, can result in prolonged PTT as well; pts w/ multiple myeloma may cause deficient vWF as well.

d. *Tx*: DDAVP or cryoprecipitate.
   i. *Mild dz*: DDAVP (vasopressin analogue) is given to release vWF from endothelium.
      - DDAVP sometimes assoc. w/ vasoactive flushing, headaches, tachycardia.
   ii. *Mod–severe dz*: cryoprecipitate or concentrated VIII-vWF should be considered.

2. *Hemophilia A* (FVIII deficiency)
   a. Second most common hereditary bleeding diathesis. Sex-linked inheritance (same for hemophilia B).
   b. Goal is to replace to 100% level of FVIII.
   c. Mild cases may be treated w/ DDAVP.
   d. May have Ab to FVIII (always screen) → rFVII successfully used.
3. *Hemophilia B*, "Christmas disease" (FIX deficiency)
   a. Do not replace > 50% of FIX—assoc. w/ thromboses.
4. *Lupus*
   a. Occasionally assoc. w/ decreased prothrombin, and occasionally FVII from antibody. More often, have thrombocytopenia.
   b. *Tx*: high-dose corticosteroids, component replacement as necessary.
5. *Platelet functional disorders*
   a. *Bernard-Soulier syndrome*: rare, AR; mild thrombocytopenia, "giant" platelets, GP Ib deficiency (binding site for vWF)—unlike vW Dz, normal VIII.
   b. *Glanzmann's thrombasthenia*: rare, AR; plts lack GP IIb-IIIa (no crosslink w/ fibrinogen). Dx by abnormal response to platelet agonists.
   c. *Uremia*: inhibits vWF, GP Ib, GP IIb-IIIa. *Tx*: dialysis, DDAVP, estrogen, recombinant factor VII.
6. *Vitamin K deficiency*
   a. Usu. from abx that decrease gut bacteria that generate vitamin K, or in TPN-dependent pts. Hepatic insufficiency will often increase PT before PTT as FVII has shortest half-life.
   b. If need to correct immediately, FFP is given. Otherwise oral or vitamin K is adequate (SQ preferred over IV as latter assoc. w/ anaphylaxis in some studies).
7. *Factor X deficiency*
   a. Amyloidosis, multiple myeloma.
8. *Acidosis and hypothermia*: correct ASAP in bleeding pt w/ priority over transfusions.

D. Hypercoagulable states

1. *Inherited disorders*:
   a. *Factor V Leiden mutation* (most common inherited cause): resistance to activated protein C.
   b. Antithrombin deficiency (treat w/ heparin and FFP).
   c. Protein C, protein S deficiencies (prone to warfarin-induced skin necrosis).
   d. Hyperhomocysteinemia (treat w/ folate supplementation).
2. *Acquired disorders*:
   a. Cancer, pregnancy
   b. Surgery, trauma
   c. Immobilization
   d. Exogenous estrogen
   e. Hypercalcemia
   f. Heparin-induced thrombocytopenia
      i. Usu. occurs w/in 3 wk of heparin administration; can result in arterial "white clots."
      ii. Due to antibodies to platelet factor 4.
      iii. *Tx*: d/c heparin, begin argatroban, lepirudin, or bivalirudin.
   g. Anticardiolipin antibody
   h. Lupus anticoagulant (actually a *pro*-coagulant antibody)

E. Mixed states

1. Disseminated intravascular coagulation DIC

a. Results from dysfunctional overactivation of coagulation cascade w/ concomitant widespread thrombosis as well as fibrinolysis.
b. Clinically manifests as diffuse bleeding; death is usu. secondary to primary process or thromboses in critical organs.
c. Laboratory abnormalities include increased PT/PTT and thrombocytopenia, as well as hypofibrinogenemia.
d. Tx is focused on removing stimulus (i.e., sepsis, amniotic embolism). Blood products (PRBC, FFP, platelets, cryoprecipitate) are administered as needed.

F. **Adjuncts to achieve hemostasis:**
1. Topical
a. *Collagen based*: e.g., Avitene® (powder, sheet).
b. *Cellulose based*: e.g., Surgicel® (oxidized, in sheet or powder).
c. *Thrombin based*: Tisseel® (human thrombin + fibrinogen + bovine aprotinin + calcium chloride).
d. *Other*: Gelfoam® (pork skin gelatin in sponge, powder).
2. Systemic
a. *Amicar®* (ε-aminoaproic acid): inhibits conversion of plasminogen to plasmin, thus inhibiting fibrinolysis.
i. Frequently used to reverse effects of urokinase.

III. ANTICOAGULATION

A. **Indication:** refer to Table 2.1.
1. *Risk factors*: pelvic fx needing surgery or bed rest > 48 h; LE fx needing surgery or bed rest > 48 h; spinal cord injury; spinal column fx (excluding transverse/spinous process); LE venous injury proximal to popliteal fossa; anatomic head injury w/ GCS < 9; obesity (BMI > 30); pregnancy; h/o DVT/PE, hypercoagulable state, CA, or estrogen use; mechanical ventilation > 48 h; femoral line placed in ED; immobilization > 48 h; CVA.
a. If planned admission for > 48 h and have any of the above, then order:
i. LE venous duplex w/in 72 h of injury, then weekly surveillance. (*Note*: not needed if have IVC filter and contraindication to heparin.)
ii. SCDs or foot pumps (SCDs preferred).
iii. Lovenox 30 mg SC q 12 h. (*Exception*: if pt waiting for operative fixation of orthopedic *or* spine injuries or if have intracranial bleed, use unfractionated heparin 5000 U SC 2–3 times per day.)
• *Contraindications to heparin/LMWH*: craniotomy/intracranial bleed (5 d), ongoing hemorrhage, coagulopathy (INR > 1.5, PTT > 1.5 × control, plt < 100 K, clinical evidence), HIT, perispinal hematoma (5 d), major pelvic hematoma or retroperitoneal bleed (either requiring transfusion w/in last 5 d).
b. If have 2 or more risk factors and contraindication to heparin IVC filter. If age < 50 yo, can d/c filter and begin Lovenox once contraindication to anticoagulation resolves.
c. DVT prophylaxis—selected recommendations from ACCP (add more–i.e., surveillance, etc.): [Geerts WH, et al., Prevention of venous thromboembolism: the seventh ACCP conference on antithrombotic and thrombolytic therapy, *Chest*. 2004;126:338–400.]

B. **Mechanical**
1. Sequential compression devices (SCDs) more effective than foot pumps. Work principally by compressing veins (pt should ambulate as soon as possible postop), preventing stasis. No proven system fibrinolytic benefit from SCDs.

C. **Pharmacologic**
1. *Heparin*
a. Potentiates antithrombin III, which inhibits thrombin and factor Xa.
b. *Unfractionated*:
i. Give as a protocol infusion.
• For intraoperative vascular surgery, generally 5000–10,000 U IV (100–150 U/kg) during clamping of vessels is appropriate.

TABLE 2.1. Summary of 2008 ACCP DVT Prophylaxis Recommendations**

Risk Level	DVT % Calf / Proximal	PE % Clinical / Fatal	Rec. Prophylaxis
Low • Minor surg • < 40 yo • No risk factors*	2 / 0.4	0.2 / < 0.01	Early mobilization alone
Moderate • Minor surg • 40–60 yo w/out risk factors • Risk factors	10–20 / 2–4	1–2 / 0.1–0.4	LDUH (2 times per day), LMWH (< 3400 U/d), GCS, or IPC
High • > 60 yo • 40–60 w/ risk factors	20–40 / 4–8	2–4 / 0.4–1.0	LDUH (3 times per day), LMWH (> 3400 U/d), or IPC
Highest • Multiple risk factors • Hip/knee arthroplasty • HFS • Maj trauma/SCI	40–80 / 10–20	4–10 / 0.2–5	LMWH (> 3400 U/d), fondaparinux, oral VKA (INR 2–3), or IPC/GCS + LDUH/LMWH

*Risk factors (other than age > 40): prior VTE, cancer, molecular hypercoagulability. LDUH (low-dose unfractionated heparin), LMWH (low-molecular wt heparin), GCS (graded compression stockings), IPC (intermittent pneumatic compression devices), VKA (vitamin K antagonist—i.e., Coumadin).
**Geerts WH, et al., *Chest*. 2008;133(6suppl):381S–453S.

- For DVT/PE dosing, follow your hospital protocol, or, if not available, consider:
  - *Initial*: 70–80 U/kg IV bolus, then 15–18 U/kg/h. Check PTT in 6 h.
    - *PTT < 36*: 80 U/kg IV bolus, increase rate by 4 U/kg/h.
    - *PTT 36–60*: 40 U/kg IV bolus, increase rate by 2 U/kg/h.
    - *PTT 60–80*: maintain infusion.
    - *PTT 81–110*: decrease rate by 2 U/kg/h.
    - *PTT > 110*: hold infusion × 1 h, then decrease by 3 U/kg/h.
  - Continue at least 5 d *and* INR goals w/ warfarin achieved.

c. *Fractionated*:
   i. Better bioavailability, more predictable dose-response.
   ii. Usu. unnecessary to follow coagulation measurements, but level of factor Xa, not PTT is the appropriate assay if desired.
   iii. *For inpt tx of DVT a/o PE*: enoxaparin, 1 mg SQ q 12 h (or 1.5 mg/kg SQ q 24 h), continue at least 5 d *and* INR goals w/ warfarin achieved.

d. Reversed by protamine, usu. given as 1 mg protamine IV (over 10 min) per 100 mg of unfractionated heparin (or per 1 mg enoxaparin).
   i. *Side effect of protamine*: possible immunologically mediated hypotension (give in ICU setting).

e. Heparin-Induced thrombocytopenia (HIT), seen in 1–5% of pts exposed to heparin, usu. manifesting sx (decreased platelets from baseline, not necessarily below normal level; thrombosis) 10–14 d after initial exposure.
   i. *Tx*: D/C heparin of all forms.
   ii. Alternate anticoagulants for pts w/ HIT:
      - *Hirudin derivatives* (Lepirudin): analog of leech salivary anticoagulant, renal clearance. Dosage = 0.1 mg/kg/h w/ goal to achieve PTT 2× normal. If exceed this, stop × 2 h, then restart at 50% prior rate. If low, decrease by 20% and check PTT 4 h later.
      - *Argatroban*: hepatic clearance, same cost as low-dose hirudin. Half-life 4 h vs hirudin's 24-h (neither has an effective reversal agent). Follow w/ aPTT. Start at 2 mcg/kg/min,

titrate to aPTT 1.5–3 × baseline—don't exceed 10 mcg/kg/min or aPTT of 100 sec. If hepatic impairment, begin at 0.5 mcg/kg/min.

   f. Safe for use in pregnancy.

2. *Warfarin* (Coumadin)
   a. Inhibits gamma-carboxylation of vitamin K-dependent coagulation factors (II, VII, IX, X).
   b. Can cause paradoxical hypercoagulable state when first administered (for several days) as half-lives of protein C and protein S (vitamin K-dependent anticoagulant factors) are shorter than procoagulant factors. Thus, heparin should be used as a "bridge" for the first several days.
   c. Reversed by vitamin K (10 U IV/IM/PO) or 2–4 U FFP.
   d. Metabolized more slowly by the elderly, Asians, and those w/ hepatic dysfunction (depends on cytochrome p450—see Chapter 24). Dietary content of green, leafy vegetables should remain relatively constant.
   e. *INR goals*: DVT 2–3; AFib 2–3; post-MI 2.5–3.5; post-prosthetic valve placement 2–3.
   f. *Contraindicated* during pregnancy—teratogenic.
3. *Clopidogrel* (Plavix)
   a. Inhibitor of ADP-induced platelet aggregation by inhibitory binding of GP IIb/IIIa complex receptor.
   b. Indicated for recent MI, recent stroke, or established peripheral vascular dz, and usu. dosed as 75 mg PO q d.
4. *Pentoxifylline* (Trental)
   a. Poorly understood mechanism w/ hemorrheologic effects (decrease viscosity); also inhibits platelet activation and adhesion. Generally given as 300 mg PO 3 times per day w/ meals.
5. *Cilostazol* (Pletal)
   a. A phosphodiesterase III inhibitor, unknown mechanism (vasodilator, platelet effects?). 45–90% ↑ claudication distance.
6. *Acetylsalicylic acid* (aspirin)
   a. Irreversibly blocks prostacyclin synthetase (cyclooxygenase inhibitor), preventing formation of thromboxane A_2, a potent platelet.

IV. ANEMIA:

A. **Begin** w/ peripheral smear and classify as macrocytic (mean corpuscular volume [MCV] < 84) or microcytic (MCV > 96). Another useful index is mean corpuscular Hgb concentration = Hgb × 10/Hct (normal = 32–36%); hypochromia < 31%.
   1. Microcytic hypochromic anemia (MCV < 83, MCHC < 31%); see Table 2.2.

TABLE 2.2. Microcytic Hypochromic Anemia

	Serum iron	TIBC	Bone Marrow Iron	Misc.
Iron deficiency	↓	↑	0	Tx w/ Fe
Chronic dz	↓	↓	++	
Thalassemia Major	↑	Normal	++++	See reticulocytosis and indirect hyperbilirubinemia
Thalassemia Minor	Normal	Normal	++	See increased fetal Hgb A, target cells, and poikilocytosis
Lead toxicity	Normal	Normal	++	RBC basophilic stippling
Sideroblastic	↑	Normal	++++	Marrow ring sideroblasts

2. Macrocytic anemia (MCV > 95)
   a. *Megaloblastic bone marrow*: vitamin B_{12} deficiency, folic acid deficiency, drug-induced DNA synthesis impairment, hereditary DNA synthesis impairment.
   b. *Nonmegaloblastic bone marrow*: hypopituitarism, hypothyroidism, aplastic/hypoplastic anemia, accelerated erythropoiesis, bone marrow infiltration.

B. Alternate approach

1. *Reticulocyte count*: normal 50–100 k/cc
   a. Low–normal → BM failure.
   b. High → hemolysis, acute loss.
2. If BM failure, then go to MCV (mean corpuscular volume)
   a. *Microcytic*: Fe deficiency, chronic dz, thalassemia.
   b. *Hypochromic microcytic*: marrow = no iron; low total Fe, high TIBC; dx = Fe deficiency marrow = + iron; high HbA_2 or high HbF; dx = beta-thalassemia marrow = ring sideroblasts; low HbA_2; dx = sideroblastic anemia.
   c. *Normocytic*: chronic dz, Fe deficiency, secondary (hepatic, renal, endocrine d/o), BM d/o (aplasia, myelodysplasia, myelofibrosis).
      i. Check folate (?folate defic.), Fe and TIBC (low in chronic dz; LFT also often abn.), creatinine (low in uremia), T_4 (low in myxedematous anemia).
   d. *Normoblastic w/ teardrops*: check marrow:
      i. Aplastic → aplastic anemia, expect pancytopenia.
      ii. Fibrosis → myeloid metaplasia, expect alkaline phoshatase to be elevated.
      iii. Infiltrated/tumor/lymphoma → myelophthisic, expect leukocytosis.
   e. *Macrocytic*: folate or B_{12} deficiency, congenital d/o, alcoholism, drugs, hepatic d/o; marrow usu. megaloblastic.
      i. Check B_{12} (h/o gastric intestinal surgery?, poss. achlorhydria?), folate.
3. *If suspect hemolysis* (high reticulocytes):
   a. Check peripheral blood smear (schistocytes/helmet cells, spherocytes, spur cells, sickle cells, target cells, Heinz bodies, tear-shaped RBCs, stomatocytes, eliptocytes).
   b. Consider other tests as indicated/needed to eval for possible hemolysis.
      i. *Unconj/indir. bilirubin*: should be increased.
      ii. *Haptoglobin*: should be decreased.
      iii. *Serum LDH*: should be increased.
      iv. *Urine hemosiderin*: may be present.
      v. *Urine Hgb*: may be present.

CHAPTER 3

ANESTHESIA

TABLE 3.1. Common Sedatives and Analgesics

Drug	Comments	Dose	Onset and Half-life
Midazolam (Versed)	BZD sedative, excellent retrograde amnesia	IV bolus: 1–5 mg over 2 min q 2–4 h prn IV infusion: 1–20 mg/h (usu. 3 mg/h) Infusion increase: bolus 5 mg, then increase rate by 1 mg/h	2–5 min and 1–4 h (up to 48 h in renal insufficiency)
Lorazepam (Ativan)	BZD sedative, longer acting	PO: 0.5–4 mg q 2–4 h prn IV bolus: 2–4 mg (0.05 mg/kg) over 2–5 min IV infusion: 1–20 mg/h (usu. 3 mg/h) Infusion increase: bolus 4 mg, then increase rate by 1 mg/h	5–20 min and 12.9 h (elderly 15.9 h—accumulates w/ time)
Morphine	Opioid analgesic	IV bolus: 1–10 mg prn q 3–4 h prn IV infusion: 1–20 mg/h, titrate by 1 mg/h	3–4 h duration
Fentanyl	Synthetic opioid w/ faster onset, shorter duration than MSO_4. Less BP and resp depression. High doses w/ chest wall tightness.	IV bolus: 25–200 mcg q 1 h prn IV infusion: 25–200 mcg/h, titrate by 25 mcg/h	1–2 h duration
Meperidine (Demerol)	Metaboline normeperidine assoc. w/ neuropsychiatric side effects	1–1.8 mg/kg (75–150 mg) up to 150 mg IM/SC/PO or slow IV q 3–4 h	depends on route of administration
Dilaudid	Potent narcotic	0.5–2.0 mg IM/SC or slow IV q 4–6 h	depends on route of administration
Propofol	Anesthetic sedative. Watch for hypotension, apnea. Stop if triglycerides > 300–400. Fat overload. Rapid tolerance to effect. Avoid if allergic to egg, soybean oil, or glycerol; given in 10% Intralipid. Useful bronchodilator.	5 mcg/kg/min, increasing by 5 q 5–10 min. Average: 25–35 mcg/kg/min Anesthetic dose: 50–100 mcg/kg/min	Onset: 9–51 sec Duration: 3–10 min Half-life: 40 min
Haloperidol (Haldol)	For delirium of refractory agitation. Watch for neuroleptic malignant syndrome. Torsades: avoid QTc > 500 msec.	IV bolus: 1–10 mg IV q 1 h prn	*Ensure no QTc > 40 msec or increase by 25+%

I. LOCAL

A. Maximum doses of common local anesthetics:

1. *Lidocaine* 1% (10 mg/cc): max dose 5 mg/kg w/out epi; 7 mg/kg w/ epi.
    a. Onset 10 min; duration 1–3 h.
    b. *Toxicity*: includes dizziness, circumoral paresthesias, a metallic taste, a/o visual changes, which may culminate in disorientation, seizures (tx w/ benzodiazepines), or even cardiovascular collapse.
2. *Bupivacaine* (Marcaine): max dose 2 mg/kg w/out epi; 3 mg/kg w/ epi.
    a. Onset 15 min, duration 3–6 h.
    b. *Toxicity*: similar to that of lidocaine, although the cardiovascular effects tend to be more significant and persistent.

TABLE 3.2. Paralytics (Neuromuscular Blockers)

	Succinylcholine (Anectine)	Pancuronium (Pavulon)	Rocuronium (Zemuron)	Cisatracurium (Nimbex)
Type	Depolarizing	Nondepolarizing	Nondepolarizing	Nondepolarizing
Dose (mg/kg)	1–2 (avg. dose 100 mg)	0.1	0.6–1.0	0.1–2.0
Time to onset	30 sec	90 sec	75 sec	90 sec
Duration	5 min	60–180+ min	30–70 min	35–80 min
Chronotrope effect		↑ HR (vagolytic effect)	↑ HR w/ high dose only	None
Miscellaneous	• Can raise K^+ by 0.5 mEg/L • Avoid if rhabdo., burn, long immobilization, etc. • Potential to cause *malignant hyperthermia*	• Prolonged effect w/ renal > hepatic failure	• Prolonged effect w/ hepatic > renal failure	• No *histamine* release (advantage over other paralytics) • Can cause ↓ BP, ↑ HR • Not affected w/ hepatic or renal failure

II. APPLICATION

A. **Rapid sequence intubation** (mix, match as appropriate).
   1. *Fentanyl* 2 mcg/kg IV (150 mcg) → *succinylcholine* 1.5 mg/kg IV (100 mg).
   2. *Etomidate* 0.3 mg/kg IV (20 mg) → *rocuronium* 1.0 mg/kg IV (70 mg).
   3. *Midazolam* 0.1 mg/kg IV (7 mg) → *rapacuronium* 1.5 mg/kg IV (100 mg).

B. **PCA orders**
   1. *Morphine*: 1 mg q 15 min, lockout dose 16 mg q 4 h, loading dose 4 mg.
   2. *Demerol*: 12.5 mg q 15 min, lockout dose 200 mg q 4 h, loading dose 25 mg.

C. **Sedation**
   1. *Etomidate*: short-acting agent providing amnesia and hypnosis w/ minimal cardiovascular depression (useful in hemodynamically unstable pts). Prolonged usage, however, is assoc. w/ adrenal insufficiency.
   2. *Ketamine*: related to PCP, induces dissociative anesthesia w/ somatic (not visceral) analgesia and amnesia. *Increases BP, HR and ICP.* Decreases bronchomotor tone, but may produce large amounts of oropharygeal secretions (often given w/ glycopyrrolate). Limited use in abdominal surgery as produces no muscular relaxation. Benzodiazepine administration helps prevent emergence dysphoria/delirium.
   3. *Versed*: see Table 3.1.
   4. *Propofol*: see Table 3.1.

D. **Paralytics (neuromuscular blockers)**
   1. *Train of four*: if overdose on paralytics, can lead to polyneuropathy.

E. **Agitation**
   1. *Haloperidol* (Haldol): 2–5 mg IM.
   2. *Lorazepam* (Ativan): 0.5–2 mg IM/IV/PO q 6–8 h, max 10 mg/d.

III. REVERSAL AGENTS

A. **Narcan** 0.4–2.0 mg IV/IM/SC/ET q 2–3 min prn; adult postop reversal 0.1–0.2 mg.

B. **Flumazenil Sed. reversal:** 0.2 mg IV over 15 sec, then 0.2 mg q 1 min up to 1 mg.

C. **OD reversal:** 0.2 mg IV over 30 sec, then 0.3–0.5 mg q 30 sec up to 3 mg.

IV. ICU SEDATION/ANALGESIA PROTOCOL

A. Begin w/ 2–10 mg MSO_4 IV q 1–2 h around the clock.

1. Use Fentanyl if hemodynamically unstable.
2. RN titrate to Ramsey 3–4.
3. All pts get a daily sedation vacation to assess mental status.

B. In addition to morphine, if anxiety persists (oriented/appropriate, but pt anxious/fearful), can augment w/ prn Ativan to Ramsey 3–4. If w/in 48 h of anticipated extubation, change to propofol. Do not use Versed—inappropriate half-life.

C. If delirious (inappropriate/disoriented), use Haldol prn.

V. MALIGNANT HYPERTHERMIA

A. Life-threatening disorder secondary to defect in calcium metabolism in sarcoplasmic reticulum. Occurs in 1:50,000 adults and more frequently in children. 30% mortality.

B. Assoc. w/ inhalational anesthetics, amide-class local anesthetics, and succinylcholine.

C. Dx:

1. May manifest w/in 30 min of exposure to agent w/ fever, tachycardia, cyanosis, a/o rigidity. Additional findings may include increased end-tidal CO_2, hyperkalemia, hypercalcemia, and metabolic acidosis.
2. Elevated CPK levels are seen, and muscle bx confirms the dx (tx should not be withheld until this is performed).

D. Tx:

1. Stop responsible agent and actively cool the pt.
2. Hyperventilate w/ 100% oxygen.
3. Dantrolene (2–10 mg/kg IVP), repeat as needed.
4. Get arterial and central venous access.
5. Consider sodium bicarbonate for metabolic acidosis.
6. Aggressively tx hyperkalemia (see Chapter 1).
7. Maintain vigorous urine output w/ IVF +/– furosemide to 2+ mL/kg/h.

VI. END-TIDAL CO_2 MONITORING

A. Abrupt decrease

1. Plugging or disconnection of tubing.
2. Venous air/gas (i.e., CO_2) embolism (laparoscopy, GI endoscopy, liver resection).
   a. *Tx*: release pneumoperitoneum; place in Trendelenburg, left side down; hyperventilate w/ 100% oxygen, consider right atrial air aspiration through central line.
3. Tension PTX.
4. MI.
5. Excess pneumoperitoneum or intraabdominal HTN → decreased venous return.

B. Increase

1. Insufficient minute/alveolar ventilation.

CHAPTER 4

INFECTIOUS DISEASE

I. PREVENTING INFECTIONS IN SURGICAL PATIENTS

A. Perioperative [Mangram AJ, et al., Guideline for prevention of surgical site Infection, *Am J Inf Cont.* Apr 1999;27(8):97–132.]

1. *Abx*
   a. Give w/in an hour of case and appropriately throughout case.
   b. Generally antibiotics can be stopped postoperatively w/in 24 h. In cases of severe contamination and significant leukocytosis (i.e., perforated diverticulitis w/ abscess), consideration may be given to continuation until afebrile w/ normal WBC.
2. *Clip hair, don't shave. Shower night before w/ chlorhexidine.*
3. *Colon preparation*:
   a. *Mechanical bowel prep*: evolving body of data suggests trend toward *increased* risk of wound infection, intraabdominal abscess, and anastomotic leak w/ mechanical bowel prep. Standard regimen is (preop day) begin Go-LYTELY (polyethylene glycol) 4 L PO over 2 h, then clear liquid diet only, then NPO after midnight. Be wary of dehydration and electrolyte abnormalities (i.e., hypokalemia), particularly in elderly pts.
   b. *Antibiotics*: traditionally, agents such as neomycin (1 g) *and* erythromycin base (1 g) have been given around 1300 h, 1400 h, and 2300 h the day before surgery. However, multiple authors have reported no additional benefit from oral abx beyond that provided by perioperative parenteral/IV agents.
4. *Periop-augmented FiO_2 may be of benefit.*
5. *Avoiding hypothermia.*

B. ICU/floor

1. Commencement of enteral feeds as soon as possible *may* help prevent translocation, bacteremia, and some infections.
2. See recommendations for prevention of ventilator-assoc. pneumonia below (section IIB2b.).

II. INFECTIOUS DISEASES BY ORGAN SYSTEM (also see Chapter 22, on medical problems of surgical patients)

A. Neurologic

1. *Meningitis*
   a. *Chronic* (> 7 d)
   b. *Subacute* (1–7 d)
   c. *Acute* (< 24 h)
      i. *Presentation/pathology*:
         - Fulminant process almost invariably from bacterial infection.
         - *Neonates*: *Streptococci* (Group G, D, non-Group B), *E. coli*, *Listeria*.
         - *Infants/children*: *H. influenzae* > *S. pneumoniae* > *N. meningitides*.
         - *Adult*: *S. pneumoniae* > *N. meningitidis* > other.
         - Headache, F/C, photophobia, seizures (~ 1/3), decreased mental status.
         - Infants may only present w/ fever, lethargy, emesis, or respiratory embarrassment.
         - *Physical exam*:
            - Nuchal rigidity, discomfort w/ passive neck flexion.
            - *Kernig sign*: neck pain w/ passive knee extension (> 130°) while pt is supine w/ hip flexed (90°).
            - *Brudzinski sign*: passive flexion of neck results in active hip and knee flexion.

- *Infants*: may become more irritable when being held than when left alone; +/– bulging fontanelle.
- *Papilledema*: relatively late finding c/w elevated ICP.

ii. *Dx*:

- Lab assays to evaluate potential causes of altered mental status warranted.
- Head CT w/ contrast or MRI w/ gadolinium useful to evaluate for abscess or mass.
- Lumbar puncture invaluable (tube #1–glucose, protein; tube #2–cell count, differential; tube #3–gram stain, culture).
- *Bacterial meningitis findings include*: increased opening pressure (> 5–15 cm H_2O); increased PMNs; (+) gram stain; decreased glucose; protein > 150.

iii. *Tx*:

- *Aseptic*: rarely nonviral . . . for leptospirosis give IV doxycycline, penicillin G, or ampicillin.
- *Acute bacterial empiric tx*:
  - *< 1 mo old*: ampicillin + either cefotaxime or gentamicin.
  - *1 mo–50 yo*: cefotaxime (or ceftriaxone or meropenenem) + dexamethasone + vancomycin.
  - *50 yo or debilitated* (i.e., chronic alcoholic): above + ampicillin.

B. Cardiothoracic

1. *Endocarditis px*:

a. *By condition*:

i. *Recommended*:

- *High risk*: prosthetic cardiac valves (including homograft), previous bacterial endocarditis, complex cyanotic congenital heart dz (tetrology of Fallot, transposition of the great arteries, etc.), surgically constructed systemic pulmonary conduits/shunts.
- *Moderate risk*: other congenital cardiac malformations not listed in "high" or "low" risk categories, acquired valvular dysfunction (i.e., rheumatic heart dz), MVP w/ regurg or thickened leaflets.

ii. *Not recommended*: isolated secundum atrial defect, h/o sx repair of ASD/VSD/PDA (and no residua after 6 mo), h/o CABG, MVP w/out regurg, physiologic/functional/innocent heart murmurs, h/o Kawasaki dz w/out valvular dysfunction, h/o rheumatic fever w/out valvular dysfunction, cardiac pacemakers and implanted defibrillators.

b. *By procedure*:

i. *Recommended*:

- *Dental*: dental extractions, periodontal procedures, dental implant, root canal, prophylactic dental cleaning if bleeding anticipated, etc.
- *GI*: esophageal varices sclerotx, esophageal stricture dilation, ERCP w/ biliary obstruction, biliary tract surgery, surgery involving intestinal mucosa.
- *GU*: prostate surgery, cystoscopy, urethral dilation.
- *Respiratory tract*: tonsillectomy/adenoidectomy, surgery involving respiratory mucosa, rigid bronchoscopy.

ii. *Not recommended*:

- *Dental*: placement of rubber drains, suture removal, local anesthetic infection (nonintraligamentary), fluoride tx, taking oral impressions, shedding of primary teeth, etc.
- *GI*: TEE, endoscopy +/– bx.
- *GU*: vag hysterectomy, vag delivery, C-section, in uninfected tissues: urethral catheterization, uterine D&C, therapeutic abortion, sterilization procedures, IUD insertion/removal IUD, circumcision.
- *Respiratory tract*: endotracheal intubation, flexible bronchoscopy +/– bx, tympanostomy tube placement.
- *Other*: cardiac cath, balloon angioplasty, implanted cardiac cath, incision or bx of surgically scrubbed skin.

c. *Prophylactic regimens* (adult doses listed below; give 1 h before procedure if PO, 30 min if IM/IV).
   i. *Dental/oral/respiratory tract/esophageal*:
      - *Standard PO*: amoxicillin 2 g.
      - *Standard parenteral*: ampicillin 2 g.
      - *PCN allergic PO*: clindamycin 600 mg/cephalexin 2 g/azithromycin 500 mg/clarithromycin 500 mg.
      - *PCN allergic parenteral*: clindamycin 600 mg/cefazolin 1 g.
   ii. *GI/GU procedures* (nonesophageal):
      - *High-risk pts*: ampicillin 2 g + gentamicin 1.5 mg/kg not exceeding 120 mg.
      - *High-risk PCN allergic*: vancomycin 1 g + gentamicin 1.5 mg/kg not exceeding 120 mg.
      - *Mod-risk pts*: amoxicillin 2 g or ampicillin 2 g.
      - *Mod-risk PCN allergic*: vancomycin 1 g. [Dajani AS, et al., *JAMA*. 1997;277:1794–1801.]

d. *Endocarditis tx—empiric*:
   i. *Native valve, no IVDA*: penicillin G (or ampicillin) + nafcillin (or oxacillin) + gentamicin; alternatively, can give vancomycin + gentamicin.
   ii. *Native valve, IVDA*: vancomycin or daptomycin.
   iii. *Prosthetic valve*: vancomycin + gentamicin + rifampin.

2. *Pneumonia*
   a. *Community acquired* (usu. manifest w/in 48 h of admission).
      i. *Empiric tx*:
         - *Outpt*: azithromycin PO or clarithromycin PO or doxycycline PO.
         - *Inpt, non-ICU*: ceftriaxone IV or azithromycin IV.
         - *Inpt/ICU not on ventilator*: gatifloxacin IV or levofloxacin IV (alt. ceftriaxone + azithromycin).
   b. *Ventilator assoc.*: most common ICU infection, responsible for most deaths (30% mortality).
      i. *Early*: w/in 48 h of admission, usu. community-acquired organisms (*S. pneumoniae, H. influenzae, M. catarrhalis*).
      ii. *Late*: after 48 h of admission, usu. nosocomial pathogens (*Pseudomonas, Acinetobacter, Enterobacter, MRSA*).
      iii. *Dx*: obtain CXR and consider other dx if no infiltrate.
         - BAL or PBC dx depends on 10^4 CFU or 10^3 CFU, respectively.
         - To guide if appropriate to perform BAL, can use "clinical pulmonary infection score" (CPIS).
         - *Temperature*: 36.5–38.4 = 0; 38.5–38.9 = 1; ≥ 39 or < 36.5 = 2.
         - *WBC*: ≥ 4K - ≥ 11K = 0; < 4K or > 11K = 1; < 4K or > 11K and ≥ 50% bands = 2.
         - *Tracheal secretions*: none: scant = 0; nonpurulent = 1; purulent = 2.
         - *Oxygenation* (PaO_2:FiO_2 ratio): > 240, ARDS or pulm contusion = 0; < 240 and no ARDS = 2.
         - *CXR*: no infiltrate = 0, diffuse/patchy infiltrate = 1; localized infiltrate = 2.
         - If total CPIS > 6, then BAL cath; if total CPIS ≤ 6 but high suspicion for VAP, BAL cath; if ≤ 6, and low suspicion for VAP, eval for other source of infection.
         - If perform BAL, place on empiric abx after completing BAL [Singh N, et al., *Am J Respir Crit Care Med*. 2000;(162):505–11.]
      iv. *Tx*: crucial to begin appropriate abx tx early.
         - For empiric VAP, provide coverage for *S. aureus* and double-coverage for GNR, particularly *Pseudomonas* (some double-cover any of the "SPACE" organisms–*Serratia, Pseudomonas, Acinetobacter, Citrobacter, Enterobacter*). No benefit in treated most cases of VAP > 8 d.
         - *Tx of choice*: imipenem IV or meropenem IV (add vancomycin or linezolid if suspect MRSA; latter has better bioavailablity in pulmonary parenchyma).

v. *Px*: preventive measures include minimizing vent circuit changes, minimizing time on vent, oral instead of nasal intubation, avoiding heated humidifiers, aggressive pulmonary toilet and drainage of subglottic secretions, and semirecumbent (HOB 30°) instead of fully recumbent positioning. Pneumonia (non-VAP), carafate instead of H_2 blockers or PPI. Placement of feeding tube to transpyloric v. in stomach does not significantly reduce aspiration risk if HOB elevated (+/–).

c. *Aspiration pneumonia*: tends to occur in right > left lung, and in upper part of middle lobe or lower part of upper lobe. Mendelson's syndrome refers to aspiration pneumonitis. Generally, gastric pH precludes bacterial contamination, but infectious complications, including abscess occur. Abx of choice is piperacillin-tazobactam.

C. Gastrointestinal

1. *Helicobacter pylori*: H_2 blocker or PPI × 2 wk, *plus* . . .
   a. Bismuth subsalicylate 525 mg PO 4 times per day × 2 wk, *plus* . . .
   b. Metronidazole 250 mg PO 4 times per day × 2 wk, *plus* . . .
   c. Tetracycline 500 mg PO 4 times per day × 2 wk.
   d. *Note*: alternate abx include combination of clarithromycin 500 mg PO 2 times per day and one of the following: tetracycline *or* metronidazole *or* amoxicillin 1000 mg PO 2 times per day. [Howden CS, Hunt RH, *AJG*. 1998;93:2336.]
2. *Appendiciitis*: pip/tazo, amp/sulbactam acceptable. If not perforated, no need to continue postop. If perforated, continue postop 7–10 d, then stopping if afebrile and normal WBC.
3. *Cholecystitis, cholangitis*: routine → amp/sulb or pip/tazo, if life-threatening imip or merop. For routine cholecystectomy (acute cholecystitis, generally give antibiotics [i.e., cefazolin] for up to 24 h postop and discontinue if afebrile). Abx unnecessary for surgery for biliary colic.
4. *Pancreatitis*: imipenem, meropenem good penetration for established infected pancreatitis–prophylaxis in cases of severe/necrotizing pancreatitis of no proven benefit.
5. *Perforated viscus*: drug of choice is piperacillin-tazobactam as increasing resistance to cefoxitin, cefotetan.
   a. Ampicillin-sulbactam is reasonable alternative. For penicillin-allergic, consider ertapenem or combination of fluoroquinolone + metronidazole.
6. *Primary (spontaneous) bacterial peritonitis*: IV cefotaxime or piperacillin-tazobactam or ceftriaxone. If penicillin-allergic, consider fluoroquinolone or carbapenem.

D. Genitourinary

1. *UTI*: most common nosocomial infection outside ICU. Gram-negative rods (*E. coli*, *Klebsiella*, *Serratia*, *Proteus*).
   a. *Dx*: > 10 WBC and colony count > 10^5.
      i. Candiduria should prompt evaluation for systemic candidiasis.
   b. *Tx*: empiric tx against gram negative bacteria.
      i. Bacterial (*uncomplicated*) → Levofloxacin or TMP-SMX DS × 3 d.
      ii. Bacterial (*complicated* . . . Foley cath., etc.) → piperacillin-tazobactam, carbapenem, or FQ × 2–3 wk.
      iii. Fungal → d/c Foley catheter if have one, repeat cx; no tx necessary if negative (40% this will occur).
      iv. If have to replace Foley, 20% will recur; tx w/ oral or IV diflucan—bladder washings w/ amphotericin are rarely necessary. Also must tx if (+) *Candida* cx elsewhere (blood, sputum, etc.) *C. albicans* usu. sensitive to fluconazole; *C. torulopsis/glabrata* often require amphotericin.
2. *Pyelonephritis* (uncomplicated): fluoroquinolone × 7–14 d.
3. *Epididymo-Orchitis*:
   a. *< 35 yo* (usu. *Chlamydia*): oflox 300 mg PO 2 times per day × 10 d, or ceftriaxone 250 mg IV × 1 + doxy 100 mg PO 2 times per day × 10 d.
   b. *> 35 yo, or homosexual males* (usu. GNR): fluoroquinolone PO 10–14 d.
4. *Prostatitis* (acute): fluoroquinolone PO × 10–14 d (specifically ofloxacin if < 35 yo). If chronic, tx for 4–8 wk.

5. *PID/TOA*:
   a. Outpt → ofloxacin PO + metronidazole PO *or* ceftriaxone IV + doxycycline IV + metronidazole IV.
   b. Inpt → cefotetan/cefoxitin + doxy.
   c. Uncommonly, TOA will be refractory to abx and require percutaneous drainage or adnexectomy.
6. *Candidiasis*: fluconazole 150 mg PO once.
7. *Trichomoniasis*: metronidazole 2 g PO once.
8. *Bacterial vaginosis* (*Gardnerella*): metronidazole 500 mg PO 2 times per day × 7 d.

E. Skin and soft tissue

1. *Early (< 48–72 h postop) wound infection*: β-hemolytic strep, *Clostridium*
   a. *Consider same tx as for necrotizing soft-tissue infection*: clindamycin 900 mg IV q 8 h + penicillin 4 M U IV q 4 h.
2. *Necrotizing fasciitis*
   a. Type I–polymicrobial vs Type II–β-hemolytic strep.
   b. *Initial management*:
      i. Do not delay getting to OR (don't wait on needle aspirates for gram stain or x-rays for gas in tissues)—this is a clinical dx of a surgical emergency.
      ii. While waiting for OR, begin high-dose penicillin G (4 M U IV q 4 h + clindamycin 900 mg IV q 8 h).
         - Clindamycin superior to other antianaerobe, metronidazoe, in that clindamycin inhibits clostridial elaboration of toxins.
3. *Bites*: usu., ampicillin/clavulanate 875/125 PO 2 times per day adequate. Consider tetanus prophylaxis as well: refer to Table 4.1.
   a. *Human*: *Streptococcus viridans*, *S. aureus*, *S. epidermidis*, corynebacterium, *Eikenella corrodens*.
      i. Usu. do *not* primarily close wound, esp. on hand.
      ii. If present w/ sx of infection, give amp/clav IV; *alternative*: clindamycin IV + fluoroquinolone IV (or + SMP-TMX IV).
   b. *Cat*: *Pasteurella multocida*; alternative abx include cefuroxime or doxycycline.
   c. *Dog*: *Pasteurella multocida*; alternative abx include clindamycin +/– TMP-SMX.
4. *Diabetic foot*:
   a. *Polymicrobial*: *S. aureus*, Gp B strep, possible colforms. Advanced cases frequently have anaerobes.
   b. *Tx*:
      i. Outpt, minimal inflammation → TMP-SMX DS + (Pen VK *or* FQ *or* 2 d/3 d gen. cephalosporin).
      ii. Inpt → (ampicillin-clavanulate + TMP-SMX DS) or (FQ + vancomycin or linezolid).
      iii. Severe infection, inpt → vancomycin (or linezolid) + (amp/sulb or carbapenem) + metronidazole.
5. *Hidradenitis suppurativa*
   a. Chronic, relapsing, suppurative, cicatrizing process thought to be secondary to superinfection of obstructed apocrine glands (limited to axilla, perineum).
   b. Medical tx w/ abx such as macrolides or tetracyclines considered standard, although w/ increased MRSA incidence, other options such as clindamycin are reasonable.
   c. Surgical options range from incision/drainage, curettage, unroofing of fistulous tracts, marsupialization of wounds, excision and grafting or local flap coverage.
6. *Tetanus prophylaxis and tx*: see Table 4.1.
7. *Rabies prophylaxis*
   a. *Preexposure prophylaxis*: (Rabies virus vaccine, Imovax® Rabies) 1 mL IM on days 0, 7, and 21 to 28. Do not shorten the interval between doses, but prolonging intervals doesn't impair ultimate immunity.

TABLE 4.1. Tetanus Prophylaxis and Treatment

Immunity Status	Clean/Low-Risk Wound	Tetanus-Prone/High-Risk Wound
	• Clean incision • Superficial graze • Scald	• Any of the following: ◦ Wound/burn older than 6 h ◦ Contact w/ soil, manure, or compost ◦ Puncture wound ◦ Compound fx ◦ Large amount devitalized tissue ◦ Animal/human bite
Completed 3 doses of tetanus immunization or booster w/in last 10 yr.	• No tx	• No tx, although a booster dose tetanus toxoid (0.5 mL IM) if no booster in last 5 yr
Last of 3-dose course or booster > 10 yr ago.	• Booster of adsorbed tetanus vaccine	• Booster of adsorbed tetanus vaccine
Not immunized or uncertain status	• Full course of adsorbed tetanus vaccine	• Full course of adsorbed tetanus vaccine *AND* Human tetanus immunoglobulin (250 U IM—peds get 4 U/kg)
Clinical dz		• Abx • Tetanus immunoglobulin up to 6000–10,000 U IM

b. *Postexposure prophylaxis*: thoroughly wash wound w/ soap, water. If not immunized before: Rabies immune globulin (Bay Rab®, Imogam®) 20 U/kg, 1/2 infiltrated at bite site if possible and the remainder IM. Follow w/ rabies vaccine, 1 mL IM, on days 0, 3, 7, 14, and 28. If have previously had postexposure rabies vaccine *or* had preexposure vaccine *or* have documented rabies AB titer that is adequate: Rabies vaccine IM on days 0 and 3 only. RIG is not indicated. Booster (ongoing risk): 1 mL IM q 2–5 yr or when AB titers are insufficient.

III. ANTIBIOTIC PROPHYLAXIS FOR SURGERY

TABLE 4.2. Antibiotic Prophylaxis for Surgery

Type of Procedure (usu. start 1 h preop, may continue 24 h postop)	First Choice	Alternate Choice(s)
Cardiothoracic (cont IV abx until d/c chest tubes)	Cefazolin or cefuroxime	Vancomycin
Upper GI	Cefazolin	Cefoxitin, cefotetan
Liver/pancreas/biliary tract	Cefazolin	Ceftizoxime
Appendix	Cefoxitin or cefotetan	FQ + metronidazole
Colorectal	See section IA3. on colon prophylaxis	
Head/neck (abx only required if contaminated)	Cefazolin	Clindamycin + gentamicin
Vascular	Cefazolin	Vancomycin
SBE prophylaxis	See section IIB1. on endocarditis prophylaxis	
Urologic procedure (abx recommended only if bacteriuria)	Cefazolin × 24 h, then nitrofurantoin or TMP-SMX; FQ for TURP	

IV. **POSTSPLENECTOMY PROPHYLAXIS**: see Chapter 18 on spleen.

V. **ANTIBIOTIC CLASSES** (for dosing information and side effects, see Chapter 23 on pharmacology and surgical pharmacopoeia)

A. **Bacteriocidal**

1. *Penicillins* (beta lactam inhibitors).
2. *Cephalosporins* (beta lactam inhibitors).
3. *Vancomycin* (binds to penicillin-binding protein, inhibits peptidoglycan synthesis).
4. *Metronidazole* (degrades DNA).
5. *Fluoroquinolones* (DNA gyrase inhibitors).
6. *Nitrofurans* (damages DNA through reactive intermediates).

B. **Bacteriostatic**

1. *Macrolides* (50s subunit).
2. *Tetracyclines* (30s subunit).
3. *Chloramphenicol* (50s subunit, reduced membrane permeability).
4. *Trimethoprim* (inhibits uptake of folic acid for thymidine, and therefore DNA, synthesis).
5. *Sulfonamides* (inhibits folic acid synthesis).

C. **Mixed**

1. *Aminoglycosides* (30s subunit).

VI. **BACTERIA BY GRAM STAIN AND RECOMMENDED EMPIRIC** [Adapted from Sanford Guide® 2010]; anaerobes in **bold**

A. **Gram-positive rods/bacilli:**

1. ***Clostridium botulinum*** (all *Clostridia* large, w/ spores) tx w/ antitoxin, supportive care.
2. ***C. difficile*** dx w/ toxin assay. Tx w/ oral metronidazole or vancomycin (IV inferior).
3. ***C. perfringens*** PCN G; alt. metronidazole, clindamycin.
4. ***C. tetani*** px w/ toxoid, metronidazole or Pen G.
5. *Listeria* cause of meningitis, found in unpasteurized milk products; AMP +/– aminoglycoside; alt. SMP-TMX.
6. *Corynebacterium diphtheriae* (diphtheroid, pleomorphic, small) erythromycin; alt. pcn.
7. *C. jeikeium* (diphtheroid, pleomorphic, small) tx w/ vancomycin; alt. PCN G.
8. *B. anthracis* (large, w/ spores) tx w/ penicillin or doxycycline.
9. *B. cereus* vancomycin, alt. clindamycin.
10. ***Actinomyces*** AMP or PCN G; alt. tetracyclines.
11. *Nocardia* TMP-SMX; alt. amikacin.
12. *Erysipelothrix rhusiopathiae* PCN G or AMP; FQ.

B. **Gram-positive cocci:**

1. *Staphylococcus* (*S. aureus* = coagulase pos., *S. epidermidis* = coagulase neg.); tx varies.
2. *Streptococcus* (*S. pneumoniae, S. pyogenes* [Gp. A], *S. agalactiae* [Gp. B], *Enterococc*).
3. Most species susceptible to PCN G.
4. ***Peptostreptococcus*** PCN G.

C. **Gram-negative rods/bacilli:** fluoroquinolones, aminoglycosides usu. effective *E. coli* varies (depends on clinical scenario; as always, check institution antibiogram)

1. *Klebsiella* (depends on clinical scenario).
2. *Proteus* AMP; alt. TMP-SMX.
3. *Acinetobacter* imipenem or meropenem; alt. Unasyn.
4. *Citrobacter* antipseudomonal PCN; alt. FQ.
5. ***Lactobacillus*** PCN G or AMP; alt. clindamycin.
6. *Brucella* Doxy + (Gent or streptomycin).
7. ***Bacteroides*** (nonfermentative) metronidazole; alt. cefoxitin.

8. *Campylobacter jejuni* erthryromycin; alt. FQ.
9. *Haemophilus influenzae* cefotaxime or ceftriaxone; alt. TMP-SMX.
10. *Pseudomonas aeruginosa* (nonfermentative) antipseudomonal PCN.
11. *Stenotrophomonas maltophila* (nonfermentative) TMP-SMX; alt. ticarcillin-clavanulate.
12. *Salmonella* FQ or ceftriaxone; alt. chloramphenicol.
13. *Vibrio cholerae* doxy or FQ; alt. TMP-SMX.
14. *Vibrio parahemolyticus* abx not diminish clinical course.
15. *Vibrio vulnificus* doxy + ceftazidime; alt. Cefotaxime.
16. *Pasteurella* PCN G or AMP or amoxicillin; alt. doxycycline.

D. Gram-negative diplococci:

1. *Neisseria gonorrhea* (pairs) ceftriaxone or cefixime; alt. spectinomycin.
2. *Neisseria meningitides* (pairs) PCN G; alt. ceftriaxone.
3. *Moraxella catarrhalis* (pairs) amoxicillin-clavanulate; alt. aztithromycin.

E. Gram-negative coccobacilli:

1. *Haemophilus ducreyi* azithromycin or ceftriaxone; alt. erythromycin.
2. *H. influenzae* cefotaxime or ceftriaxone; alt. TMP-SMX.

CHAPTER 5

RENAL

I. RENAL PHYSIOLOGY/DIURETICS

A. Physiology

1. *Avg. net urine output 1–2 L/d.*
2. *Creatinine is neither secreted nor absorbed, thus useful for calculating GFR*:
   a. $GFR = [(150 - age) \times (\text{total wt in kg})]/(72 \times Cr_{plasma})$
3. *Hormonal components*:
   a. *Renin*: produced by juxtaglomerular apparatus in afferent arterioles in response to decreased hydrostatic pressure in afferent arteriole, decreased sodium concentration at macula densa (distal tubule), and increased sympathetic tone.
      i. Cleaves angiotensinogen to angiotensin I.
      ii. *Angiotensin I* converted to angiotensin II in the lung.
      iii. *Angiotensin II*:
         - Peripheral arterial vasoconstrictor.
         - Particularly potent on renal efferent arteriole, increasing sodium reabsorption in proximal tubules.
         - Stimulates adrenal zona glomerulosa to elaborate aldosterone (further increasing sodium reabsorption and potassium excretion–in collecting duct).
   b. *Atrial natriuretic factor*: polypeptide secreted by atrium in when stimulated by stretch or elevated plasma sodium. Induces renal loss of sodium and water, peripheral vasodilation, and inhibits renin secretion as well as ADH (see c. below) activity.
   c. *Antidiuretic hormone* (ADH): secreted by posterior pituitary, usu. in response to increased osmolarity. Increases permeability of collecting duct to water, facilitating increased reabsorption.
      i. *SIADH*: inappropriate ADH secretion w/ concentrated urine and hyposmolar plasma.
      ii. *Diabetes insipidus*: lack of, or insensitivity of kidneys to ADH, leading to hypotonic urine, and hyperosmolar plasma.

B. Diuretics

1. *Loop diuretics*
   a. Furosemide (Lasix); other loop diuretics include bumetanide, ethacrynic acid, and torsemide.
      i. *Mechanism*:
         - Inhibits $Na^+/K^+/2Cl^-$ coupled transport system in thick ascending loop of Henle, reducing reabsorption of NaCl. Also decreases reabsorption of Na^+ and Cl^- and increases K^+ excretion in distal renal tubule.
         - Loop diuretics also have a direct effect to dilate renal vasculature and increase systemic venous capacitance. More effective if given as continuous IV infusion (1–9 mg/h) than as boluses of 20–40.
      ii. *Most useful* for hypertension, CHF, cirrhotic ascites, and pulmonary edema.
      iii. *Side effects*:
         - *Electrolyte disorders*: hyponatremia, hypokalemia, hypomagnesemia, hypocalcemia, hypochloremia.
         - Prolonged use can lead to metabolic (contraction a/o hypochloremic) alkalosis.
         - Ototoxicity (usu. reversible) and allergic reactions in persons sensitive to sulfonamides.
2. *Thiazide diuretics*
   a. Hydrochlorothiazide

i. Inhibits Na^+ reabsorption in distal tubules, leading to net loss of water and Na^+ as well as K^+ and H^+.

ii. Thiazide diuretics may increase serum Ca^{++}.

3. *Potassium-sparing diuretics*

a. Spironolactone other potassium-sparing diuretics include amiloride.

i. Competes w/ aldosterone receptors in distal renal tubules increasing excretion of Na^+ and Cl^- but conserving K^+ and H^+. Can also block aldosterone effects on vascular smooth muscle.

ii. Useful in managing cirrhosis w/ ascites/edema.

b. Triamterene

i. Interferes w/ Na^+/K^+ active exchange in distal tubule, collecting tubules, and collecting ducts. Decreases Ca^{++} excretion but increases Mg^{++} loss.

4. *Carbonic anhydrase inhibitor diuretics*

a. Acetazolamide (Diamox)

i. Reversibly inhibits carbonic anhydrase resulting in decreased H^+ secretion at renal tubule and increased renal excretion of Na^+, K^+, HCO_3^-, and water.

ii. Usage can lead to metabolic acidosis. Also used to treat altitude sickness in part by counteracting respiratory alkalosis. May be used to alkalinize urine as well.

5. *Osmotic diuretics*

a. Mannitol

i. Increases glomerular filtrate osmotic pressure, inhibiting tubular reabsorption of water.

ii. Watch serum osmolarity if prolonged/repeated usage.

II. OLIGURIA

A. < 400 cc/24 h

B. W/u:

1. *UA w/ microscopy*: abundant tubular epithelial cells w/ epithelial cell casts → ATN. WBC casts → interstitial nephritis. Pigmented casts → myoglobinuria.

2. *Urine spot sodium*: < 20 suggests prerenal azotemia (dry) as kidneys appropriately try to conserve Na^+. > 40 suggests intrinsic renal problem (i.e., ATN), but may be inaccurate in face of diuretic usage, or in elderly who may have difficulty conserving Na^+ (mixed d/o).

3. *Fractional excretion of sodium* (FENa): not valid if received diuretics in prior 24 h.

a. FENa = (Urine Na^+/Plasma Na^+)/(Urine creatinine/Plasma creatinine) × 100.

i. FENa < 1% indicates prerenal azotemia (usu. hypovolemia or heart failure).

ii. FENa > 2% suggests intrinsic renal dysfunction (usu. ATN).

4. *Fractional excretion of urea* (FEUr): useful when FENa is not accurate (i.e., recent diuretic usage).

a. FEUr = (Urine urea × Plasma creatinine)/(Plasma urea × Urine creatinine) × 100.

i. FEUr ≤ 35% suggests prerenal azotemia.

ii. FEUr > 35% suggests intrinsic renal dysfunction (usu. ATN).

5. *Prerenal*: hypovolemia, cardiac dysfunction, drug-induced renal vasoconstriction (i.e., NSAIDs).

a. UNa < 20, FENa < 1%.

6. *Renal*: acute tubular necrosis (ATN), acute interstitial nephritis (AIN), glomerulonephritis.

a. UNa > 40, FENa > 2% (3% is more convincing).

b. *ATN* (most common): can be from sepsis, circulatory shock, nephrotoxins (aminoglycosides, radiocontrast dye, myoglobin, etc.). End result from ischemia or inflammatory cells is often obstruction of tubules. Often accompanied by other organ injury.

c. *AIN*: often from complicated UTIs resulting in papillary necrosis and sloughing. Tx w/ abx as appropriate. Cessation of nephrotoxic (i.e., NSAIDs) agents imperative. Other implicated drugs have included PCN, sulfa, and phenytoin. Frequently assoc. w/ diabetes mellitus important to achieve good control of that disease.

d. *Glomerulonephritis*: most often from diabetes and immunologic renal pathology; results in changes in glomerular permeability and selectivity while 90% have granular deposits on u/a; the finding of RBCs in the urine are considered "the hallmark" of glomerulonephritis (*Note*:

RBCs in urine should prompt consideration of sarcoidosis, PAN, lupus, endocarditis, and Goodpasture's in addition to urolithiasis and tumors).

7. *Postrenal*: acute looks like prerenal; chronic looks like renal.
   a. Papillary necrosis, retroperitoneal tumors, prostatism, urethral strictures.
8. *Management*:
   a. Optimize hemodynamics
      i. *Filling pressures*: if CVP > 4 or PCWP > 8, infuse to CVP of 6–8 a/o PCWP of 12–15.
      ii. *Cardiac output*:
         - If CO still low after doing above, give IVF until CVP at 10–12 and PCWP near 20.
         - *If CO still low, consider inotropes for goal of CI > 3 L/min/m²*:
            - If normal BP → dobutamine at 5 mcg/kg/min
            - If low BP → dopamine at 5 mcg/kg/min
      iii. Low-dose dopamine is not protective for ARF in setting oliguria. Fenoldopam at low dose (0.03 mcg/kg/min → higher dose up to 1.6 mcg/kg/min) shouldn't lower blood pressure but will increase renal blood flow; while not renal protective, can convert oliguric to nonoliguric renal failure, making the complication of volume overload less problematic.

III. ACUTE RENAL FAILURE

TABLE 5.1. Lab Findings in Acute Renal Failure

	Hypovolemia	ATN	Acute Interstitial Nephritis	Glomerulonephritis	Obstruction
Sediment	Bland	Broad, brown, granular casts	WBC, eosinophils, cellular casts	RBC, RBC casts	Bland or bloody
Protein	0–low	0–low	Minimal, possibly increased w/ NSAIDs	Increased, > 100 mg/dL	Low
Urine Na^+	< 20	> 30	> 30	< 20	< 20 (acute) > 40 (days)
Urine osm	> 400	< 350	< 350	> 400	< 350
FENa % ($[U_{Na}/P_{Na}]/[U_{Cr}/P_{Cr}]$)	< 1	> 1	Variable	< 1	< 1 (acute) > 1 (days)

A. General: usu. from ischemia or toxins, and lasts 7–21 d. Mortality from community acquired is 10–30%, but obstetric < 15%, highest in ICU pts. Major cause of death in ARF pts is infection. Predictors of poor outcome include oliguria, poor nutritional markers, mechanical ventilation, acute MI or CVA or SZ, and chronic immunosuppression.

B. Dx:

1. Rise in serum Cr 0.5 (or 50%) or more above baseline; reduction in calculate creatinine clearance of at least 50% from normal.
2. *Creatinine clearance*:
   a. *Normal*: males 97–137 mL/min/1.73 m²; females 88–128 mL/min/1.73 m².
   b. *Calculation* (requires 24-h urine): (Urine Cr × Urine volume in mL)/(Serum Cr × 1400).
   c. Increased w/ pregnancy, exercise. Decreased w/ renal insufficiency, increasing age (decreases 1 mL/min/yr > 30), certain medications (cimetidine, procainamide, various abx, quinidine).
   d. Alternately, can gauge renal function w/ GFR (unless pt is vegetarian, uses creatine supplement, is malnourished, or an amputee).
      i. GFR (male) = (140 – age) × (wt in kg)/(Serum Cr × 72)
      ii. GFR (female) = (140 – age) × (wt in kg) × 0.85/(Serum Cr × 72)

C. Tx:

1. *Dietary restrictions*: avoid high-phosphorus foods, carefully monitor K^+.

D. Prophylaxis

E. Dye Nephropathy for high-risk pts (diabetics, CRI, etc.)

1. *Sodium bicarbonate*:
   a. 1 h prior to procedure give 3 cc/kg (max 330 cc) over 1 h of 3 amps (150 mEq $NaHCO_3$/1 L D5W or sterile water).
   b. Postscan continue infusion as 1 cc/kg (max 110 cc/h) for 6 h. [Merten GJ, *JAMA*. 2004;291(19): 2328–34.]
2. *N-acetylcysteine* (Mucomyst):
   a. 600 mg PO 2 times per day preprocedure day and 600 mg PO 2 times per day on day of procedure.
   b. Also give 1/2 NS at 1 cc/kg × 12 h pre- and postprocedure [Tepel M, *N Engl J Med*. 2000;343(3): 180–4.]
3. Fenoldopam is a selective renal dopamine D-1 agonist (no effects on other dopamine or adrenergic receptors). Although its use may result in augmented renal perfusion, natriuresis, and urine output, data do not suggest any consistent renal protective effects.

IV. DIALYSIS

A. Dialysis indications: hyperkalemia, acidosis, volume overload, sx uremia (n/v, anorexia, encephalopathy, sz, asterixis, pericarditis, bleeding).

B. Types of dialysis

1. *Peritoneal*: safe, effective for ESRD, but rarely used for ARF (need to place catheter, fluid leaks, surgical wound, poor peritoneal blood flow while hypotensive, negative effect of abdominal fluid on respiratory mechanics).
2. *Hemodialysis* (CVAHD, CVVHD)
   a. Corrects electrolyte abnormalities.
   b. Avoid subclavian access if possible (IJ preferred).
   c. Intermittent hemodialysis or ultrafiltration can be done at bedside or special unit, lasting 3–4 h, and can remove 3–5 kg of volume/session.
      i. Preferred means if pt is hemodynamically stable or has life-threatening electrolyte derangements.
      ii. Continuous renal replacement therapy (CRRT) performed at bedside over 24 h (equiv. of 3–4 hemodialysis sessions).
      iii. Ideal if hemodynamically unstable and acute hemodialysis not tenable due to hypotension.
         - Spontaneous/arteriovenous vs pumped/venovenous.
      iv. CRRT preferred over IHD for ARF in pts at risk for cerebral edema because of fluid shifts but unsuitable for life-threatening hyperkalemia or exogenous toxemia.
         - For CVVHD, 1000–2000 U heparin is given into arterial limb, then run at 500 U/h, to PTT 1.5–2.0 normal.
         - If heparin contraindicated, or recurrent system clotting, regional citrate anticoagulation may be used (requires modification of dialysate and IV calcium infusion).
      v. Ultrafiltration (slow continuous ultrafiltration/SCUF; hemofiltration/CAVH/CVVH; hemodiafiltration CAVHDF, CVVHDF).
      vi. Only removes excess volume.
      vii. Complications of CRRT (Bleeding—pt's get *heparinized*, line disconnection, hematoma, hypotension, filter clotting, access infection, access malfunction).

CHAPTER 6

SURGICAL INTENSIVE CARE UNIT

I. AIRWAY AND BREATHING (VENTILATION)

A. Airway

1. *Intubation criteria*
   a. *Inadequate, unprotected, or threatened airway*: i.e., GCS < 9, vomiting, inhalation injury, etc.
   b. RR > 35 (or significantly increasing work of breathing).
   c. $PaCO_2 > 50$ mm Hg.
   d. Respiratory acidosis w/ pH < 7.25.
   e. $PaO_2 < 60$ mm Hg.
   f. $SaO_2 < 85\%$.
   g. $PaO_2/FiO_2 < 250$.
2. *Rapid sequence intubation* (see Chapter 3).
3. *Equipment*
   a. MacIntosh blade is curved, placed in vallecula to lift epiglottis.
   b. Miller blade is straight, placed over/across the epiglottis.
   c. Most adults require a #3 (less commonly #4) blade of either MacIntosh or Miller.
      i. Premature infants, #0 Miller; other infants, #1 Miller; children, #2 Miller.
   d. *Tube size*: adult males 7.5–8.0; adult females 7.0–7.5.
      i. *Children*: ETT width same as 5th fingernail, or use size = (4 + age yr)/4.
   e. In (most) adult males, place tube at 23 cm (incisors or angle of mouth); only go to 21 cm in females. CXR should show tip 2–5 cm above carina in all cases.
      i. Children depth = (age yr/2) + 12.
   f. For tracheostomy, most adults should get a #8 Shiley tracheostomy tube or a 6-0 ETT.

B. Breathing

1. *Pulmonary physiology*
   a. *Transmural pressure*: alveoli in healthy lungs transmit pressure equally in all directions, but alveoli in decreased compliance parenchyma transmits w/ disproportionate distension against the capillaries, compressing them. Because of this, excessive pressure will increase dead-space ventilation, and further hypoxia. This is one of the reasons for limited volume in ARDS pts. Further, w/ ARDS, pathology is not uniformly distributed, and relatively healthy, easily distended alveoli may get overinflated, leading to volutrauma. Additionally, remember PEEP does not so much recruit alveoli as it does prevent alveoli w/ critically low volumes from collapsing during expiration.
   b. *Peak and plateau pressures*: peak pressure is a function of resistance to inflowing air as well as elastic recoil of lungs (P_{peak} ~ resistance × elasticity). Plateau pressure, however, is proportional only to elasticity of lungs and chest wall (air has already flowed into the lungs → $P_{plateau}$ ~ elasticity). Resultingly, airway resistance ~ $P_{peak} - P_{plateau}$. Remember that peak pressure (normal < 50 cm) correlates w/ luminal obstruction, whereas plateau pressure (normal < 35) corresponds w/ chest/lung compliance.
      i. *Evaluating pathophysiology w/ peak and plateau pressures*:
         - *P_{peak} increased, but $P_{plateau}$ normal/unchanged*:
           - Indicates increased airway resistance → ETT obstruction, excess secretions in airway, bronchospasm, etc. Mandates suctioning, possible bronchodilators.
         - *P_{peak} and $P_{plateau}$ both increased*:

- Indicates decreased distensibility of lungs a/o chest wall → pneumothorax, thoracic eschar, lobar atelectasis, pulmonary edema, pneumonia, ARDS, increased abdominal pressure, chest muscle contraction (dyssynchronous breathing), auto-PEEP.
- Note that PEEP will increase plateau pressure as well (subtract PEEP from $P_{plateau}$ when evaluating compliance).

- *P_{peak} decreased*:
  - Indicates likely tubing disconnection or air leak → inflate lungs w/ BVM and listen for cuff leak during inflation. Hyperventilation from pt may also generate sufficient NIF to pull air into lungs.
- *P_{peak} unchanged, but acute respiratory deterioration*:
  - Consider PE or extrathoracic process.

c. *Pulmonary gas exchange and oxygen delivery*:

i. *Oxygen delivery = cardiac output (L/min) × CaO_2 × 10*:

- Normal = 0.9 – 1.1 L/min *or* 520 – 600 mL/min/m^2.
- Arterial O_2 content (CaO_2): (1.34 × Hgb × SaO_2) + (0.003 × PaO_2).
  - Normal PaO_2 ~ 90 mm Hg; normal PvO_2 ~ 40 mm Hg.

ii. *A-a PO_2 gradient* (PO_2 difference between alveolar gas and alveolar blood):

- Affected by age, altitude/barometric pressure, and FiO_2.
- In general, A-a gradient ~ 2.5 + 0.21 × age. Upper limits of normal by age, on room air (i.e., 20 yo → 17, but 80 yo → 38).
- Gradient increases ~ 6 mm Hg for every 10% increase in FiO_2.
- In a healthy young person w/ FiO_2 1.0, A-a gradient should be 25–65, and PaO_2 600 mm Hg.

iii. *Evaluating hypoxemia*:

- *Hypoventilation* (excess narcotic, weakness, etc.): A-a PO_2 normal, PvO_2 normal.
- *V/Q mismatch* (pneumonia, ARDS, PE, pulmonary edema): A-a PO_2 ↑, PvO_2 normal.
  - Shunt (V/Q < 1) results in no increase in PaO_2 w/ supplemental oxygen.
- *DO_2/VO_2 imbalance* (low cardiac output, anemia, hypermetabolic state): A-a PO_2 ↑, PvO_2 ↓.

2. *Mechanical ventilation*

a. *General principles*

i. *Effect of positive-pressure ventilation*: decreases venous return to heart and thus right ventricular filling (decreases preload); augments left ventricular systolic function (effectively decreases afterload, increases stroke volume). Overall effect is to generally increase cardiac output in normovolemic pts while decreasing cardiac output in volume-depleted pts.

ii. *Volutrauma*: recent studies suggest that excessive *volume* is more injurious to alveoli than increased pressure, and may be responsible for releasing inflammatory cytokines.

iii. *PEEP*: functions to increase functional reserve volume and recruit alveoli or diminish atelectasis. Improves P:F ratio. Effects on cardiac output are the same as for positive-pressure ventilation (see i. above). Another maneuver to increase oxygenation is inverting the I:E ratio. Potential risk is breath-stacking or auto-PEEP, which can raise pCO_2; it is also uncomfortable for the pt and requires heavy sedation.

b. *Ventilation modes*

i. *Assist control*: a form of volume-cycled ventilation where the ventilator delivers a complete cycle when triggered by pt inspiration; will also give breaths if rate of breathing is below a set threshold. Main risks w/ this mode are auto-PEEP a/o respirator alkalosis in pts w/ relatively unimpaired respiratory drive.

ii. *IMV/SIMV*: delivers a ventilatory cycle if pt does not meet minimum threshold spontaneous breathing rate. Spontaneous breaths may or may not be supported w/ pressure support, depending on settings. In SIMV, the intermittent ventilation breaths are synchronized w/ the spontaneous breaths.

iii. *Pressure-regulated volume control*: similar to volume control ventilation, but adjusts flow rate to avoid exceeding a programmed peak pressure; useful in decreased lung compliance (i.e., ARDS).

iv. *Bilevel ventilation* (functionally same concept as *airway pressure release ventilation [APRV]*): essentially a mode of inverse I:E ratio IMV utilized to reduce PIP while maintaining mean airway pressure. Ventilator cycles between 2 different levels of CPAP. Higher level facilitates oxygenation while lower level provides improved ventilation. Hypercapnia is accepted to achieve oxygenation goals.

v. *Pressure support*: all breaths are initiated by pt and pressure is delivered to augment the breath w/out specifying a particular volume. Generally one can titrate the pressure so that the pt autoregulates minute volume w/ a respiratory rate of 12–20.

vi. *CPAP* (continuous positive airway pressure): when referring to non-intubated pts, acts as PEEP, and is administered through tightly sealed face or nasal masks. Most often used for pts w/ obstructive sleep apnea.

vii. *High-frequency percussive ventilation*: uses small tidal volumes w/ rates of 3–8 Hz (adults). Sets baseline pressure control rate, upon which the oscillatory breaths are superimposed. Also known as volumetric diffusive respiration (VDR), which was initially described as a means to "internally percuss" the lungs. Most frequently used in inhalation injury.

c. *Initial ventilatory settings*

i. If paralyzed or no respiratory drive → A/C: FiO_2 1.0, RR 12, PEEP 5, Vt 6 cc/kg (~ 500).

ii. If have respiratory drive → SIMV: similar settings as above.

iii. Vt should almost never be > 8 cc/kg, and 4 cc/kg is usu. desirable to avoid stretch injury physiology.

iv. *Oxygenation*: PaO_2 increases/decreases *pari passu* w/ FiO_2 and PEEP.

- As described above, one may also increase oxygenation w/ increased I:E ratios, adopting a strategy of permissive hypercapnea; respiratory acidosis (even w/ $PaCO_2$ > 100) is better tolerated than hypoxia. See entry vi. below for more information.

v. *Ventilation*: $PaCO_2$ changes inversely w/ minute ventilation, which is the product of Vt and respiratory rate.

vi. Mechanical ventilation for pts w/ ALI/ARDS [Arnato MB, et al., *N Engl J Med.* 1998;338(6): 347–54; The Acute Respiratory Distress Syndrome Network, *N Engl J Med.* 2000;342(18): 1301–8]:

- ALI = acute onset PaO_2:FiO_2 < 300 w/ bilateral infiltrates and no evidence of hydrostatic pulmonary edema (i.e., PAWP ≤ 18 mm Hg).
- ARDS = acute onset PaO_2:FiO_2 < 200 w/ bilateral infiltrates and no evidence of hydrostatic pulmonary edema (i.e., PAWP ≤ 18 mm Hg).
- Work toward a volume of (not exceeding) 6 mL/kg of predicted body wt in conjunction w/ the goal of maintaining end inspiratory plateau pressures ≤ 30 cm H_2O.
- Permissive hypercapnia can be tolerated in pts w/ ALI/ARDS if required to minimize plateau pressures and tidal volumes. The use of hypercarbia is limited in pts w/ preexisting metabolic acidosis and is contraindicated in pts w/ increased intracranial pressure. Sodium bicarbonate infusion may be considered in select pts to facilitate use of permissive hypercarbia (only if pH < 7.15).
- In facilities w/ experience, prone positioning should be considered in ARDS pts requiring potentially injurious levels of FIO_2 or plateau pressure who are not at high risk for adverse consequences of positional changes.

d. *Maintenance and weaning*

i. First priority, get FiO_2 < 60%. Once at 50%, can reprioritize.

ii. Increasing PEEP can help accomplish. Will decrease preload, but assist w/ afterload.

iii. *Maintain FiO_2*: PEEP ratio 5:1 or less (i.e., pt w/ FiO_2 of 0.50 [50%] should have PEEP of at least 10).

iv. One efficient way to wean is to go to PSV. PSV good for decreasing resp alkalosis, as is SIMV.

- Set FiO_2 and PEEP for oxygenation, then order titrate PS for RR of 12–28 (pt usu. autoregulates to maintain adequate minute ventilation).
- Goal is to get to 10/5 PSV w/ FiO_2 0.40–0.50.

- Once at PSV goal or minimal SIMV (i.e., rate of 4), try T-piece w/ blow-by oxygen (CPAP of 10–15/5).
- *Predictors of successful extubation*:
  - Daily sedation holidays combined with spontaneous breathing trials.
  - *Rapid shallow breathing index* (RSBI) (RR/Vt in liters): < 105 generally OK, < 80 better, < 60 very high likelihood of success.
  - Another predictor is NIF more negative than 25 cm H_2O.

v. *Preparing to wean*: diurese pt as much as tolerated, elevate head of bed. Consider cuff leak test. Consider having BiPap nearby. Aggressive suction, nebs, IS after extubation. Not uncommon for pts to spontaneously diurese after extubation. Make sure good nutrition, PO_4, pt rested, obeying commands.

vi *Sedation*: protocols should be used for sedation of critically ill mechanically ventilated pts, predetermined end points and w/ daily interruption/lightening of continuous infusion sedation w/ awakening and retitration.

e. *Extubation criteria*

i. Gold standard in past has been 2 h of CPAP. W/ this in mind, many hospitals are going to standard protocol of daily CPAP/SBT trials.

ii. *Consider extubation if tolerates 2 h SBT and*:

- $FiO_2 < 0.5$
- PEEP < 8 cm H_2O
- RR < 30
- Minute ventilation (VE) < 12 L/min
- pH 7.35–7.47
- $PaO_2 > 65$
- $PaCO_2$ 33–49
- Condition that led to intubation improved and hemodynamically stable, off pressor/inotrope drips
- Able to obey commands, initiate breaths, clear secretions
- Cuff leak present
- ICP < 20
- RSBI < 105
  - Most accurate method has been to calculate rapid shallow breathing index (RSBI) = resp rate/vol (in liters). < 105 should be able to extubate. < 60 definitely worth a trial.
- Inspiratory force more negative than 25 cm H_2O.

iii. 10–15% reintubation rate acceptable.

f. *Indications for tracheostomy*

i. Upper respiratory tract obstruction (in emergency, use cricothryroidotomy or jet insufflation).

ii. Mental status unable to maintain long-term airway.

iii. Anticipated need for mechanical ventilation > 3 wk.

iv. Inadequate strength or vital capacity.

v. Uncontrolled secretions.

II. CIRCULATION (SHOCK, RESUSCITATION, AND CRITICAL CARE MAINTENANCE)

A. Inflammatory response states

1. *SIRS* (systemic inflammatory response syndrome):

a. *Dx requires 2 of the following 4 criteria*:

i. *Temperature*: ≤ 36°C or ≤ 38°C

ii. *Heart rate*: ≤ 90 bpm

iii. *Respiration*: ≤ 20 breaths/min *or* $PaCO_2$ < 32 mm Hg

iv. *WBC*: ≤ 12,000 or ≤ 4000 cells/mm^3 or > 10% bands

2. *Sepsis*: SIRS secondary to identified infectious source.
3. *Severe sepsis*: sepsis assoc. w/ at least 1 organ system dysfunction.
4. *Septic shock*: refractory hypotension/hypoperfusion despite fluid optimization and vasopressors.
5. *MODS*: multiple organ dysfunction syndrome.

B. Shock

1. *Types*
   a. *Hypovolemic* (e.g., hemorrhage)
   b. *Distributive* (e.g., neurogenic—different than "spinal shock," which denotes spinal arreflexia after trauma, septic)
   c. *Cardiogenic* (e.g., MI)
   d. *Obstructive* (e.g., cardiac tamponade, tension pneumothorax)

C. Resuscitation

1. Give crystalloids, PRBCs until CVP 15 and hct of 30. If still unstable (HR > 120, SBP < 90, BD > 6), possible cardiac problems → insert PA catheter, consider echo.
2. Give fluids until PCWP 15.
   a. If still unstable, bolus 500 cc of crystalloid, until CI (goal 3.8) decreases by 0.3. Consider the PCWP just before the decrease in CI to be optimal PCWP.
3. If CI < 3.8 after reaching "optimal" PCWP or PCWP of 25, consider inotrope support (i.e., dobutamine, milrinone).
4. If hypotension (MAP < 60) persists w/ CI < 3.8, consider inotrope w/ vasopressor activity (dopamine, levophed, epinephrine).
5. If hypotension still present w/ CI > 3.8, consider pressor (levophed, phenylephrine).
6. *Serum markers for resuscitation*:
   a. *Base deficit*: > 6 worrisome.
   b. *Lactate*: > 2 abnormal, but > 4 is clinically significant.
      i. Marker for anaerobic metabolism.
      ii. *Can also be elevated from*:
         - *Hepatic insufficiency*: decreased clearance by liver.
         - *Thiamine deficiency*: B_1 a cofactor for pyruvate dehydrogenase, needed for pyruvate entry into mitochondria.
         - *Alkalosis*: stimulates glycolysis.
         - *Enteric microbe production* (D-lactic acid): note, endotoxin can also inhibit pyruvate dehydrogenase.
         - *Epinephrine infusion*: can lead to increased glycogenolysis.
         - *Nitroprusside toxicity*: can cause cyanide accumulation.
   c. Bicarbonate equivalent on chemistry panel.

D. Central venous, PA catheters, and arterial catheters

1. *Central lines*:
   a. Generally place a central line no longer than 15–16 cm.
   b. U/S guidance rapidly becoming considered standard of care.
   c. *Depth guide for subclavian line*:
      i. Insert to 15 cm on right and 18 cm on left.
   d. *Depth guide for internal jugular line*:
      i. Insert to 9 cm on right and 12 cm on left.
2. *Arterial lines*: document Allen's test before proceeding.
3. *Pulmonary artery catheters and shock states*:
   a. May be used to help guide fluid management in pts who are difficult to assess.
      i. No proven mortality benefit from the use of PA-catheters in critically ill pts, however.
   b. *Hemodynamic parameters* (indexed parameters are preferred where appropriate):

i. *Central venous pressure* (CVP): 1–6 mm Hg.
ii. *Cardiac index* (CI): 2.4–4.0 L/min/m^2.
iii. *Pulmonary capillary wedge pressure* (PCWP): 6–12 mm Hg.
iv. *Left ventricular stroke work index* (LVSWI): 40–60 g m/M^2.
v. *Right ventricular ejection fraction* (RVEF): 46–50%.
vi. *Right ventricular end diastolic volume index* (REDVI): 80–150 cc/m^2.
vii. *Systemic vascular resistance index* (SVRI): 1600–2400 dynes.sec.m^2/cm^5.
viii. *Pulmonary vascular resistance index* (PVRI): 200–400 dynes.sec.m^2/cm^5.
ix. *Oxygen delivery* (DO_2) = CI × 13.4 × Hgb × SaO_2: 520–570 cc/min.m^2.
x. *Mixed venous oxygen saturation* (SVO_2): 70–75%.
xi. *Oxygen uptake* (VO_2) = CI × 13.4 × Hgb × (SaO_2 – SvO_2): 110–160 cc/min.m^2.
xii. *Oxygen extraction ratio* (O_2ER) = VO_2/DO_2 (×100): 20–30%.

TABLE 6.1. Hemodynamic Parameters for Normal and Shock States

Shock Type	CVP	PA	PCWP	CI	SVR
Normal	0–6	25/6–12	6–12	> 2.5	700–1300
Hypovolemic	0–2	15–20/0–2	2–6	< 2.0	> 1500
Cardiogenic	> 8	50/35	> 25	< 2.0	> 1500
Septic	0–2	15–20/0–6	< 6	> 2.5	< 1500
Major PE	8–12	50/12–15	< 12	< 2.0	> 1500
Tamponade	12–16	25/12–16	12–16	< 2.0	> 1500
Neurogenic	0–2	15–20/0–2	6–12	> 2.5	< 700

c. *Heart failure patterns*
   i. *Right heart failure*: high CVP, low CI, high PVRI
   ii. *Left heart failure*: high PCWP, low CI, high SVRI
d. *Hypotension patterns*
   i. *Hypovolemic*: low CVP, low CI, high SVRI
   ii. *Cardiogenic*: high CVP, low CI, high SVRI
   iii. *Vasogenic*: low CVP, high CI, low SVRI
e. *Valvular/wall patterns*
   i. *Tamponade* (equal diastolic pressures): CVP = PADP = PAWP
   ii. *Mitral stenosis* (increased "a" wave): PAWP = LAP > LVEDP
   iii. *Mitral regurgitation* (increased "v" wave): PAWP = LAP > LVEDP
   iv. *Aortic regurgitation*: LVEDP > LAP = PAWP

III. ADDITIONAL NOTES FOR MANAGEMENT OF SPECIFIC TYPES OF SHOCK

A. Hypovolemic

1. Aside from fluid administration and mechanical control of bleeding (surgery), consider possible need for blood replacement products and adjunctive maneuvers a/o medications to aid hemostasis (see Chapter 2).

B. Septic: outlined are key *portions* of recommendations from the Surviving Sepsis Campaign. [Dellinger RP, et al., *Crit Care Med.* 2004;32(3):858–73, Surviving Sepsis Campaign guidelines for management of severe sepsis and septic shock.]

1. *Initial resuscitation*
   a. Hyperlactasemia suggests hypoperfusion even if not hypotensive. Goals for first 6 h of resuscitation include:

   i. *CVP*: 8–12 mm Hg
   ii. *MAP*: ≥ 65 mm Hg
   iii. *UOP*: ≥ 0.5 cc/kg/h
   iv. *Central venous (superior vena cava) or mixed SvO_2*: ≥ 70%

b. For pts on ventilator (and pts w/ intraabdominal hypertension), a higher CVP of 12–15 mm Hg is recommended.

c. During the first 6 h of resuscitation, if central venous oxygen saturation or mixed SvO_2 of 70% not achieved w/ fluid resuscitation to a central venous pressure of 8–12 mm Hg, transfuse packed RBCs to achieve a hematocrit > 30% a/o titrate dobutamine gtt (up to 20 mcg/kg/min) to achieve this goal.

2. *Dx*
   a. Obtain cultures of appropriate body fluids/sites before beginning abx, preferably at least 2 blood cultures, w/ at least 1 drawn percutaneously and 1 drawn through each vascular access device, unless the device was recently (< 48 h) inserted.
3. *Antibiotic therapy*
   a. Start IV abx w/in 1 h of severe sepsis dx, after cx have been obtained. In severe sepsis or septic shock, broad empiric coverage warranted until can be directed by cx results.
   b. No evidence exists that for an appropriately identified pathogen, combination therapy is more effective than monotherapy, though some advocate combination tx for *Pseudomonas* (authors' note: others recommend mnemonic "SPACE" or "SPICE" organisms be provided w/ double-coverage—*Serratia*, *Pseudomonas*, *Acinetobacter*, indole-positive *Proteus*, *Enterobacter*).
   c. 7–10 d is typically appropriate and should be guided by clinical response. Most would use combination therapy for *neutropenic* pts w/ severe sepsis or septic shock for duration of neutropenia.
4. *Source control*
   a. Identify and remove infectious foci (lines [probably most common source], necrotic tissue, etc.) ASAP.
5. *Fluid therapy*
   a. No data consistently suggest advantage to crystalloid vs colloid resuscitation.
   b. Boluses (500–1000 cc crystalloid or 300–500 cc colloid over 30 min) may be repeatedly given if BP, UOP suggest benefit w/out untoward effects of hypervolemia.
6. *Vasopressors*
   a. Begin vasopressors when appropriate fluid challenges fail to meet goals; may also be required transiently to sustain life and maintain perfusion in the face of life-threatening hypotension, even when a fluid challenge is in progress and hypovolemia has not yet been corrected.
   b. Norepinephrine or dopamine (through a central catheter as soon as available) is the first-choice vasopressor agent to correct hypotension in septic shock (over epinephrine [potential tachycardia, possibly disadvantageous effects on splanchnic circulation] and phenylephrine [decrease in stroke volume]). Phenylephrine ↓ risk tachycardia. Dopamine ↑ MAP and CO (as inotrope and chronotrope). Norepinephrine primarily vasoconstrictor, little change in heart rate and less increase in stroke volume compared w/ dopamine—more potent than dopamine and may be more effective at reversing hypotension in pts w/ septic shock. Dopamine may be particularly useful in pts w/ compromised systolic function but causes more tachycardia and may be more arrhythmogenic.
   c. Consider vasopressin if refractory to fluids, high-dose vasopressors; administered at 0.01–0.04 U/min (higher doses assoc. w/ MI, decrease in CI, cardiac arrest). May decrease stroke volume. A direct vasoconstrictor w/out inotropic or chronotropic effects, may result in decreased CO and hepatosplanchnic flow. Discourage use if cardiac dysfunction, particularly if CI is ≤ 2.5.
   d. Place arterial catheter as soon as practical to help guide pressor titration.
7. *Inotropic therapy*
   a. If low CI despite adequate fluid resuscitation, consider use of dobutamine. If used in the presence of low blood pressure, combine w/ vasopressor therapy. Hypotensive pts w/ severe sepsis may have low, normal, or increased CI. Therefore, tx w/ a combined inotrope/vasopressor such as norepinephrine or dopamine is recommended if unable to measure CI. Once able to monitor cardiac output in addition to blood pressure, a vasopressor such as norepinephrine and an inotrope such as dobutamine may be used separately to target specific levels of mean arterial pressure and cardiac output. [Dellinger RP, et al., *Crit Care Med.* 2004;32(3): 858–73.]

b. Increasing CI to achieve an arbitrarily predefined elevated level is not recommended; goal of resuscitation should instead be to achieve adequate levels of oxygen delivery or avoid flow-dependent tissue hypoxia.

8. *Steroids*
   a. Hydrocortisone 200–300 mg/d, for 7 d in 3 or 4 divided doses or by continuous infusion, recommended in pts w/ septic shock who, despite adequate fluid replacement, require vasopressor therapy to maintain adequate blood pressure.
   b. Relative adrenal insufficiency defined as post-ACTH cortisol increase > 9 mcg/dL. Some would use 250-mcg ACTH stimulation test to identify responders (> 9 mcg/dL increase in cortisol 30–60 min post ACTH administration) and discontinue therapy in these pts.
   c. Do not wait for ACTH stimulation results to administer corticosteroids.
   d. Consider administering a dose of dexamethasone until ACTH stimulation test performed because dexamethasone, unlike hydrocortisone, does not interfere w/ the cortisol assay.
   e. One study showed hemodynamic and immunologic rebound effects after abrupt cessation of corticosteroids.
   f. Some would add fludrocortisone (50 mcg orally 4 times per day) to this regimen.
9. *Recombinant human activated protein C* (rhAPC)
   a. *rhAPC (Xigris) recommended if*: APACHE II > 25, sepsis-induced multiple organ failure, septic shock, or sepsis-induced ARDS w/ no absolute contraindication related to bleeding risk or relative contraindication.
   b. *Contraindications include*: active internal bleeding; recent (w/in 3 mo) hemorrhagic stroke; recent (w/in 2 mo) intracranial or intraspinal surgery, or severe head trauma; trauma w/ an increased risk of life-threatening bleeding; presence of an epidural catheter; intracranial neoplasm or mass lesion or evidence of cerebral herniation.
10. *Blood product administration*
    a. In absence of hypoperfusion/lactic acidosis, CAD, hemorrhage, or coronary artery disease, RBC transfusion should be limited to Hgb < 7.0 g/dL (< 70 g/L) to target a Hgb of 7.0–9.0 g/dL.
    b. RBC transfusion in septic pts increases oxygen delivery but does not usu. increase oxygen consumption.
    c. This transfusion threshold contrasts w/ the target of a hematocrit of 30% in pts w/ low SvO_2 during the first 6 h of resuscitation of septic shock.
    d. In severe sepsis, transfuse platelets if < 5000/mm^3, regardless of apparent bleeding.
    e. Consider transfusion when 5000–30,000/mm^3 and there is a significant risk of bleeding.
    f. Higher platelet counts than 50,000/mm^3 are typically required for surgery or invasive procedures.
11. *Bicarbonate therapy*
    a. There is no evidence to support the use of bicarbonate therapy in the tx of hypoperfusion-induced acidemia assoc. w/ sepsis—outcomes w/ hemodynamic variables or vasopressor requirements w/out evidence of benefit.

C. Cardiogenic

1. Generally requires PA catheter monitoring and appropriate fluid and inotrope/pressor management, as described in Chapter 7.

D. Neurogenic

1. Generally limited w/ spinal cord injury above level of T5.
2. Loss of sympathetic tone results in hypotension w/ relatively warm extremities (similar to septic shock), but w/ relative bradycardia. Manage w/ fluids and appropriate alpha agonist (i.e., phenylephrine, norepinephrine, etc.).
3. "Spinal shock" is a different entity, referring to usu. transient arreflexia after blunt spinal trauma.

IV. PROPHYLAXIS

A. DVT/PE: see Chapter 2 on hematology.

B. Upper GI bleeding (usu. related to stress-related mucosal bleeding).

1. *Efficacy*: H_2 blocker (ranitidine, etc.) ~ PPI (omeprazole, etc.) > Carafate.
2. Prophylaxis geared toward preventing clinically significant bleeding.
3. *Biggest risk factors*: mechanical ventilation and coagulopathy.

C. Infection

1. *Intravascular catheters* [O'Grady NP, et al., Guidelines for the prevention of intravascular catheter-related infections, *MMWR*. Aug 9, 2002;51, RR-10]:
   a. *Observations and recommendations from NIH and Centers for Disease Control and Prevention*:
      i. Coagulase-negative *Staph* accounts for almost 40% of all nosocomial bloodstream infections, w/ tie for second w/ *S. aureus, Enterococcus*, and gram-negative rods (all species together). *Candida* infections ~ 8%, w/ non-*albicans* species increasing in proportion.
      ii. Teflon, silicone, polyurethane catheters more resistant to infection than PVC or polyethylene.
      iii. *Rate of infection by site* (lowest > highest): subclavian, femoral, jugular.
         - *Note*: femoral lines also assoc. w/ thromboembolism in ICU pts. Right (then left) jugular is line of choice for pt who will need hemodialysis.
      iv. Full sterile barrier precautions indicated.
      v. No infectious risk difference found between transparent semipermeable dressings and gauze dressings.
      vi. Catheters w/ chlorhexidene or silver sulfadiazeine cuffs or coatings demonstrated to reduce risk of infection.
      vii. Peripheral IVs should be changed every 72–96 h to avoid phlebitis.
      viii. Central lines do *not* need to be changed routinely—no demonstrated decrease in infectious risk.
         - Burn pt units often have policies of routine changing every 72 h; however, central lines placed in emergency situations should be replaced w/in 48 h in a different site.
         - In pts w/ bacteremia/sepsis, use clinical judgment and cultures to guide decision to leave/replace catheter. Remove if pt hemodynamically unstable and line is suspected. If removing for infectious reasons, guide-wire replacement is not indicated.
         - Purulence at infection site is indication for replacement (at different site). *Note*: many authorities add local erythema and tenderness as indications for replacement.
      ix. Hemodialysis should use AV fistulas/grafts and not rely on catheters. However, if a catheter is used, it should be cuffed if anticipated to be left for > 3 wk.
2. *Glucose control*
   a. Although tight glycemic control (80–110 mg/dL) in SICU pts was shown to reduce morbidity and mortality in 2001 [van den Berghe, et al., *N Engl J Med*. Nov 8, 2001;345(19):1359–67], the NICE-SUGAR study [Finfer S, et al., *NEJM*. 2009;360:1283–97] demonstrated higher mortality w/ tight control and recommended no tx for glucose < 180. However, select groups of surgical pts may benefit from tighter control, which may be achieved w/ continuous infusion of insulin and glucose, monitoring glucose (every 30–60 min) and on a regular basis (every 4 h) once the blood glucose concentration has stabilized.
3. *Lungs*
   a. Maintain HOB > 300, particularly if receiving tube feeds.
   b. Maintaining good oropharyngeal hygiene.
   c. Maintenance of normal gastric pH.
   d. Application of antimicrobial paste to oral mucosa.

V. ABG INTERPRETATION AND ACID-BASE PROBLEMS

A. ABG normal values

1. *Normal pH*: 7.35–7.45
2. *pCO_2*: resp alkalosis < 35–45 < resp acidosis
3. *HCO_3*: met acidosis < 22–26 < met alkalosis

B. **ABG interpretation**

1. *First step*: is the pH high, low, or normal?
2. *Second step*: is the pCO_2 high, low, or normal?
3. *Third step*: is the degree of compensation (CO_2 or HCO_3) expected, more, or less?
   a. **pH < 7.35**
      i. If pCO_2 low or normal, then primary **met acidosis**.
         - *Check anion gap*: $AG = Na - (Cl + HCO_3) \rightarrow$ normal < 12. (*Note*: hypoalbuminemia can falsely lower AG.)
           - If AG > 12, then gain of acid is responsible (generally a *medical* problem except for lactic acidosis in trauma, bowel infarction, etc.).
             - *"MUD PILERS:"* methanol, uremia, DKA/starvation, paraldehyde, isopropyl alcohol/INH, lactic acidosis, ethanol/ethylene glycol, rhabdomyolysis, salicylates.
             - *DKA tx*: start insulin drip at 0.1 U reg insulin/kg/h; continue insulin until gap is gone, then add dextrose once glucose < 250. To correct Na^+, add 1.6 to Na^+ level for every 100 mg/dL the glucose is over 100 mg/dL.
             - mmol/L HCO_3 = (base deficit × kg body wt) (0.3).
           - If AG < 12 (normal), then loss of HCO_3 is responsible (often a surgical issue, such as fistulas, surgical drains, etc.)
             - *Check urine pH and urine anion gap*: UAG = Na + K – Cl.
             - UAG = –10 to +10.
             - UAG < –10 = extrarenal non-AG metacidosis.
             - UAG > +10 = renal non-AG metacidosis.
             - In general, urine pH > 6 suggests renal cause, urine pH > 6 suggests GI cause.
             - *If urine pH < 5.5 and UAG is negative* (often surgical issue): etiology: diarrhea, surgical drains, fistulas, ureterosigmoidostomy/ileal bladder/ileal ureter, cholestyramine. If none of these exists and pt is hypokalemic, consider Type 2 RTA.
             - *If urine pH < 5.5 and UAG is positive, w/ hyperkalemia*: type 4 RTA (hyperaldosteronism—hyperkalemia prevents ammoniagenesis, which lowers H^+ excretion). Tx hyperkalemia w/ kayexylate or diuretics.
             - *Other causes of normal AG w/ hyper- or normokalemia*: early renal failure, other renal dz (amyloidosis, hydronephrosis, sickle cell nephropathy), acidifying agents (ammonium chloride, calcium chloride, arginine), sulfur toxicity.
             - *If urine pH > 5.5 and UAG is positive, pt usu. hypokalemic*: type I RTA ("distal:" no distal H^+ excretion). Tx w/ 1–2 mEq/kg/d of bicarb.
             - *But*: w/ variable urine pH and UAG that is negative, but w/ hypokalemia (may be confused w/ first scenario listed—r/o if no diarrhea, surgical drains, fistulas, etc.): Type 2 RTA ("proximal"). Tx w/ 10–20 mEq/kg/d of bicarb.
             - *Other causes of normal AG w/ hypokalemia*: mineralocorticoid deficiency (angiotensin deficiency/liver failure, ACEi, renin deficiency, aging, extracellular volume expansion, lead, beta blockers, prostaglandin inhibitors, methyldopa, acetazolamide, mafenamide, post-hypocapnia).
         - Check difference between measured and expected pCO_2 to identify a superimposed respiratory d/o.
           - *Met acidosis*: change pCO_2 = change HCO_3 × 1.3.
             - pCO_2 too high, concurrent resp acidosis.
             - pCO_2 too low, concurrent resp alkalosis.
      ii. If pCO_2 high, then primary **resp acidosis**.
         - Pneumonia, narcotic OD, COPD, neuropathy/myopathy.
         - Check change in pH to determine acute vs chronic and if superimposed metabolic d/o is present.

- *Acute resp acidosis*: change HCO_3 to change pCO_2 should be 1:10.
  - HCO_3 too high, concurrent met alkalosis.
  - HCO_3 too low, concurrent met acidosis.
- *Chronic resp acidosis*: change HCO_3 to change pCO_2 should be 3:10.
  - HCO_3 too high, concurrent met alkalosis.
  - HCO_3 too low, concurrent met acidosis.

b. **pH > 7.45**

i. If pCO_2 high or normal, then primary **met alkalosis**.

- Check measured vs expected $PaCO_2$ to see if assoc. resp d/o present. Change pCO_2 = change $HCO_3 \times 0.7$.
  - PCO_2 too high, concurrent resp acidosis.
  - PCO_2 too low, concurrent resp alkalosis.
- *Check urine chloride*:
  - Urine $Cl^- < 20$ mEq/L *(chloride responsive)*.
    - *NGT suctioning, vomiting, diuretics, excess LR, TPN, blood transfusions* (usu. > 8), colonic villous adenoma, correction of chronic resp acidosis (conversely, in primary metabolic alkalosis, body will decrease rate to retain acid, which may make vent weaning difficult), CF pt sweating, *volume contraction* (renin-aldosterone retains Na^+, balanced electrically w/ Cl^- and HCO_3 retention. H^+, K^+ lost in urine in exchange. Cl^- preferentially follows H^+, K^+, thus HCO_3 is retained comparably more. Must tx by volume expansion w/ emphasis on Na^+, K^+, and Cl^- replacement. Chronic high-dose steroid use results in the same effect).
  - Urine $Cl^- > 20$ mEq/L *(chloride resistant)*.
    - *Normotensive*: hypokalemia, hypercalcemia, hypomagnesemia, hypoparathyroidism, refeeding carbs after fasting, milk-alkali syndrome, Bartter syndrome.
    - *Hypertensive*: hyperreninism (renal artery stenosis, primary hyperaldosteronism, Cushing syndrome, congenital adrenal hyperplasia, pseudohyperparathyroidism).

ii. If pCO_2 low, then a primary **resp alkalosis**.

- Check change in pH to see if d/o is acute vs chronic, or if superimposed metabolic d/o is present.
- PE, pregnancy, anxiety, endotoxemia, altitude, fever.
  - If altitude, consider acetazolamide.
  - If on vent, change from CMV or SIMV, consider rate. Change from CMV to SIMV (neuro picture concern for apnea) or PSV.
- *Acute resp alkalosis*: change HCO_3 to change pCO_2 should be 2:10.
  - HCO_3 too high, concurrent met alkalosis.
  - HCO_3 too low, concurrent met acidosis.
- *Chronic resp alkalosis*: change HCO_3 to change PCO_2 should be 4:10.
  - HCO_3 too high, concurrent met alkalosis.
  - HCO_3 too low, concurrent met acidosis.

c. **pH normal**

i. If pCO_2 high, mixed resp acidosis, met alkalosis.

ii. If pCO_2 low, mixed resp alkalosis, met acidosis.

iii. If pCO_2 normal, a mixed d/o may still exist.

- Check anion gap if elevated or normal.

iv. Mixed d/o also exists if $PaCO_2$ is abnormal, but pH is unchanged or normal, or if pH is abnormal and the $PaCO_2$ is unchanged or normal.

CHAPTER 7

CARDIAC AND EKG

I. CARDIAC

A. Anatomy

1. *3 main arteries*: left main (left anterior descending artery w/ septal perforators and diagonals + circumflex w/ obtuse marginals); right main w/ acute marginal; and posterior descending.

B. Physiology

1. $V = IR$ (Ohm's law): V is blood pressure, which the body wants to maintain as constant. I is left ventricular output (LVEDV × EF), R is systemic arterial constriction (SVR). If I falls, R must increase (cold extremities, weak pulse). If R falls, I must increase (warm extremities, strong pulse).
2. $CO = HR \times SV$.
3. *Right heart failure* (more common in ICU pts): fluid cannot be driven forward to lungs, backs up in IVC, leads to JVD, hepatic congestion, LE edema.
    a. CVP > 15 mm Hg and CVP ≥ PCWP.
    b. May mimic pericardial tamponade.
    c. Right ventricular EF and RVEDV measured by PA catheter are best measures.
        i. A decrease in RVEF and increase in RVEDV is seen.
    d. Echocardiogram can be useful as well.
    e. If PCWP < 15 mm Hg, give volume until PCWP or CVP increases by 5 *or* either one reaches 20 mm Hg.
    f. If RVEDV is less than 140 cc/m^2, give volume until there.
    g. If PCWP > 15 or RVEDV is 140 or higher, give dobutamine at 5 mcg/kg/min.
4. *Left heart failure*: fluid cannot be driven forward, leads to pulmonary congestion:
    a. *Above all think*: fluids/preload → if low PCWP, infuse volume.
        i. If colloid osmotic pressure normal (20–25 mm Hg), aim for PCWP of 20 mm Hg.
        ii. Once at goal wedge pressure:
            - If low BP → dopamine (3–10 mcg/kg/min).
            - If normal BP → dobutamine (3–15 mcg/kg/min), amrinone (5–10 mcg/kg/min).
            - If high BP → nitroprusside (0.3–2 mcg/kg/min—no more than 10 mcg/min for 10 min), nitroglycerine (1–50 mcg/min for venodilation, > *50 mcg/min* for arterial dilation).
            - High PCWP but low CO → dobutamine, amrinone (NOT dopamine).
            - High PCWP, normal CO → nitroglycerine, consider furosemide.
5. *New York Classification of CHF*
    a. *Class I*: no sx.
    b. *Class II*: sx w/ significant exercise.
    c. *Class III*: sx w/ routine activity.
    d. *Class IV*: sx at rest.

C. Acquired disease

1. *Coronary artery disease*
    a. *CABG indications*:
        i. Significant 3-vessel (LAD, circumflex, right main) dz w/ LV dysfunction.
        ii. Significant 3-vessel dz, good LV function, and 1+ important proximal stenoses.
        iii. Significant 2- to 3-vessel dz w/ severe angina, regardless of LV function.
        iv. Left main stenosis > 50%, even if asymptomatic.

v. 2-vessel dz w/ severe proximal LAD stenosis or LV dysfunction.

b. *Bypass conduits*: vein grafts 10-yr patency 50–60%, usu. affected by atherosclerosis. IMA grafts more resistant to atherosclerosis w/ 90% 10-yr patency. Radial artery more spastic than IMA; patency > vein grafts but < than IMA.

c. *Complications of CAD/myocardial infarction*: ventricular aneurysm, myocardial rupture, ruptured papillary muscle, VSD, chronic mitral insufficiency; last three can cause postop pulmonary edema (listen for new murmurs, consider ECHO, Swan).

d. *Post CABG hypotension/heart failure*:

i. Volume.

ii. Mediastinal hematoma.

iii. MI.

- Papillary muscle rupture w/ MR.
- Ventricular septal defect.
- Ventricular aneurysm.
- Free wall rupture.

e. *Signs of ventricular dysfunction/heart failure*:

i. First, otherwise unexplained increase in PCWP.

ii. Next, an increase in heart rate and decrease in stroke volume.

iii. Last, decrease in cardiac output.

- End diastolic volume best measure for systolic/diastolic heart failure.

2. *Valvular heart disease*

a. *Mitral valve*: indications for operation (balloon mitral valvuloplasty, mitral commisurotomy, valve replacement).

i. *Stenosis*:

- Sx (i.e., evidence of pulmonary hypertension, endocarditis, systemic embolization).
- Valve area < 1 cm^2.

ii. *Insufficiency*:

- Symptoms refractory to medical management (ACE inhibitor tx of choice).
- Pulmonary hypertension.
- Severe mitral regurgitation w/ structural abnormality.
- LV ejection fraction < 60%, or LV end-systolic diameter > 45 mm.

b. *Aortic valve*: indications for operation.

i. *Stenosis*:

- *Sx*: angina, syncope, CHF.
- Pressure gradient transvalvular velocity > 4 m/sec.
- Transvalvular gradient 50 mm Hg or valve area < 1 cm^2.

ii. *Insufficiency*: (try medical afterload reduction w/ nifedipine a/o ACEi first.) Class II (or greater) CHF. If asx, criteria include LV dilation (left ventricular end-systolic dimension 50–55 mm).

c. *Endocarditis*: generally 4–6 wk of abx is adequate tx.

i. *Indications for operation*: valve insufficiency contributing to CHF, persistent bacteremia after abx therapy, gram-negative infection, valve annulus abscess, recurrent emboli, mobile vegetations > 1 cm.

II. EKG ANALYSIS

A. EKG basics

1. *Rate*: 300, 150, 100, 75, 60, 50, etc.
2. *Rhythm*: regular, irregular, irregularly irregular, etc.
3. *Axis*

a. *Approximating*:

i. Normal = I^+, AVF^+

ii. LAD = I^+, AVF^-

iii. RAD = I^-, AVF^+
iv. Extreme LAD = I^-, AVF^-

b. *Hemiblocks*:
   i. *Left anterior*: shows LAD, but no LVH. (I^+, AVF^-, often II^-.)
   ii. *Left posterior*: shows RAD, but no RVH. (I^-, AVF^+.)

B. EKG waves and segments

1. *P wave*
   a. *Amplitude*: > 2.5 mm in II suggests RAE.
   b. *Duration*: > 0.12 sec in II suggests LAE.
   c. *Biphasic*: biphasic in V_1 w/ terminal component > 1 mm, 0.4 sec suggests LAE.
   d. *Relationship to QRS*: present before all QRS.
      i. Progressive distance between QRS then dropped QRS = Mobitz I (Wenckebach).
      ii. Fixed interval and fixed ratio of dropped QRSs = Mobitz II.
      iii. No relation between P and QRS = 3rd-degree (complete AV) block.
2. *PR segment*
   a. *Short*: < 0.12 sec may be WPW or LGL.
   b. *Long*: > 0.20 is 1st-degree AV block.
3. *Q wave*
   a. Significant if > 0.04 sec duration and amplitude > 1/3 QRS complex.
4. *QRS complex*
   a. Prolonged (> 0.12) suggestive of BBB.
   b. *RBBB*: look for "rabbit ears" (R') in V_1 a/o V_2.
   c. *LBBB*: look for notched appearance in V_5 a/o V_6.
5. *R and S amplitude*
   a. *Left ventricular hypertrophy*: $RV_1 > SV_1$ and $RV_6 < SV_6$.
   b. *Right ventricular hypertrophy*: $RV_{5\text{ or }6} + SV_{1\text{ or }2} > 35$ mm *or* AVL > 12 mm.
6. *ST segment*
   a. *Elevation*: suggests infarction or pericarditis if in all leads.
   b. *Depression*: suggests subendocardial ischemia, or if present in precordial leads w/ elevated R waves indicates strain pattern. *Note*: an upsloping depressed ST segment usu. not worrisome, but horizontal or downsloping ST segments are.
7. *T wave*
   a. *Peaked*: hyperkalemia or early ischemia.
   b. *Flat*: hypokalemia.
   c. *Inverted*: later ischemia.
   d. Generally positive when net QRS positive, negative when net QRS negative.
8. *U wave*
   a. Hypothermia

TABLE 7.1. EKG Analysis

Region	Leads	Coronary Artery	Infarct Assoc. W/
Anterior	V_{1-4}	LAD	
Lateral	I, AVL, V_{5-6}	LCx	
Inferior	II, III, AVF	R	Bradycardia
Posterior		R	

TABLE 7.2. Inotropic and Vasoactive Medications

Drug Type and Name(s)	Dose	Indications	Caveats/Miscellaneous
Inotropes			
Dopamine	5–20 mcg/kg/min	• Hypotensive heart failure	• Dopamine, then beta, then alpha • Can lead to myocardial ischemia, tissue hypoxia/necrosis and decreased UOP w/ high doses • Assoc. w/ tachyarrhythmias
Dobutamine (Dobutrex)	5–20 mcg/kg/min	• Normotensive heart failure	• Like intermediate dopamine, see increased HR and SV, but get decreased SVR (opp. of intermed-high-dose dopamine) • Assoc. w/ tachyarrythmias, myocardial ischemia, hypotension
Milrinone (Primacor)	50 mcg/kg over 10 min, then 0.375–0.75 mcg/kg/min	• Normotensive heart failure	• Increased SV, but decreased SVR like dobutamine, but little effect on HR • Rare tachyarrhythmia; mycocardial ischemia, hypotension
Epinephrine	1–10 mcg/min; 1 mg q 3–5 min for resuscitation	• Cardiac arrest • Anaphylaxis • Post-CABG	• Tachyarrythmias, myocardial ischemia, tissue hypoxia/necrosis, hyperglycemia
Norepinephrine (Levophed)	0.5–1 mcg/min may require up to 8–30 mcg/min	• Septic shock, cardiogenic shock, PE	• Increased SVR and SV • Can lead to myocardial ischemia, tissue hypoxia / necrosis, hyperglycemia, oliguria
Vasoconstrictors			
Phenylephrine (Neo-Synephrine)	100–180 mcg/min, then 40–60 mcg/min	• Neurogenic shock, septic shock, anesthesia-induced hypotension	• Myocardial ischemia, tissue hypoxia/necrosis
Norepinephrine (Levophed)	0.5–1 mcg/min may require up to 8–30 mcg/min	• Septic shock, cardiogenic shock, PE	• Increased SVR and SV • Can lead to myocardial ischemia, tissue hypoxia / necrosis, hyperglycemia, oliguria
Vasopressin (Pitressin)	0.01–0.04 U/min; 40 U once for resuscitation	• Septic shock, cardiac arrest	• Increases SVR • Myocardial ischemia, tissue hypoxia/necrosis, hyponatremia
Vasodilators			
Hydralazine	5–20 mg q 20–30 min	• Hypertension	• Arteriolar dilator, not good for MI, ischemia, or aortic dissection • Onset 10–30 min • Duration 2–4 h
Nitroglycerine	5–100 mcg/min	• Hypertension	• Venous > arteriolar dilator • Onset 2–5 min • Duration 5–10 min • Good for cardiac ischemia, but poss. unpredictable BP response

(Continues)

TABLE 7.2. Inotropic and Vasoactive Medications *(Continued)*

Drug Type and Name(s)	Dose	Indications	Caveats/Miscellaneous
Nitroprusside	0.25–10.0 mcg/kg/min	• Hypertension	• Arteriolar > venous dilator • Fast onset (seconds) • Duration = 3 min • Cyanide toxicity w/ prolonged use
Calcium Channel Blockers			
Diltiazim	Load 20 mg, drip	• Afib/Aflutter rate control	
Nicardipine	Begin at 5 mg/h	• Hypertension	• Increase 2.5 mg/h q 5 min up to max of 15 mg/h
Beta Blockers			
Esmolol (Brevibloc)	250–500 mcg/kg/min for 1 min, then 50–300 mcg/kg/min	• Afib/Aflutter rate control • Hypertension	• Pure beta blocker • Onset < 5 min • Duration 10–20 min (half-life 9 min) • Good for aortic dissection or postop hypertension
Metoprolol	5 mg IV push		
Labetalol (Normodyne)	20 mg, then 20–80 mg q 10 min or 2 mg/min Max 300 mg	• Hypertension	• Alpha and beta blocker • Onset 5–10 min • Duration 3–6 h • Not indicated if bronchospasm, 1st-degree heart block, cardiogenic shock, or severe bradycardia
Glycoside			
Digoxin		• CHF • Afib/Aflutter rate control and conversion	
PDE-Inhibitor			
Amiodarone	Load: 150 mg over 10 min, can repeat once, then 1 mg/min over 6 h (if Vfib 300 mg) Maintenance: 0.5 mg/min	• Afib/Aflutter rate control and conversion • Ventricular arrythymias	• Hypotension, bradycardia, phlebitis, prolongs PR/QRS/QT • Pulmonary fibrosis, hypothyroidism

III. HYPOTENSION AND CARDIAC PHARMACOPOEIA (ALL DOSAGES INTRAVENOUS)

A. Congenital disease

1. *Fetal/perinatal circulation*
   a. 2 umbilical arteries (blood to placenta, relatively unoxygenated), 1 umbilical vein (blood from placenta, relatively well oxygenated).
   b. *Ductus arteriosus*: from left pulmonary artery to descending aorta; blood thus bypasses lungs in utero.
   c. *Ductus venosus*: from portal vein to IVC; shunts blood from liver in utero.
2. *Cyanotic*
   a. Right → left shunt.
   b. Cyanosis may result in polycythemia, endocarditis, hypertrophic osteoarthropathy, and CVA.
   c. CXR and echocardiogram good starters for evaluation.

d. *Examples*:
   i. *Simple defects*
      - Pulmonic stenosis w/ right → left shunt
   ii. *Complex lesions*
      - Tetrology of Fallot
         - *Comprised of*: overriding of aorta; pulmonary stenosis, VSD, right ventricular hypertrophy
      - Transposition of the great arteries
      - Truncus arteriosis
      - Tricuspid atresia
      - Total anomalous pulmonary venous return

3. *Noncyanotic*
   a. Left → right shunt.
   b. Increased pulmonary congestion leading to Eisenmenger syndrome from prolonged pulmonary HTN.
   c. *Examples*:
      i. *Septal defects*
         - *ASD (ostium secundum)*: isolated ASDs represent the most common congenital heart anomaly. 80% spontaneously close in infancy.
         - *VSD*: more frequently symptomatic (failure to thrive, tachypnea, cardiomegaly) in infancy than ASDs. Repair usu. advocated if sx or by 1 yo.
         - *AV canal defect* (endocardial cushion defect, includes ostium primum ASDs): frequently assoc. w/ trisomy 21.
      ii. *Patent ductus arteriosus*
         - Ductus arteriosus comes from confluence of left and main pulmonary artery, and empties into arch just beyond left subclavian artery origin. Patency (increased incidence w/ prematurity) beyond 3 mo postpartum requires intervention to interrupt left → right shunt w/ resultant left heart overload as well as potential endocarditis, obstructive pulmonary vasculopathy, a/o aneurysm development.
         - *Presentation*: failure to thrive, pulmonary congestion common in neonates; machinery murmur.
         - *Dx*: Echocardiography.
         - *Tx*:
            - *Medical*:
               - *Indomethacin*: inhibits prostaglandin synthesis; first-line tx for neonates to close PDA.
            - *Surgical*:
               - Percutaneous catheter closure appropriate after neonate period or if significant pulmonary HTN.
               - Open ligation/clipping via left posterolateral thoracotomy appropriate in poor candidates for catheter closure.
      iii. *Coarctation*: most commonly seen in males and in up to 30% of pts w/ Turner syndrome; results in relative HTN in proximal aorta and upper extremities. CXR classically shows notched ribs from enlarged intercostal arteries. Untreated, can cause CHF, hemorrhagic CVA, endocarditis, a/o rupture of aorta. Resection and grafting is traditional tx.

CHAPTER 8

THORACIC AND ESOPHAGUS

I. THORACIC

A. Anatomy and physiology

1. *Anatomy*
    a. Right lung 55% volume (3 lobes), left lung 45% volume (2 lobes).
    b. Azygous vein on right side, empties into SVC. Thoracic duct begins on right, crosses to left (at approx T6) to empty to left subclavian at confluence w/ internal jugular vein.
    c. Phrenic n. anterior (to hilum) but vagus n. posterior (to hilum).
    d. *Pneumocytes*: type I (> 95%) involved in gas exchange; type II (< 5%) produce surfactant.
2. *Physiology*
    a. *Functional adequacy for resection*:
        i. Need postop $FEV_1 > 0.8$ (or ≥ 40% predicted value).
            - Can assay relative contribution of FEV_1 from planned resection portion w/ V/Q scan preop.
        ii. Need predicted postop FVC > 1.5 L.
        iii. Need preop (room air) $pCO_2 \leq 45$ or $pO_2 \geq 50$.
        iv. Need preop VO_2 max ≥ 10 cc/min/kg.
        v. Desired DLCO ≥ 11–12 cc/min/mm Hg CO (≥ 50% predicted value).
    b. *Ventilation volumes* (also see Chapter 6, section I. on ventilation).
        i. *FVC* (forced vital capacity): if decreased, suggests restrictive dz. FVC < 2 L (or < 50%) concerning for postop complications. Vital capacity refers to volume of air in maximal expiration after maximal inspiration.
        ii. *FEV_1* (forced expiratory volume in 1 sec): if decreased, suggests obstructive dz. $FEV_1 < 0.8$ L concerning for postop complications.
        iii. *FEV_1/FVC*: low number suggests obstructive dz.
        iv. *MVV* (maximal voluntary ventilation): < 50% predicts moderate postop risk.
        v. *FRV* (functional residual volume/capacity): amount of air left in lungs after normal expiration. This volume is increased w/ PEEP, stemming from alveolar recruitment.
        vi. *TV* (tidal volume): volume of air in normal expiration after normal inspiration.
        vii. *TLC* (total lung capacity): total maximum volume of lungs (i.e., measured at maximum inspiration, and including residual volume).

B. Pathology

1. *Abnormal lesions*
    a. *Malignant*
    b. *Solitary pulmonary nodule*
        i. Asymptomatic mass, well-circumscribed, < 3 cm diameter.
        ii. *Excisional bx indicated unless*:
            - No radiographic change in 2 yr.
            - Calcification pattern c/w hamartoma.
            - Clear evidence of infectious process (i.e., tuberculosis).
            - Prohibitive operative risk (→ FNA).
            - Strong clinical suspicion for small cell carcinoma (→ FNA).
        iii. *If hx of previous cancer, ddx changes*:
            - *Prior h/o sarcoma or melanoma*: lesion most likely a met.
            - *Prior h/o GI or GU cancer*: lesion equal chance of met or lung primary.

        - *Prior h/o head/neck or breast CA*: lesion more likely lung primary.

   c. *Pulmonary sequestrations*: aberrant lung tissue not connected to bronchial tree, receiving systemic (not pulmonary) arterial blood flow (usu. thoracic aorta). Tx = resection.
      i. *Intralobar*: w/in a lobe, more likely to drain into pulmonary vein, more commonly diagnosed in adults.
      ii. *Extralobar*: outside a lobe, more likely to drain into systemic vein, more commonly identified in children.
   d. *Cystic adenoid malformation*: see Chapter 20 on pediatrics.
   e. *Bronchogenic cysts*: most common mediastinal cysts; no connection w/ bronchial system. Tx = resection.
   f. *Thymoma*
      i. 50% malignant, 50% symptomatic, 50% have myasthenia gravis.
         - Conversely, only 10% of pts w/ myasthenia gravis (Ab to acetylcholine receptors) have a thymoma.
            - *Myasthenia gravis sx*: weakness, ptosis, diplopia.
            - *Myasthenia gravis tx*: anticholinesterase meds, plasmapheresis, steroids. 80% of all cases improve w/ thymectomy, even if no evident thymoma present.
      ii. All thymomas should be resected.
   g. *Mediastinal masses* (neurogenic most common overall)
      i. *Anterior* (most common site)
         - Thymoma (most common)
         - Thyroid mass (much less commonly, parathyroid)
         - Teratoma/germ-cell tumor
         - Lymphoma (see Chapter 12 on oncology and Chapter 13 on endocrine)
      ii. *Middle* (heart, trachea, etc.)
         - Cysts (bronchogenic, pericardial, enteric)
         - Lymphoma
      iii. *Posterior* (esophagus, descending aorta, etc.)
         - Neurogenic tumors
         - Enteric cysts
         - Lymphoma

2. *Infectious pathology*
   a. *Empyema*
      i. Infected pleural fluid, most often secondary to pneumonia, but may result from trauma or systemic infection as well. Uncomplicated, can lead to invasion of chest wall (empyema necessitatis), bronchopleural fistula, spread to pericardium, rib osteomyelitis, a/o general sepsis: *3 phases*:
         - *Exudative*: thin fluid, low cell count.
            - *Tx*: IV abx and (almost always) large-bore chest tube.
         - *Fibrinopurulent*: fibrinous deposition on pleura, abundant PMNs, may begin to loculate.
            - *Tx*: IV abx and open vs video-assisted decortication. VATS contraindicated if evidence of stage III dz (thickened rind/peel, contracted hemothorax, possibility of abscess or malignancy).
         - *Organizing/chronic*: thick exudate, heavy sedimentation. Empyema wall organizes w/ fibroblast proliferation and angiogenesis. Lung will not spontaneously reexpand after simple evacuation.
            - *Tx*: IV abx and open decortication.
               - Empyema tube(s) placed through partially resected rib bed may be appropriate if extensive amounts of thick pus/loculations.
               - Eloesser flap refers to marsupialization of a thoracostomy to drain the empyema, achieved by suturing skin to parietal pleura to create a controlled drainage sinus.

- Clagett technique refers to open drainage, pleural cavity irrigation w/ abx (short or long term), and subsequent closure of chest wall w/ tube left in place to continue abx irrigation. Most often done for fistulas resulting from empyema.

b. *Abscess*
   i. Usu. from aspiration (followed by pneumonia, lung cancer, septic emboli, etc.), located in superior segment RLL > posterior segment RUL > superior segment LLL > elsewhere. Consider in ddx bronchiectasis and carcinoma. Aspiration abscesses most often involve anaerobes whereas pneumonic cases are usu. from *S. aureus.*
   ii. *Dx*: CXR and bronchoscopy. Latter can get washings for cx and cytology, removal of FB (if present), and drainage.
   iii. *Tx*:
      - Initially tx w/ abx (8 wk standard, some advocate 16 wk) and bronchoscopic drainage—95% effective.
      - Percutaneous drainage may be attempted as adjunctive therapy.
      - Surgery reserved for failure of medical management, significant hemorrhage, possibility of malignancy. Resection is preferred over pneumonostomy/pneumonotomy. For poor surgical candidates, a Mondaldi catheter/tube may be placed for drainage, but requires presence of pleural adhesions for adequate seal.

c. *Fungal*
   i. *Aspergillosis*: opportunistic infection, can cause solid or cavitary lesions; relatively resistant to antifungals; voriconazole more effective than amphotericin B. Surgery may be required for refractory cases.
   ii. *Coccidioidomycosis*: antifungals recommended only if persistent sx (i.e., fever, fatigue for several wks). Appropriate agents include fluconazole, itraconazole, or amphotericin B.
   iii. *Histoplasma*: antifungals recommended only for moderate (itraconazole) or severe (liposomal amphotericin B).

d. *Other*
   i. *M. tuberculosis.*
   ii. *Nocardia*: aerobic, gram (+), variably acid-fast filamentous rods; can present as multiple abscesses, and may invade chest wall, producing draining sinuses. *Tx of choice*: TMP-SMX, although linezolid is growing in popularity.
   iii. *Actinomyces*: anaerobic to microaerophilic, gram (+), non-acid-fast filamentous rods; generally spreads to thorax from oropharyngeal source, w/ potential to erode into chest wall, w/ abscesses and draining sinuses. Characteristically produce sulfur granules. *Tx of choice*: PCN (ampicillin → amoxicillin *or* penicillin G → penicillin V).
   iv. *Paragonimus*: lung flukes, which can cause pulmonary nodules a/p cavitary lesions. Tx w/ praziquantel is generally adequate; surgery usu. reserved for extrapulmonary manifestations (i.e., in CNS).
   v. *Entamoeba*: from direct extension or blood-borne spread of hepatic abscess of *E. histolytica*. Metronidazole (10 d) or tinidazole (5 d) followed by oral paromomycin (7 d). Surgery rarely needed, although chest tube may be indicated.

3. *Other*
   a. *Pneumothorax*: see Chapter 9 for injury-related.
      i. *Spontaneous*: 20% recur after 1st event, 60% after 2nd, 80% after 3rd.
         - More common on right.
         - Initial tx w/ chest tube, w/ surgery indicated for recurrence, large apical blebs (see on CT), air leak > 7 d, failure to reexpand, or in high-risk professions (divers, pilots).
         - *Surgery*: usu. VATS mechanical pleurodesis +/– resection of blebs.

TABLE 8.1. Pleural Fluid Analysis

	Transudate	Exudate
Pleural fluid protein : serum protein	< 0.5	> 0.5
Pleural fluid LDH : serum LDH	< 0.6	> 0.6
Absolute pleural fluid LDH	< $^2/_3$ upper limit of normal for serum	> $^2/_3$ upper limit of normal for serum

b. *Hemothorax*: see Chapter 9.

c. *Chylothorax*: milky-white character w/ increased lymphocytes and triacylglycerols; fat stained by Sudan red; defined by pleural fluid w/ > 110 mg/dL triglycerides.

   i. Lesion *above* T5–6 → left side chylothorax.

   ii. Lesion *below* T5–6 → right side chylothorax.

   iii. Conservative tx if < 700–1000 cc/d; up to 4 wk chest tube, low-fat diet or TPN, octreotide.

      - Failure of conservative management → ligate thoracic duct on right, low in mediastinum for isolated lesion. If due to malignant dz, try pleurodesis (mechanical or chemical/talc); lower success rate.

d. *Pleural effusion*:

   i. *Etiology*: most common reason for bilateral effusion is CHF. Divide into transudative and exudative w/ Light's criteria below (need 1 criterion to call exudates; need all 3 to call transudate).

      - *Transudate*: CHF, infection/empyema, cirrhosis, Meigs syndrome.
      - *Exudate*: malignancy, catamenial hemothorax, chylothorax.

   ii. *Management*:

      - Medical management of systemic issues (i.e., CHF, cirrhosis).
      - Thoracentesis (diagnostic and therapeutic).
      - Chest tube or Pleur-X catheter.
      - *Pleurodesis*:
         - *Chemical*: tetracycline, talc, bleomycin, and others have been used.
         - *Mechanical*: sponge pad or other abrasive means is effective.

e. *Chest tubes*:

   i. *Indications*: pneumothorax, hemothorax, chylothorax; subcutaneous emphysema in trauma pt. PTX seen on chest CT but not CXR (occult PTX) usu. does *not* need intervention.

   ii. If placed for traumatic reason, should cover w/ 1st-generation cephalosporin for no longer than 24 h (per Eastern Association for the Surgery of Trauma guidelines at www.east.org).

   iii. See Chapter 9 for management of retained hemothorax or massive air leak w/ subcutaneous emphysema in trauma setting.

   iv. Place initially on suction (usu. 20 cm water wall suction) for 24 h. Change to water seal after that. If CXR 6 h after the change to water seal demonstrates no ptx, and pt has no air leak or significant drainage (> 200 cc/24 h), consider removing chest tube. Repeat CXR 6 h after d/c CT.

   v. If placed for pleural effusion, limit drainage to no more than 1 L/d to avoid reexpansion pulmonary edema.

   vi. *Chest tube drainage system* (Pleur-evac by Teleflex): has 3 reservoirs, evolved from older 3-bottle system. Facing the Pleur-evac, from right to left, the chambers are (note, the order of the first and second reservoirs are reversed in the old bottle system):

      - *First reservoir* collects the draining fluid (collection chamber).
      - *Second reservoir* is the air trap. Fluid here allows air to egress from pleural space, but not return. Fill to 2 cm of water level through the suction tube (large tube at top left of box).
      - *Third reservoir* is the suction control chamber, which acts to regulate the amount of pressure from wall suction. Wall suction above the level set here will suck air through a vent; bubbles in this setting do NOT indicate an air leak. Fill w/ water (usu. 20 cm) through the atmospheric vent (rubber flap at top left of box).

   vii. Check for air leak in the air leak meter located between the suction control chamber and the collection chamber. Small air leaks may also be suggested by holding a U of tubing up and observing the column of fluid. If it is of symmetric height, that is normal, but if the column is displaced away from the pt (i.e., the level is higher on the distal arm), then an air leak may be present (called the meniscus sign).

f. *Thoracic emergencies*

   i. *Hemoptysis*

      - *Etiologies*: bronchiectasis, neoplasm, embolism (including septic), PA rupture.
      - *Tx*: depends on etiology.

  - In general, first maneuver is turned to side w/ bleeding side down if known, give 100% O_2 and check coags, CBC, T&C, etc.
  - In OR, perform rigid bronchoscopy and suction.
  - If from left bronchus, place #8 Fogarty catheter in bronchus and inflate, then intubate trachea.
  - If from right bronchus (too short for Fogarty), replace rigid w/ flexible bronchoscope, then intubate left bronchus over scope w/ ETT.
  - Consider a-gram and selective bronchial artery embolization, but if deteriorates, will need thoracotomy and resection.

ii. *Pulmonary embolism* (PE)

- Physiological insult from embolized venous thrombus w/ pulmonary vascular occlusion and shunt resulting from cytokine-mediated increased vascular resistance and edema. In pts w/ patent foramen ovale, paradoxical embolus may occur as well.
- Primary risk factor is iliac DVT; more peripheral DVTs—unknown risk increase.
- *Presentation*:
  - May be asymptomatic or present w/ dyspnea, chest pain, hypoxemia, normal, low, or high $PaCO_2$, or be hemodynamically unstable. Signs of right heart failure (present to some degree in more than 1/3 of pts) such as JVD or enhanced second heart sound suggest significant process.
  - *Most common EKG finding*: sinus tachycardia. Right heart strain pattern, RBBB, anterior T-wave inversion less common. $S_1Q_3T_3$ frequently mentioned, rarely seen.
  - *CXR*: may be normal or demonstrate Hampton's hump (focal consolidation at costophrenic angle or lateral pleural edge), Westermark's sign (diminished peripheral pulmonary vasculature markings), or Palla's sign (enlarged right descending pulmonary artery).
- *Dx*:
  - Significant index of suspicion should prompt CT angiogram of chest. The traditional gold standard of pulmonary arteriography is rarely needed.
  - V/Q scan largely supplanted by chest CT, although, if obtained, a "high-probability" study (decreased perfusion w/ normal ventilation) should prompt intervention.
  - D-dimers may be elevated due to a number of conditions (including recent surgery), but a normal D-dimer suggests dx other than PE.
- *Tx*:
  - Immediate intervention when PE is suspected includes analgesia (morphine preferred), supplemental oxygen, and airway maintenance.
  - In pts w/out contraindications to heparinization, begin IV unfractionated heparin w/ bolus of 80 U/kg (5000–10,000 U) followed by drip of 18 U/kg/h (no greater than 1600 U/h), titrating to keep PTT 1.5–2.5× > control. Some institutions are allowing therapy w/ low-molecular wt heparin instead; no titration needed.
  - Long-term anticoagulation w/ warfarin should be bridged w/ concomitant heparin/warfarin for 3–5 d, followed by warfarin alone w/ INR of ~ 2 (to avoid paradoxical thrombosis or warfarin-induced skin necrosis), continuing for 3–6 mo. Low-molecular wt heparin possible, but requires parenteral administration.
  - IVC (level ~ L3) filter reserved for pts w/ known DVT and contraindications to heparinization.
    - Provides no therapeutic benefit for established PE, but 95% effective at preventing further emboli.
  - Life-threatening hemodynamic instability may warrant more extreme measures such as catheter-based thrombolytics or embolectomy (venous/suction or open method).

iii. *Air embolism*

- Can occur from venous trauma, improper technique in managing central lines, or laparoscopic surgery.
- *Classic sx*: hypotension, bradycardia, or "mill wheel" murmur. Possible. cardiac arrest or convulsions.

- *Dx*: suggested by hx and physical, definitive dx w/ esophageal echocardiogram.
- *Tx*:
  - Do not delay intervention waiting for definitive dx (i.e., echocardiogram).
  - Usu. should put pt head-down, left side down. Attempt to aspirate air via central line from heart.
  - If due to pulmonary trauma, place in Trendelenburg, occlude hilum of affected lung, aspirate air from left ventricular apex/aorta, and perform open cardiac massage.
    - *Alternate recommendations*:
      - If suspect air still in right side of system, place head-up, right side up; attempt to aspirate w/ central venous catheter from right atrium.
      - If suspect left-sided emboli (often present w/ cardiac arrest), address w/ thoracotomy after placing pt in Trendelenburg to trap air in left ventricle.
  - Neuro deficits may be successfully treated w/ hyperbaric oxygen therapy.

iv. *Fat embolism*

- Attributable signs a/o sx may be seen in up to 2% of pts w/ long bone fx and up to 10% of pts w/ unstable pelvic fx. Vast majority of pts are symptomatic w/in 48 h of injury. Etiology may in part be due to release of tissue thromboplastin and other biologically active substances.
- Triad of confusion, dyspnea, and petechiae (esp. of upper trunk and subconjunctiva) considered classic. Fever, seizures, coma, right-sided heart failure, dysrhythmia, and other sx may occur.
- *Dx*: clinical. Thrombocytopenia often reported. Fat in urine is neither sensitive nor specific for dx.
- *Tx*: aggressive hemodynamic and ventilatory support are the only interventions of proven benefit. Early fx stabilization helps avoid the syndrome.

v. *Sudden change in end-tidal CO_2.*

- *Increase*: malignant hypethermia (see Chapter 3).
- *Decrease*: PE, airway disconnection, right main stem intubation.

II. ESOPHAGUS AND DIAPHRAGM

A. Esophageal anatomy and physiology

1. *Length*: male 40 cm, females 37 cm. Comprised of inner layer of circular muscle and outer layer of longitudinal muscle. No serosa. Upper 1/3 is striated, w/ progressively more smooth muscle distally.
2. *3 points of narrowing*: cricopharyngeus (most narrow), aortic arch/left main stem bronchus, GE junction/diaphragmatic hiatus.
3. *Blood supply*:
   a. Cervical = inferior thyroid artery.
   b. Thoracic = bronchial arteries.
   c. Abdominal = left gastric and inferior phrenic arteries.
4. Thoracic duct is dorsal to esophagus, crossing from right → left in upper 1/3 of chest, entering neck posterior to left SC vein. Vagus nerve lies on both sides, and forms 2 plexi—right vagus → posterior, left vagus → anterior.
5. *Three types of peristaltic waves*:
   a. *Primary*: normal antegrade waves assoc. w/ voluntary swallowing.
   b. *Secondary*: normal antegrade waves not assoc. w/ voluntary swallowing, often in response to irritation or distension.
   c. *Tertiary*: spontaneous, abnormal waves.

B. Benign pathology

1. *Congenital*
   a. *Tracheoesophageal fistula*
      i. (Gross classification) Type C "common type:" 87%, proximal atresia w/ distal fistula.
      ii. Type A (isolated atresia) and Type B ("H"), each 5–7%.
      iii. 50% of cases w/ other VACTERL (vertebral, anorectal, cardiac, tracheoesophageal, renal, limb) defects.

iv. *Acquired TEF* occurs rarely, usu. from ET tube cuff erosion.

v. *Tx*:

- Place feeding gastrostomy tube (and low-pressure ET tube cuff distal to fistula if still requiring ventilatory support).
- Divide fistula through cervical approach and close esophagus in 2 layers.
- Resect involved portion of trachea and primarily close (generally possible w/ up to 5-cm gap), and interpose pedicled muscle flap between esophagus and trachea.

2. *Infectious*: thrush–white plaques that can be scraped off, tx options:
   a. *Fluconazole*: 200 mg PO, once.
   b. *Itraconazole (solution)*: 200 mg PO q d × 1 wk.
   c. *Nystatin*: 500,000 U, swish and swallow 4 times per day × 2 wk.
3. *Mechanical/trauma*:
   a. *Esophageal perforation*: most often iatrogenic. Thoracic > cervical > abdominal.
      i. *Dx*: initial test should be Gastrografin (*not* barium—has particulate matter that binds to bacteria) swallow. If nondiagnostic, then consider barium study.
      ii. *Tx*: (see Chapter 26 on key steps for key operations for more operative details)
         - If pt not septic *and* Gastrografin drains back into esophagus from cavity, can treat w/ careful observation, NPO, and abx × 7–10 d.
         - Perforation at thoracic inlet or midesophagus w/ leakage → right thoracotomy drainage +/– patch.
         - Perforation in lower esophagus w/ leakage into abdomen → left thoracotomy a/o celiotomy drainage and patch/repair.
         - If presents > 24 h, debride lesion, and drain internally w/ T tube or Malecot tube; drain externally w/ mediastinal/chest tubes.
         - May resume feeding if repeat esophagogram after tx demonstrates healing.
      iii. *Caustic injury*:
         - *Acid*: coagulative necrosis limits penetration.
         - *Alkali*: liquefactive necrosis frequently causes full-thickness injury.
         - *Acutely*: maintain airway. CXR, AXR.
            - *If suspect perforation*: see section 3a. above on esophageal perforation.
            - *If do not suspect perforation*:
               - Esophagoscopy to grade injury. If ulceration or necrosis (2nd or 3rd degree), admit to ICU, make NPO, give IVF, abx, PPI. Steroids may be given to prevent strictures, but may also mask signs of perforation. Gastrografin swallow at 24 h.
                  - Feeding gastrostomy and retrograde passage of string for subsequent dilatation is commonly recommended. Otherwise, for 2nd- or 3rd-degree burns, endoscopic stent placement (for 3–4 wk) can help maintain patency. A final option is TPN or feeds via Dobhoff tube.
                  - Maintain pt NPO until can swallow saliva w/out pain. EGD at 3 wk, 3 mo, and 6 mo.
                     - Stricture typically occurs 1–2 mo post-injury. Generally begin tx w/ dilatations w/ completion of re-epithelialization.
                     - TE fistula, hiatal hernia, achalasia, and carcinoma are less common long-term sequelae.
                  - Alternately, some authors advocate exploratory celiotomy for 2nd- or 3rd-degree injury, w/ esophagogastrectomy, cervical esophagostomy, and feeding jejunostomy.
   b. *Boerhaave syndrome*
      i. Refers to tear in distal esophagus from vigorous retching/emesis, usu. resulting in longitudinal *left* posterolateral tear several cm cephalad to GE junction.
      ii. *Mackler triad*: h/o vomiting, abrupt-onset lower thoracic pain, SC emphysema in base of neck.

c. *Mallory-Weiss tear*: tear in GE junction from mechanism similar to Boerhaave (above). Generally self-limited, although endoscopic management (heater probe, epinephrine injection, etc.) often useful adjunct. Surgery rarely needed to oversew lesion.

d. *Foreign body ingestion*:

i. *Tends to get caught in 3 locations*: cricopharyngeus, aortic arch/left main stem bronchus, diaphragmatic hiatus. Rigid esophagoscopy indicated for removal.

ii. If passes into stomach, almost always passes spontaneously, and can be managed expectantly following serial x-rays and clinical exam. Some advocate early celiotomy for batteries, however, given risk of caustic injury.

4. *Diverticula*

a. *False* (pulsion)

i. *Zenker's (cricopharyngeal)*:

- Due to hypertonic/uncoordinated cricopharyngeus, mucosa bulges above that muscle and under lower pharyngeal constrictors (through Killian's triangle) most often on left posterolateral side behind SCM.
- Classic sx dysphagia, regurgitation of undigested food, halitosis. Dx w/ barium swallow, not endoscopy (perforation risk).
- *Tx*: myotomy of cricopharyngeus and (if large) diverticulectomy, via left cervical incision between carotid sheath and trachea. High-risk pts may be managed w/ diverticulopexy +/– cricopharyngeal myotomy.

ii. *Epiphrenic*: like Zenkers, these lack muscular layer. Evaluate, r/o GERD (endoscopy), achalasia (BE, manometry). Tx w/ diverticulectomy via left thoracotomy or VATS stapling. If LES pressure elevated, consider myotomy. Surgical area can be reinforced w/ flap or fundoplication as appropriate.

b. *True*

i. *Traction*: usu. small and in midthorax. Result from adjacent inflammatory process (usu. LN, often from TB), which draws wall out. Generally asymptomatic, not requiring tx.

5. *Strictures*

a. *Plummer-Vinson syndrome*: also known as sideropenic dysphagia, refers to cervical dysphagia in setting of chronic iron-deficiency anemia, usu. from *upper* esophageal web, although pharyngeal/esophageal dysmotility may also contribute to problem. Assoc. w/ atrophic oral mucosa, glossitis, and spoon-shaped fingernails (koilonychia). 10% develop SCCA of hypopharynx, oral cavity, or esophagus. *Tx*: correction of iron supplementation and esophageal dilatation as needed.

b. *Schatzki ring*: a *lower* esophageal web or ring, found at the squamocolumnar junction, and almost invariably in conjunction w/ a hiatal hernia. Generally asymptomatic if lumen is > 20 mm, but almost always symptomatic if < 13 cm. Ring only involves mucosa and submucosa, and often responds to dilatation and medical tx for GERD. Surgical resection should not be done w/out concominant correction of hiatal hernia.

6. *Motility disorders*

a. *Achalasia*: *sine qua non* = increased resting pressure of lower esophageal sphincter.

i. *Dx*: GI swallow—see "beak-like" tapering in distal esophagus. F/u w/ upper endoscopy (look for esophagitis, CA, Bx [decreased/absent ganglion cells in Auerbach's plexus]) and manometry (*need*: usu. aperistalsis; incomplete EGS relaxation; high resting pressure [usu. > 30 mm Hg]).

ii. *Standard*: esophagus has little to no peristalsis.

iii. *Vigorous*: esophagus has normal or exaggerated peristalsis.

iv. *Tx*:

- *Medical*: calcium channel blockers, nitrate, endoscopic botulinum toxin.
- *Surgical*: Heller myotomy: perform laparoscopically or through left chest, extending from lower pulmonary vein to 1–2 cm onto stomach. If pt has reflux, do a Dor or loose Nissen (abdominal approach) or partial wrap such as Belsey-Mark IV (thoracic approach).
- *Other*: dilation: contraindicated in children or vigorous achalasia. Reasonable initial results in up to 3/4 of pts, but often transient in effect.

b. *Nutcracker esophagus*

c. *Diffuse esophageal spasm*: often mimics cardiac chest pain assoc. w/ dysphagia. Barium gives "corkscrew" appearance. Manometry reveals significant amount of tertiary, nonpropulsive contractions and normal LES pressure.

i. *Medical tx*: ameliorating life stressors, nitroglycerine or isosorbide (relax smooth muscle), calcium channel blockers.

ii. *Surgical tx*: extended myotomy of thoracic esophagus, approached through right chest—rarely necessary.

7. *Gastroesophageal reflux* (including Barrett esophagus)

a. *Dx*: suggested by sx such as heartburn, regurgitation, chest pain, etc. Gold standard for confirmation is 24-h pH probe (i.e., pH < 4 for > 7% of the time definite evidence of dz). **MUSE** score used to classify extent: **M**etaplasia, **U**lcer, **S**tricture, **E**rosions. Each component scored 0–3 pts.

b. *Tx*:

i. *Medical*: lifestyle modification (elevate HOB 6–10" w/ blocks, lose wt, cease smoking, reduce EtOH, avoid late evening meals, limit chocolate/fat/peppermint/caffeine/acid) and H_2 blockers/PPI.

ii. *Surgical*:

- *Indications for partial fundoplication*: poor esophageal motility; severe aerophagia; previous gastrectomy or other reason to have insufficient fundus for loose total fundoplication; planned Heller myotomy for achalasia.
- *Specific repairs*:
  - *Nissen fundoplication*: 360° fundal wrap (the only nonpartial wrap)
  - *Dor fundoplication*: 150° to 200° anterior wrap
  - *Belsey-Mark IV*: transthoracic 270° anterior wrap
  - *Hill repair*: 90° lesser curve plication and pexy to medial arcuate ligament
  - *Toupet fundoplication*: 270° posterior wrap
  - *Watson*: 120° anterolateral wrap
  - *Collis gastroplasty*: tubularization of distal stomach for foreshortened esophagus

c. *Barrett esophagus*

i. Premalignant condition, most frequently found in white males, found 10–15% of pts w/ symptomatic GERD. 9–45% of pts w/ Barrett have concurrent esophageal adenocarcinoma.

ii. *Dx*: endoscopic bx demonstrates usual squamous epithelium replaced by columnar ("intestinal") epithelium. Subsequent endoscopy (surveillance) should bx every 2 cm from GE junction to Z-line (squamo-columnar junction).

iii. *Tx*: endoscopic surveillance at least every 2 yr results in slightly lower stage dz at dx of cancer.

- Antireflux surgery/fundoplication reserved for GERD refractory to medical management.
- *Low-grade* dysplasia → options include ablation w/ laser, photodynamic tx, etc.
- *High-grade* dysplasia → esophagectomy (nearly indistinguishable from carcinoma in situ, and 1/3 of pts w/ high-grade dyplasia have carcinoma somewhere in the esophagus).

8. *Hiatal hernias*:

a. *Type I* (sliding): esophagus slides up through hiatus into thorax.

b. *Type II* (paraesophageal): esophagus stays intraabdominal, but fundus of stomach slides through defect lateral to left phrenoesophageal ligament into thorax.

i. Risk is incarceration a/o volvulus of stomach. Manage by laparoscopy or celiotomy, reduction of hernia, repair of crural defect, and gastropexy via Stamm gastrostomy tube or Nissen fundoplication. After reduction and repair, almost half of pts develop GERD sx postop, adding to rationale for fundoplication. Poor operative candidates may be managed w/ endoscopic reduction and PEG placement w/ fixation to stomach in 2 places.

c. *Type III* (paraesophageal): coexistence of type I and type II hiatal hernias.

d. *Type IV*: viscera or intestine herniated into thorax.

III. <u>NEOPLASMS</u>: see Chapter 12 on oncology.

CHAPTER 9

TRAUMA, BITES, AND STINGS

I. RESUSCITATION PRIORITIES

A. Airway

1. *Chin lift or jaw thrust initially w/ c-spine control.*
   a. *Nasopharyngeal airway* can be used if pt spontaneously breathing and w/out if midface trauma. 7.0 ETT for men, 6.0 ETT for women.
      i. Pass through nose, listening for air movement, then pass through vocal cords as pt inspires.
   b. *Oral airway* appropriate for unconscious or altered mental status unable to protect airway. First ensure no airway protection.
      i. Preoxygenate before RSI (etomidate 0.2 mg/kg IV + succinylcholine 1 mg/kg—often give 20 and 100, respectively). Do not use succinylcholine if risk of hyperkalemia (renal failure, CVA, or other debilitating neuro d/o > 48 h old, burns > 48 h old). 8.0 ETT for men, 7.0 for women.
   c. Consider cricothyroidotomy (see Chapter 25) if unable to place ETT. 5.5–6.0 ETT (men), or #5–6 Shiley tracheostomy tube (men). Slightly smaller size usu. appropriate for women.
   d. Needle/jet insufflation may be a useful temporizing measure (up to 45 min) in children (cricothyroidotomy contraindicated in children).
   e. ETT contraindicated if suspect laryngeal fx (feel crepitus or see on laryngoscopy); *tracheostomy*, not cricothyroidotomy, indicated in this instance.
   f. Combitube used by some EMT in the field. Consists of dual-lumen tube w/ 2 balloons.
   g. Placement of NGT usu. indicated to prevent aspiration, but is controversial and contraindicated if suspect esophagus or penetrating cervical vascular injury.

B. Breathing

1. Check if can talk, cyanotic, respiratory rate, volume, chest symmetry, JVD distension, tracheal deviation. Auscultate and percuss; also palpate for subcutaneous emphysema and bony stability.
2. *THINK and RULE OUT—if present, TREAT IMMEDIATELY*:
   a. *Open pneumothorax*
      i. Cover w/ occlusive dressing; place chest tube at separate site.
      ii. Historically, small lesions treated by taping dressing on 3 sides to create flutter valve.
         - United States military experience in Iraq suggests no need for flutter valve (just place dressing).
   b. *Hemothorax*
      i. Ipsilateral decreased breath sounds and decreased percussive resonance.
      ii. Drain w/ chest tube.
      iii. Pleural space can hold up to 3 L of blood each hemithorax.
      iv. Immediate output of 1500 cc *or* 4+ consecutive hours of > 200 cc/h *or* 800 cc/4 h indication for thoracotomy.
   c. *Tension pneumothorax*
      i. Hypotension, tracheal deviation, distended neck veins, ipsilateral decreased breath sounds, and increased percussive resonance.
      ii. First decompress w/ 14-g needle in midclavicular line, 2nd intercostal space.
      iii. F/u w/ chest tube.
   d. *Pericardial tamponade*
      i. Like tension PTX, hypotension, distended neck veins. Distant heart sounds.
      ii. Pericardial window preferred over pericardiocentesis.

e. *Flail chest*
   i. 2 or more fxs in 2 or more adjacent ribs; paradoxical chest movement w/ respiration is pathognomonic.
   ii. Problems include decreased respitory excursion from pain and underlying pulmonary occlusion.
   iii. Treat rib pain w/ rib blocks or epidural anesthesia.
   iv. Treat contusion by carefully titrating fluids, supplemental oxygen, intubate as necessary.

C. Circulation

1. *Establish 2 large-bore IVs; give fluid bolus*:
   a. *Adults*: 1–2 L
   b. *Children*: 20 cc/kg
   c. Evaluate response via BP, HR, mental status, capillary refill, urinary output.
2. *Estimations of blood loss.*
   a. *Degrees*
   b. *Orthostatics* (not generally noted in a trauma pt)
      i. Check vitals in supine position, then sit pt up w/ legs hanging for 5 min. Pulse increase of > 20 bpm or decrease in SBP > 10 mm Hg suggests 20+% blood loss.
3. *Trauma CPR and ED thoracotomy.* (*Note*: resuscitative thoracotomies occur in OR and have expanded indications.)
   a. Key issues
      i. *Electrical activity?* If none, pronounce dead.
      ii. *Blunt mechanism w/ electrical activity.*
         - If unable to resuscitate via ACLS/ATLS, pronounce dead.
         - If resuscitated, proceed as usual.
      iii. *Penetrating mechanism w/ electrical activity*
         - Resuscitate w/ ACLS/ATLS; possible resuscitate thoracotomy.
         - If unable to resuscitate, pronounce dead.
         - If able to resuscitate, proceed, consult CVTS.
   b. See Chapter 26 for details.

II. DISABILITY

A. Glasgow Coma Scale: like vital signs, reassess frequently.

1. *Eyes*
   a. 4—open spontaneously
   b. 3—open to voice
   c. 2—open to pain
   d. 1—do not open
2. *Verbal*
   a. 5—oriented
   b. 4—confused
   c. 3—inappropriate words
   d. 2—unintelligible words
   e. 1—no speech
3. *Motor* (the most important component)
   a. 6—obeys commands
   b. 5—localizes pain
   c. 4—withdraws from pain
   d. 3—decorticate posturing (abn flexion)
   e. 2—decerebrate posturing (abn extension)
   f. 1—unresponsive

III. <u>EXPOSURE</u>: undress pt and evaluate entire body, but provide coverage and warmth as soon as possible.

IV. <u>SECONDARY SURVEY</u>: complete physical exam, fast exam; may introduce radiological exams and DPL.

V. HEAD, NECK, AND SPINAL CORD

A. Head

1. *Get head CT if loss of consciousness or focal neurologic deficits.*
2. *Increased cerebral pressure may be reduced by*:
    a. Elevating head of bed
    b. Mannitol (0.25–1.0 g/kg IV)
    c. Intubation w/ mild hyperventilation (keep pCO_2 around 35)
    d. Barbituates
3. *Epidural hematoma*: accoc. w/ parietal bone fx, infrequently see "lucid interval." Lenticular shape on noncontrast CT.
4. *Subdural hematoma*: assoc. w/ dural tears. Crescent shape on CT.
5. For intracranial hemorrhage after blunt head trauma, load pt w/ fosphenytoin (Cerebyx) as 1 g IV, followed by phenytoin (Dilantin) as approximately 100 mg PO 3 times per day. More precisely, can load phenytoin equivalent as 10–20 mg/kg depending on severity of risk, followed by 5–6 mg/kg phenytoin IV or PO q d, holding TF for 2 h before and after dosing. See Chapter 24 for sliding-scale dosing and related information.
6. *Diffuse axonal injury* (DAI).

B. Spinal cord

1. *Blunt injury may be treated w/ IV methylprednisolone*:
    a. Bolus w/ 30 mg/kg over 15 min.
    b. Follow w/ 5.4 mg/kg/h given over the next 23 h.
2. *Neck*:
    a. C-spine
        i. Upper (C1–C2)
            - Distance from anterior ring of C1 to odontoid.
                - Adults ≤ 2.5 mm.
                - Peds ≤ 4.5 mm.
            - Prevertebral soft tissue (airway to ant-inf margin of C2).
                - ≤ 7mm.
        ii. Lower (C3–C7)
            - Airway to ant-inf margin of C6.
                - Adults ≤ 22 mm.
                - Peds ≤ 14 mm.
            - Alignment
                - 3 mm or more displacement unusual in adults, most often happens C4–C7. C2–C4 may normally occur in peds up to teens.
    b. Vasculature
        i. *Indications for CTA a/o angiogram*:
            - Neurologic sx not explained by head CT.
            - Seat belt mark across neck.
            - Bruit in young person.
            - Fx involving foraminal canal.
            - Severe cervical hyperextension/hyperflexion.
            - Near-hanging or strangulation.
            - C-spine fx of vertebral body, pedicle, or transverse process.

- Basilar skull fx involving carotid canal or petrous bone.
- GCS ≤ 8 w/out CT or MRI findings in brain to explain.
- LeFort II or III fx.

ii. *Incision*

- *If unable to localize preop* → anterior sternocleidomastoid.
- *For innominate or proximal right subclavian* → median sternotomy +/– supraclavicular.
- *For proximal left subclavian* → left thoracotomy +/– supraclavicular.

C. Neck

1. *Penetrating neck injury*

a. Remember that *airway* control is paramount—stridor, hoarseness, hemoptysis, tracheal deviation, a/o expanding hematoma may herald loss of airway. Emergent intubation, cricothyroidotomy, or even emergent tracheostomy (if laryngeal injury) may be required.

b. If suspect possible esophageal injury or possible cervical vascular injury, do not place NGT as may worsen perforation or dislodge clot, either directly or by stimulating retching.

c. Regardless of location in neck, pts w/ airway problems, expanding hematoma, or other evidence of active bleeding should go straight to the OR.

d. Less overtly injured pts have traditionally had their injury management defined by zones:

i. *Zone I* (thoracic inlet to cricoid cartilage)

- CT angiogram (arteriogram a/o esophagram/esophagoscopy if CTA abnormal); +/– tracheobronchoscopy.

ii. *Zone II* (cricoid cartilage to angle of mandible)

- *Surgical exploration* or CTA (possible arteriogram a/o esophagram/esophagoscopy if CTA abnormal); pharyngoscopy/laryngoscopy (not tracheobronchoscopy).

iii. *Zone III* (angle of mandible to skull base)

- CT angiogram (arteriogram if CTA abnormal); pharyngoscopy (no tracheobronchoscopy or esophagoscopy).

iv. *Note*: w/ the advent of high-resolution CT scanners, an increasing body of data suggests that in the absence of obvious indications for operative exploration, multislice helical CT angiography may be appropriately used *in lieu* of operative exploration or other modality to identify injury, regardless of zone of injury [Inaba K, et al., *J Trauma*. Jul 2006; 61(1):144–9.]

e. If injury identified in any of 4 cervical vessels, must evaluate all vessels *as well as* intracranial circulation.

f. *Penetrating cervical vascular injury*:

i. See Chapter 26 on key steps in key operations for exposure of specific vessels. In general, however, neck explorations are carried out through incisions over anterior SCM. Although one should avoid ligating B jugular veins, veins may generally be sacrificed w/ impunity, or used as patch graft for the arterial system. Vertebral artery injury is generally best managed by embolization.

g. *Penetrating cervical esophageal injury*:

i. Typically approach retracting carotid sheath laterally (going medial to carotid; left-sided approach easier if no concerns on the right neck). To fully expose, must divide omohyoid, middle thyroid vein, +/– inferior thyroid artery. May approach lateral to carotid if hematoma precludes medial approach. If NGT present, palpate to find esophagus.

ii. *Dx*: due to lack of serosa, may be challenging to identify small injury. Can insufflate esophagus through NGT brought to level of injury while operative field flooded w/ saline (look for bubbles). Alternately, consider contralateral exploration, mobilization and encircling w/ Penrose drain, or intraoperative esophagoscopy.

iii. *Tx*:

- Debride to healthy mucosa and muscularis, then repair in 1 (i.e., PDS) or 2 layers.
- Interpose healthy muscle flap between suture line and other neck structures or suture lines.
- Drain uncontrolled leaks if esophagus is inaccessible. Fistula should close w/ time. Lateral esophagostomy is other option for large defects. Drains may be placed in tract or, prefererably, "purse-stringed" into esophageal defect.

2. *Blunt neck injury*
   a. *Suspect cerebrovascular lesion if*: severe cervical hyperextension/rotation or hyperflexion; near-hanging or strangulation; basilar skull fx involving carotid canal or petrous bone fx; C-spine fx involving vertebral body, pedicle, or transverse process; GCS ≤ 8 w/out evident cerebral lesion on CT or DAI; LeFort II or III fx; lateralizing neuro deficit w/out CT findings to explain; cerebral infarct on head CT; massive epistaxis; anisocoria/Horner syndrome; seat belt sign above clavicle; cervical bruit or thrill. [Biffl WL, Moore EE, Offner PJ, Burch JM, *World J Surg*. 2001;25:1036–43.]
   b. *Any of the above findings should prompt*:
      i. Standard 3-view plain films of cervical spine.
      ii. CT angiogram of head/neck (as good as 4-vessel angiogram for dx).
   c. *Management of carotid/vertebral injuries* [by grading system of Biffl WL, et al., *J Trauma*. 1999;47(5):845–58.]
      i. *Grade I*: luminal irregularity or dissection w/ < 25% luminal narrowing; hemodynamically insignificant.
         - Consider systemic fractionated or unfractionated heparin a/o ASA/antiplatelet tx.
      ii. *Grade II*: dissection or intramural hematoma w/ > 25% luminal narrowing, intraluminal thrombus, or raised intimal flap. May progress to pseudoaneurysms/thrombotic occlusions.
         - Systemically anticoagulate and repeat angiography.
      iii. *Grade III*: pseudoaneurysm—risk of thrombosis a/o rupture.
         - Repair if accessible (open or endovascular).
      iv. *Grade IV*: occlusion; very high stroke rate.
         - Systemically heparinize.
      v. *Grade V*: transaction w/ free extravasation; rare, usu. lethal.

VI. THORAX

A. Lungs

1. CXR can detect as little as 200 cc in hemithorax.
2. 85% problems corrected w/ chest tube.
3. All pts w/ pneumothoraces must have chest tube before beginning mechanical ventilation.
4. Subcutaneous air or sx of tension pneumothorax in an unstable trauma pt merits a chest tube *before* CXR.
   a. Chest tubes placed for trauma should receive 1 dose 1st-generation IV cephalosporin.
   b. Retained hemothorax traditionally treated w/ second chest tube to prevent empyema and fibrothorax, but early VATS often result in earlier discharge from hospital. [Meyer DM, Jessen ME, Wait MA, Estrera AS, Early evacuation of traumatic retained hemothoraces using thoras-copy: a prospective, randomized trial, *Ann Thorac Surg*. 1997;64:1396–401.]
5. *Indications for thoracotomy*:
   a. Immediate output of 1500 cc from chest tube.
   b. > 2 h of > 200 cc blood from chest tube.
   c. Hemopericardium/tamponade.
   d. Expanding hematoma at thoracic outlet.
   e. Exsanguinating hemorrhage from supraclavicular penetrating wound.
   f. Radiographic evidence of thoracic great vessel injury.
6. *Emergency Department Thoracotomy (EDT)* [Cothren CC, Moore EE, *World J Emerg Surg*. 2006;1:4; Powell DW, Moore EE, *J Am Coll Surg*. 2004;1999:211–5.]
   a. *Indications*:
      i. *Cardiac arrest*:
         - Witnessed penetrating trauma w/ < 15 min prehospital CPR.
         - Witnessed blunt trauma w/ < 5 min prehospital CPR.
      ii. *Persistent severe hypotension (SBP ≤ 60) secondary to*:
         - Pericardial tamponade.

- Hemorrhage (thoracic, abdominal, extremity).
- Air embolism.

b. *Contraindications*:
   i. Penetrating trauma w/ > 15 min CPR and no signs of life (papillary reflexes, spontaneous respiration, or motor activity).
   ii. Blunt trauma w/ > 5 min of CPR and no signs of life or asytole.

c. *Goals (6)*:
   i. Decompress pericardial tamponade.
   ii. Control cardiac bleeding.
   iii. Control intrathoracic bleeding.
   iv. Temporarily occlude descending thoracic aorta.
   v. Perform open cardiac massage/defibrillation.
   vi. Evacuate massive air embolism.

d. *Technique*: see Chapter 26 on key steps in key operations.

e. *Other*: overall survival < 1.4%. Better for penetrating trauma (particularly stab wound to heart w/ pericardial tamponade) than blunt trauma.

7. *Incisions*
   a. *Left anterolateral thoracotomy*: most thoracic great vessel injuries and proximal left subclavian artery injury.
   b. *Left posterolateral thoracotomy*: descending aorta, proximal left carotid artery.
   c. *Median sternotomy*: thoracic vena cava, ascending aorta and arch, innominate artery, intrathoracic left carotid artery, proximal right subclavian artery, pulmonary arteries/veins.
   d. *MS + neck extension*: thoracic outlet injury.
   e. *Right posterolateral*: azygous vein, distal right pulmonary vein, thoracic esophagus.

8. *Tracheobronchial injury*
   a. Suggested by hemoptysis, mediastinal emphysema, and persistent air leak.
   b. First maneuver should generally be bronchoscopy to confirm and localize (usu. w/in 2 cm of carina).
   c. Double-lumen ETT may be indicated in some cases.

B. Cardiac

1. *Tamponade*
   a. If stable w/ (+) pericardial effusion/tamponade, most begin w/ pericardial window, then extend to median sternotomy if (+). If pt unstable, begin w/ emergent left lateral thoracotomy, dividing pericardium anterior to phrenic nerve, which may be visible or obscured by assoc. overlying fatty tissue.

2. *Laceration*
   a. If partial thickness, repair w/ staples or pledgeted sutures.
   b. If full thickness, first occlude hole to prevent exsanguination. May use finger initially, then consider other such as Foley catheter. Repair w/ pledgeted sutures, taking care not to entrap/occlude coronary arteries; if near one, can repair w/ horizontal mattress stitches passed under the vessel.

C. Noncardiac

1. *Great vessels*
   a. Findings assoc. w/ aortic rupture or other significant injury:
      i. Widened mediastinum most accurate (> 8 cm).
      ii. Fx of scapula or first 2 ribs (controversial).
      iii. Loss of pulmonary window a/o aortic knob.

2. *Mediastinal traversing injury*
   a. If unstable, immediate chest tube, followed by CXR, OR.
   b. If indication for extrathoracic surgery, need to evaluate cardiothoracic system, the thoracic aorta, and aerodigestive tract. Can be accomplished via celiotomy for other indication; pericardial window; esophagoscopy; bronchoscopy; aortography (postop).

c. If no indication for any surgery, can w/u via CXR w/ chest tube as indicated; arteriography; esophagography; echocardiography.

3. *Blunt aortic injury*
   a. *CXR risk factors*: widened mediastinum (> 8 cm), indistinct aortic knob, indistinct AP window, indistinct descending aorta, apical cap, deviation of NGT/trachea to right, depression of left main stem bronchus, fx of ribs 1 a/o 2, or scapula.
   b. *Once pt stabilized, obtain spiral CT of thorax to further screen.*
      i. *If normal, no further w/u necessary.*
      ii. *Abnormal*:
         - Anterior mediastinal hematoma → no further w/u or tx necessary.
         - Periaortic hematoma/pseudoaneursym/intimal flap → CVTS consult to determine need for aortography.
   c. *Aortography*
      i. *If normal, no further w/u necessary.*
      ii. *Abnormal*:
         - If operative candidate, should go to OR.
         - If not operative candidate (traumatic CHI, etc.), need aggressive medical control of rate-pressure product. Maintain SBP below 100–110 mm Hg, ideally w/ short-acting beta blocker such as esmolol, which is also a negative inotrope. Additional control may be gained w/ nitroprusside if beta blocker ineffective. Obviously, in pts w/ CHI, there will be conflicting goals for BP, which will require close cooperation of specialty services and ICU team.
4. *Blunt cardiac injury*
   a. *If suspect*, get EKG.
   b. *If unstable*, get emergent echocardiography, admission to ICU, invasive monitoring, and aggressive resuscitation.
   c. *If stable* w/ normal EKG, no further w/u. If stable w/ abnormal EKG → telemetry monitoring × 24 h. Tx arrhythmias if symptomatic.
5. *Pneumothorax/hemothorax*
   a. If pt unstable w/ clinical indications of PTX/HTX, perform emergent tube thoracostomy before CXR.
   b. If stable, mechanism is blunt, and CXR is normal, no further w/u necessary.
   c. If stable, mechanism is penetrating, and CXR is normal, repeat CXR in 6 h for latent PTX.
      i. Occult PTX (PTX seen on CT but not on CXR) does not need decompression.
   d. Hemothorax or PTX (non-occult) require chest tube.
   e. Persistent PTX requires placement of additional tube directed at PTX.
   f. If still have PTX or persistent air leak, need bronchoscopy to evaluate for tracheobronchial injury. CVTS consult.
      i. Airway injury requires thoracotomy.
   g. Persistent HTX should be managed w/ right angle tube in posterior sulcus or VATS/thoracotomy.
   h. Chest tubes placed outside of OR are indication for 24 h of abx (i.e., 1st-degree cephalosporin).
6. *Thoracoabdominal injury*
7. *Trauma CPR*
   a. If no electrical activity, pronounce pt dead.
   b. If blunt mechanism and electrical activity, perform ACLS/ATLS until dead or to OR/ICU.
   c. If penetrating mechanism and electrical activity, perform ACLS/ATLS. If aortic cross-clamp and pericardiotomy successful (ED thoracotomy), take to OR and consult CVTS.
8. *Rib fx/pulmonary contusion*: ensure adequate analgesia, including possible thoracic epidural. ICU monitoring necessary if respiratory embarrassment.
9. *Esophageal injury* (not from transthoracic trauma): see Chapter 8.

VII. ABDOMEN

A. General principles

1. *Penetrating abdominal trauma* (count numbers of holes—should be even if missile not in body)
   a. *GSW to abdomen or trauma to abdomen w/ pneumoperitoneum*:
      i. All go to OR.
   b. *Stab wounds to abdomen*:
      i. 1/3 of stab wounds to abdomen do not penetrate peritoneum; another 1/3 cause no significant harm.
         - *To OR if*: peritonitis, bowel evisceration (omental evisceration only → admit for serial exams), or evidence of intraabdominal bleeding.
         - *Otherwise, locally explore*:
           - "Positive" = tract penetrates posterior fascia or peritoneum.
           - "Positive" or equivocal cases get DPL unless ex lap indicated.
             - *Positive DPL criteria*:
               - Aspiration of 10 cc gross blood
               - > 100,000 RBC/mm^3
               - > 500 WBC/mm^3
               - Bile or vegetable matter
2. *Blunt abdominal trauma*
   a. *To OR if*: evisceration, peritonitis, or (+) FAST and hemodynamic instability.
      i. Only items needed before OR are CXR, pelvis film, and T&C.
   b. If no immediate indication for OR, all get at least examination, FAST, CXR, and pelvic x-ray.
      i. *FAST (+)*:
         - To OR if hemodynamically abnormal (see a. above).
         - To CT scan if hemodynamically normal.
           - If no solid organ injury, perform DPL (may represent ruptured bowel, mesenteric bleed, etc.). Additionally (or in selected pts, instead) serial abdominal exams if pt can undergo reliable abdominal exams (no drugs/EtOH, distracting injury, or GCS < 15).
      ii. *FAST (–)*:
         - If hemodynamically abnormal, consider other source (chest, scalp, long bones, pelvis, retroperitoneum, cocaine/other drugs).
           - Reexamine pericardium.
           - Examine midaxillary lines ("FAST + 2" to exclude hemothorax).
           - Examine CXR (evaluate ET tube, exclude PTX).
           - *Consider limitations of FAST*:
             - Morbidly obese (2.7 MHz transducer may be useful for deeper penetration).
             - Subcutaneous emphysema precludes effective exam.
             - Left hemothorax limits sensitivity of pericardial examination.
         - *Indications for CT scan of abdomen/pelvis in pts w/ (–) FAST*:
           - Pelvic fx.
           - Persistent abdominal tenderness (not peritonitis).
           - Persistent HR > 110 (to eval intraparenchymal bleeding, etc.).
           - Gross hematuria or > 50 RBCs/HPF (include CT cystogram).
           - FAST limited by morbid obesity, subcutaneous emphysema, or other factor.
           - T-spine or L-spine fx.
         - If hemodynamically normal, observe.
3. *Damage control celiotomy*
   a. *Indication to get out of operation and to ICU for resuscitation* ("the lethal triad/triangle"):

i. *Hypothermia* (< 34°C)
- *Passive rewarming*: BAER hugger, warm blankets, etc.
- *Active rewarming* (preferred): warmed IV fluids, CAVR, warmed bladder/NGT lavage, warmed DPL fluid, warmed fluid lavage of thorax through chest tubes; warming of pt's blood and reintroducing it to body via pump (Gentilello technique).

ii. *Acidosis* (< 7.2) or other evidence of profound shock (e.g., BD < –7, lactate > 5)

iii. *Coagulopathy*

b. *Steps*:

i. *Control hemorrhage*! If involves liver, *pack*.

ii. *Control enteral spillage*: staple off bowel, leave in discontinuity, or occlude w/ clamps.

iii. *Control GU injury*: ligate ureters, etc.

iv. *Temporary closure of the abdomen* (i.e., close skin w/ nylons or towel clips, or VAC, etc.).

v. *Planned return to OR in ~ 24 h*, after resuscitation in the ICU.

4. *Stab wounds to back and flank*

a. Peritoneal sx, shock, or evisceration → OR.

b. Otherwise, locally explore wound to determine direction (for flank), and depth/end of tract.

i. If clearly ends w/out entry into abdomen, debride wound. *Otherwise*, see below:
- *Flank wounds*: if tracks toward peritoneal cavity and penetrates fascia → DPL. If tracks toward retroperitoneum → CT (w/ rectal contrast if concern for colorectal injury).
- *Back wounds* → CT scan (w/ rectal contrast if concern for colorectal injury).
- (+) DPL or suggestion of injury on CT scan → OR.

5. *Suspected rectal injury*:

a. Perform proctosigmoidoscopy if blood on rectal exam or if suspect colorectal injury. If abnormal, do retrograde cystourethrogram as well.

B. Abdominal vascular injury

1. 5–10% of blunt trauma celiotomies. 10% of stab wound celiotomies. 10–25% of gunshot wound celiotomies.
2. Open abdomen, pack in all quadrants and then remove lower packs, then LUQ, then RUQ.
3. Hematoma in midline *supramesocolic* area → *left* medial rotation (Mattox maneuver) including colon, kidney, pancreatic tail, gastric fundus.

a. If supramesolic area actively bleeding, apply aortic compression, then divide the lesser omentum, retract esophagus to left, and open aortic hiatus.

b. Small aortic defects repaired w/ running transverse 3-0 polypropylene.

c. Celiac axis injuries are ligated.

d. SMA repaired w/ 5-0 polypropylene, or grafted w/ saphenous vein or PTFE.

e. SMV should be repaired if possible. Follow ligation w/ vigorous IVF.

4. Hematoma/hemorrhage in midline *inframesocolic* area → *right* medial rotation (Cattell-Braasch maneuver) including transverse colon, midgut, w/ proximal infrarenal aortic control inferior to left renal vein.

a. If aorta not injured, expose IVC by Kocher maneuver w/ elevation of right colon. Repair w/ running 5-0 polypropylene transversely if possible. If ligation of IVC necessary, give vigorous IVF, wrapping B LE w/ elastic bandages, elevation of lower extremities for 7–10 d.

C. Diaphragm

1. Always warrant primary closure; mesh may be used for extensive defects. F/u w/ chest tube.
2. If hemothorax or gastric/intestinal spillage, irrigate thoracic cavity through chest tube or red rubber catheter placed through defect. Incidence of empyema highest after gastric spillage followed by colonic spillage.

D. Distal esophagus and stomach (as for all penetrating trauma, should generally have even number of holes)

1. *Distal esophagus*: Mobilize GE junction (see section 2. on stomach below).

a. In damage-control situations, large defects can be managed w/ drain placed into the hole and brought out through skin.
b. *Definitive repair*:
   i. *Simple defect*: debride, close in 1 layer (i.e., PDS), drain. If possible, bring up antrum to create serosal patch (Thal patch).
   ii. *Destruction of GE junction*: typically has significant assoc. injuries. Staple esophagus and stomach, drain, then come back later for anastomosis.

2. *Stomach*:
   a. *Examine entire stomach*: divide gastrocolic omentum to enter lesser sac and visualize posterior stomach. Mobilize GE junction (take down left triangular ligament of liver, retract left lobe, and open peritoneum).
   b. Most injuries can be managed w/ stapled wedge resection, although more extensive gastrectomy may be occasionally necessary.

E. Pancreas

1. *Anatomy/physiology/epidemiology*
   a. *Dx*: essential to have high index of suspicion based upon mechanism of injury and any of the following: worsening abdominal exam; CT scan w/ peri-pancreatic hematoma or parenchymal filling defect. FAST exam and DPL (amylase) not very sensitive as pancreas is retroperitoneal. Consider structures that are commonly injured along w/ pancreas (head/body = biliary tree, duodenum, portal vein, liver right kidney, SMA/SMV, L-1; tail = spleen, proximal jejunum, left kidney). Elevated serum amylase/lipase not specific, but absence of these means likely no significant pancreatic injury (+/–).
   b. *Tx*:
      i. *Minor* contusion or laceration w/out duct injury (*grade I*): externally drain.
      ii. *Major* contusion or laceration w/out duct injury (*grade II*): externally drain.
      iii. *Distal* (left of SMA/SMV) injury w/ duct injury (*grade III*): distal pancreatectomy is generally recommended w/ drainage and oversewing of duct +/– splenectomy. Stapling thought by some to be not as good an option as fishmouth hand-sewn resection.
      iv. *Proximal* (right of SMA/SMV) inury +/– papilla injury (*grade IV*):
         - *Intraoperative pancreatogram*: can perform duodenotomy and cannulate ampulla, but to avoid additional potential morbidity, recommend performing high-pressure cholangiogram via needle in cystic duct.
         - *Consider*:
            - Resection and external drainage.
            - External drainage and endoscopic ductal stent.
            - Internal drainage using Roux-en-Y limb (rarely used).
         - *Pancreatic head injury*: can usu. be managed w/ ample drainage via closed silastic catheters, but complex, massive damage (*grade V*; esp. if duodenum also injured) may Whipple in 2 stages (resection and subsequent reconstruction; rarely actually performed—normal/soft pancreatic parenchyma high risk for leak).
      v. *Additional thoughts*:
         - In a sick pt w/ a nonbleeding pancreatic injury, nothing else *really* has to be done immediately beyond external drainage to convert to controlled pancreatic fistula. Oversewing stump or distal pancreatectomy are relatively rapid other maneuvers.
         - For bleeding injuries in the head, control w/ local pressure, packing, or sutures. Significant hemorrhage generally belies an underlying (dorsal) vascular lesion.
         - *Exposure*:
            - *Head*: perform Kocher maneuver. Realize IVC is directly under C-loop.
            - *Body/tail*:
               - Open lesser sac through a hole in an avascular section of the left gastrocolic omentum.
               - For wider exposure, detach greater omentum from transverse colon.

F. Small intestine

1. *Duodenum*
   a. *Anatomy/physiology/epidemiology*:
      i. Between L1 and L3, first segment (duodenal bulb) intraperitoneal; the remainder is retroperitoneal. Ampulla of Vater separates 2nd, 3rd segments. SMA divides 3rd, 4th portions.
      ii. 5–10 L/d pass through duodenum.
      iii. Injured in 3–5% abdominal injuries, 75% from penetrating trauma. Blunt injury most often from "handlebar" compression/"blowout" or deceleration.
   b. *Dx*: essential to have high index of suspicion based upon mechanism of injury and any of the following: worsening abdominal exam; KUB w/ retroperitoneal air; (+) FAST; DPL w/ bile; CT w/ right-sided contrast leak or periduodenal hematoma; upper GI contrast study w/ leak or intraluminal filling defect. Consider structures that are commonly injured along w/ duodenum (D1/D2 = stomach, pancreas, biliary tree, liver, kidney, portal vein; D3/D4 = SMA/SMV, proximal jejunum, kidney, L1 vertebral body or transverse processes).
   c. *Tx*:
      i. Nonperforated (*grade I*): may be managed nonoperatively.
      ii. < 50% circumferential laceration (*grade II*): primary repair (transversely/obliquely to avoid stenosis).
      iii. > 50% circumferential laceration (*grade III*):
         - Pyloric exclusion and gastrojejunostomy
         - Duodenal diverticulization
            - Perform antrectomy and gastrojejunostomy IV
      iv. 75% circumferential laceration + CBD/ampulla injury (*grade IV*):
         - Roux-en-Y bypass
      v. *Complex pancreaticoduodenal injury*:
         - Pancreaticoduodenectomy
2. *Jejunum, ileum*: small full-thickness injury is easily managed w/ running 4-0 absorbable suture, followed by 3-0 silk Lembert sutures; close transversely if possible to avoid luminal narrowing. Otherwise, resect area and perform primary anastomosis.

G. Colon

1. 15–39% penetrating abdominal trauma; rare in blunt trauma.
2. Can usu. resect injured area and perform primary anastomosis (if too edematous to staple, then hand-sew).
3. *Indications for diversion instead of primary anastomosis*:
   a. Destructive lesions (> 50% bowel wall or devascularization of bowel segment) *and*...
      i. Hemodynamic instability (pre- or intraop SBP < 90), *or*...
      ii. Significant comorbidities, *or*...
      iii. Significant assoc. injuries (PATI < 25, ISS < 25, Flint grade < 11), *or*...
      iv. Peritonitis
4. Several recent studies have challenged the above and suggest more liberal guidelines for primary anastomosis [Nelson R, Singer M, Primary repair for penetrating colon injuries, *Cochrane Database Syst Rev*. 2003;(3):CD002247, and Dente CJ, et al., Ostomy as a risk factor for posttraumatic infection in penetratinc colon injuries: univariate and multivariate analyses, *J Trauma*. Oct 2000;49(4): 628–37.]
5. Majority of trauma ostomies can be taken down at 2 wk (not if local wound sepsis, unstable, etc.). Obtain contrast enema to ensure distal healing beforehand.

H. Rectum

1. Rare (3–5% colon injury), but prone to disaster.
2. 4 traditional linchpins of management (debride, dilute, divert, drain [presacral]) have been challenged recently by authorities. Several studies have questioned the need for presacral drainage.

3. If able to easily identify and repair injury, do so; protect repair/anastomosis (intraperitoneal portion) w/ diverting ostomy. Otherwise, if suspect extraperitoneal rectal injury, perform diverting loop ostomy, and consider presacral drainage.

I. Liver

1. *Injury scale* (similar to spleen scale)
   a. *Hematoma/vascular*
      i. *Grade I*—subcapsular, nonexpanding, < 10% SA
      ii. *Grade II*—subcapsular, nonexpanding, 10–50% SA
      iii. *Grade III*—subcapsular, > 50% or expanding, ruptured subcapsular actively bleeding, intraparenchymal > 2 cm or expanding
      iv. *Grade IV*—ruptured intraparenchymal hematoma actively bleeding
      v. *Grade V*—juxtahepatic venous injuries (i.e., retrohepatic vena cava or major hepatic veins)
      vi. *Grade VI*—hepatic avulsion
   b. *Laceration*
      i. *Grade I*—capsular, nonbleeding, < 1 cm deep
      ii. *Grade II*—capsular, bleeding, 1–3 cm deep, < 10 cm long
      iii. *Grade III*—> 3 cm deep
      iv. *Grade IV*—25–50% lobar disruption
      v. *Grade V*—> 50% lobar disruption
2. Most commonly injured abdominal organ w/ blunt trauma, but vast majority is relatively minor, not requiring operative intervention.
3. Given unique vascular supply, many hepatic injuries can be managed through interventional radiology.
4. Intraoperative maneuvers to obtain hemostasis include first taking down falciform ligament, bimanual compression, Pringle maneuver, taking down triangular and coronary ligaments (contraindicated if massive retrohepatic bleeding), shunt, total hepatic vascular isolation, finger fx and ligation, insertion of red rubber catheter w/ side holes, and overlying Penrose.
5. *Hemobilia*: classically, this manifests as triad of RUQ pain, jaundice, and upper GI bleed occurring ~ 2–3 wk after hepatic trauma. Results from fistula between hepatic arterial supply and biliary system. Confirmatory dx and tx are angiographic.
6. *Bile leak*: manifests as RUQ discomfort, sx of ileus or gastric obstruction, and jaundice. Evaluate w/ U/S or CT. CT-guided drainage w/ ERCP to localize source (and, if more significant than cystic duct leak after cholecystectomy, treat via stenting) is generally sufficient tx.

J. Spleen

1. Most common *significantly* (requiring operative intervention) injured organ in blunt trauma.
2. Rupture may manifest as falling hct and rising WBC.
3. *Injury scale* (similar to liver scale)
   a. *Hematoma/vascular*
      i. *Grade I*—subcapsular, nonexpanding, < 10% surface area
      ii. *Grade II*—subcapsular, nonexpanding 10–50% SA
      iii. *Grade III*—subcapsular, > 50% or expanding, ruptured subcapsular actively bleeding, intraparenchymal > 2 cm or expanding
      iv. *Grade IV*—ruptured intraparenchymal hematoma actively bleeding
      v. *Grade V*—major bleeding
   b. *Laceration*
      i. *Grade I*—capsular, nonbleeding, < 1 cm deep
      ii. *Grade II*—capsular, bleeding, 1–3 cm deep but not involving trabecular vessels
      iii. *Grade III*—> 3 cm deep or involving trabecular vessel(s)
      iv. *Grade IV*—involves segmental or hilar vessels w/ > 25% splenic devascularization
      v. *Grade V*—shattered/pulpified spleen, hilar disruption, devascularized or avulsed fragments
4. *Indications for operation in pts w/ splenic rupture*:

a. Need for blood transfusion.
b. Peritonitis.
c. Inability to follow exam (i.e., head injury).
d. Failed embolization of pseudoaneurysm.

5. *Splenorrhaphy vs splenectomy* (see Chapter 26 for technical aspects)
   a. *Salvage may be considered if*:
      i. < 500 cc (or 1/3 pt volume) lost or if pt hemodynamically stable.
      ii. No hilar involvement.
      iii. No coagulopathy.
      iv. Minimal assoc. injuries.
   b. *Splenic salvage may be attempted w/*: electrocautery, argon beam laser, hemostatic gel, polyglycolic mesh (to keep multiple shattered segments together), debridement/suture repair, partial splenectomy (stapler or suture w/ pledgets), etc.
   c. Must retain 30–40% of spleen and hilar blood flow architecture to preserve immune function.
6. *Pseudoaneurysm*
   a. Suggested by blush on CT.
   b. Initial management may be attempted by interventional radiology if no other indications for operation.
7. *Pediatric* (< 2 yo better than < 6 yo better than adult) spleen more elastic; more often can be managed nonoperatively.
8. *Postsplenectomy, watch for*:
   a. Howell-Jolly bodies (normal).
   b. WBC and platelet rise (normal).
   c. Atelectasis, pneumonia, pleural effusion, subphrenic abscess.
   d. Pancreatitis.
   e. Gastric injury or necrosis of greater curvature (peritonitis, fistula).
   f. OPSS.
      i. 80% of cases in children—most often w/in first 2 yr.
      ii. Mortality 50–80%, worse in children.
      iii. From decreased tuftsin, properdin, IgM, loss of RES stroma to clear encapsulated bacteria.
      iv. Pneumococcus, *H. influenzae*, Meningococcus worst culprits.
         - Give Pneumovax (covers 80% of variants) ASAP, repeat q 4–5 yr.
         - *H. influenzae*, Meningococcus vaccines also available.
   g. Most common complication is LLL atelectasis, followed by subphrenic abscess. Placement of drain in splenic fossa unnecessary (unless pancreatic injury/leak), and contributes to risk of subphrenic abscess.

K. **Great vessels**
1. *Retroperitoneal zone I hematoma* (Zone I = between renal hila)
   a. Explore all.
2. *Retroperitoneal zone II hematoma* (Zone II = lateral to renal hila)
   a. Explore if penetrating trauma or expanding or pulsatile.
3. *Retroperitoneal zone III hematoma* (Zone III = pelvis)
   a. Explore if penetrating trauma or expanding or pulsatile.

L. **Abdominal compartment syndrome** (watch for decreased UOP):

M. **Genitourinary**
1. *Initial management*
   a. Most trauma pts require Foley catherization. However, blood at meatus, high-riding prostate, or palpable bladder suggest urethral injury and warrant retrograde urethrogram. Perform by instilling 10 cc of contrast through catheter inside urethral meatus.

b. Gross hematuria warrants evaluation w/ CT cystogram or retrograde cystogram w/ ~ 300 cc of contrast in bladder.

c. Microscopic hematuria warrants imaging only if penetrating injury *or* h/o hypotension (SBP < 90 mm Hg) *or* in pediatric pts.

d. Unstable pts can be evaluated in OR w/ "one-shot" IVP using 2 mg/kg IV contrast 10 min before plain radiograph.

2. *Specific injuries*

a. *Kidney*: recent literature suggests vast majority of injuries can be managed nonoperatively. Operative principles of repair include debridement of nonviable tissue, water-tight repair of collecting system, coverage w/ renal capsule or omentum. Nephrectomy indicated in unstable pt w/ expanding or pulsatile perinephric hematoma.

TABLE 9.1. Grading Intraabdominal Hypertension

Grade	cm H_2O	mm Hg
I	10–15	7–11 (normal)
II	15–25	11–18 (close watch)
III	25–35	18–26 (+/– decompress)
IV	35	> 26 (nec. decompress)

b. *Ureter*:

i. Most often iatrogenic.

ii. Management depends on level of injury.

- *Upper third*:
  - Primary ureteroureterostomy tx of choice.
  - Renal autotransplantation or bowel interposition less-favored options.
- *Middle third*:
  - Primary ureteroureterostomy tx of choice.
  - Transureteroureterostomy is alternative.
- *Lower third*:
  - Bladder reimplantation w/ psoas hitch to decrease anastomotic tension is preferred.
    - Requires division of urachus and contralateral medial ligament, followed by incising the bladder anteriorly to create antireflux anastomosis from within. Avoid injuring genitofemoral nerve when suturing to psoas.
  - Primary ureteroureterostomy acceptable if no loss of length and no pelvic sepsis or urinoma.
  - Boari flap (tubularization of portion of bladder to anastomose to ureter).
  - Transureteroureterostomy.

iii. In a damage-control situation, one can ligate the ureter and place a nephrostomy tube using a red rubber catheter.

c. *Bladder*:

i. 10% of pelvic fx assoc. w/ bladder injury. 80+% of bladder injuries assoc. w/ pelvic fx. 50% extraperitoneal, 30% intraperitoneal, 20% combined.

ii. *Extraperitoneal*:

- Can be managed w/ catheter drainage alone for 2 wk.

iii. *Intraperitoneal*:

- Managed w/ 2 layers of running suture (chromic gut preferred, esp. for inner layer, to decrease risk nidus for stone formation) and catheter drainage for 8–10 d.

d. *Urethra*:

i. 5% of pelvic fx assoc. w/ urethral injury, usu. at junction of prostatic and membranous portions.

ii. Do not place Foley if suspect injury, unless urethrogram normal.

iii. Blunt injury managed initially w/ suprapubic cystostomy. Depending on location and nature of injury, urethral voiding and possible urethroplasty schedules vary.

VIII. EXTREMITIES

A. **Mangled extremity severity score (MESS):** consider amputation if total score > 7. *Note*: the original article that reported this threshold was retrospective. Prospective data suggest that up to 1/3 of "non-salvageable" limbs may in fact be salvageable w/ reasonable outcome.

B. **Gustilo classification for open fx** (initially developed for tibia fx):

1. *Gustilo II*: moderate soft-tissue injury and stripping.
2. *Gustilo IIIA*: high-energy, but adequate soft tissue despite laceration or undermining.
3. *Gustilo IIIB*: extensive soft-tissue injury and periosteal stripping, usu. gross contamination.
4. *Gustilo IIIC*: Gustilo B w/ limb ischemia.

TABLE 9.2. Mangled Extremity Severity Score (MESS)*

Skeletal soft tissue injury	Low energy	1 point
	Medium energy (open fx)	2 points
	High energy (military gsw)	3 points
	Very high energy (gross contamination)	4 points
Limb ischemia (2× if > 6 h isch.)	Near-normal	1 point
	Pulseless, decreased cap. refill	2 points
	Cool, insensate, paralyzed	3 points
Shock	SBP always > 90 mm Hg	0 points
	Transient hypotension	1 point
	Persistent hypotension	2 points
Age (years)	< 30	0 points
	30–50	1 point
	> 50	2 points

*Johansen, et al., *J Trauma.* 1990;30(5):568–72.

C. **Contraindications for salvage of Gustilo IIIC injury in lower extremity:**

1. Preexisting severe comorbidity
2. Severed limb
3. Tibial loss > 8 cm
4. Ischemia > 6 h
5. Severance of posterior tibial nerve in adults, or sciatic nerve in anyone (increasingly controversial)

D. **Extremity vascular injury** (see Chapter 11 for exposures):

1. *Hard signs of vascular injury* (mandate exploration in OR)
   a. Circulatory deficit
   b. Ischemia
   c. Pulse deficit
   d. Bruit
   e. Expanding or pulsatile hematoma
   f. Arterial bleeding
2. *Soft signs of vascular injury* (generally mandate further w/u such as angiography)
   a. Small or stable hematoma

b. Adjacent nerve injury
c. Otherwise unexplained shock
d. Proximity to major vessel (< 1 cm)
e. ABI < 0.9 or difference of > 0.15 from uninjured side

E. Revised trauma score:

1. *RTS* = 0.9368 GCS + 0.7326 SBP + 0.2908 RR
2. *Chance of survival*: 0 → 2.7%, 1 → 7.1%, 2 → 17.2%, 3 → 36.1%, 4 → 60.5%, 5 → 80.7%, 6 → 91.9%, 7 → 96.9%, 8 → 98.8%

TABLE 9.3. Revised Trauma Score

GCS	SBP	RR	Value
13–15	> 89	10–29	4
9–12	76–89	> 29	3
6–8	50–75	6–9	2
4–5	1–49	1–5	1
3	0	0	0

IX. NORTH AMERICAN BITES/STINGS

A. Human: always leave open if involve hand. Cover for anaerobes. *Eikenella corrodens.*

B. Dog: rarely get infected.

C. Cat: frequently become infected. *Pasteurella multocida.*

D. Venomous reptiles:

1. *Crotalid*
   a. *Resuscitate* (ABCs): consider albumin after initial crystalloids.
   b. *Labs*: CBC w/ diff and smear, fibrinogen, coags, fibrin split products, T&C, chem 7, u/a, CK.
   c. Measure, follow extremity circumference and pulse exam (q 15 min for 24 h).
   d. Wound care, tetanus px, abx.
   e. Classify envenomation.
      i. *No envenomation*: no local, systemic reactions.
      ii. *Minimal*: local swelling and pain, no systemic sx.
      iii. *Moderate*: swelling beyond area of bite, systemic sx (N/V, paresthesias, orthostasis); mild coag abn or hemoconcentration.
      iv. *Severe*: severe extremity swelling, ecchymoses, markedly abn coags, thrombocytopenia, hematuria, proteinuria, elevated CK.
      v. If no sx of envenomation w/in 6 h of envenomation, and vitals and labs all normal, can be d/c'd after 12–24 h observation. Clean, débride wounds as indicated. Give abx as indicated, esp. if human saliva exposure; include anaerobe coverage. *Tetanus* prophylaxis for all. Keep extremity *below heart level* until antivenin, then may raise it after that to help edema. Fasciotomy as for any trauma indications. Skin grafting may be necessary.
   f. *Equine-based antivenin* (Wyeth, USA)
      i. Horse immunoglobulin providing polyvalent cross-reactivity using 4 pit viper species.
      ii. *Indications/dosage*:
         - No envenomation → no antivenin
         - Minimal → 0–5 vials
         - Moderate → 10–20 vials
         - Severe → 20+ vials
            - *Caveats*: immediate, anaphylaxis; delayed, serum sickness.
            - Optimally given w/in *4–6 h*, but may be of benefit up to 72 h out in severe cases.

        - Children dosed larger mg/kg dosing.
        - Mojave rattlesnakes often require more antivenin than intended; copperheads rarely require any.

   iii. *Adverse reactions*

      - Anaphylaxis
        - Some advocate skin testing for anaphylaxis (type I rxn), but this generally wastes time and doesn't change management.
        - Be prepared w/ 0.3–0.5 cc of 1:1000 *epinephrine* SQ.
        - F/u w/ volume, antihistamines, corticosteroids prn.
        - For large doses, consider preemptive antihistamines and steroids.
      - Serum sickness (type IV rxn) may occur 1–4 wk later w/ urticaria, rash, arthralgias, a/o fever; up to 75% of pts w/ some sx. Treat w/ prednisone.

g. *Ovine-based antivenin* (CroFab™: Savage Laboratories, USA)

   i. Sheep polyvalent immune Fab.

   ii. No cases of anaphylaxis in premarketing trials. Serum sickness rare (2–3%); skin testing "not required."

   iii. Targeted for North American crotalids (Mojave rattlesnake, eastern diamondback, western diamondback, water moccasin).

   iv. *Dosage*:

      - Initially 4–6 vials, initially infused at 25 cc/h until sx (local sx, coags, etc.) normalize.
      - Therafter 2 vials q 6 h for up to 3 additional doses (18 h); an additional 2 vials may be considered in severe cases.
      - Use w/in 4 h of reconstitution.

h. *Elapid envenomation*

   i. Eastern coral snake, *Micrurus fulvius* (NC to west Texas), can be lethal; effective antivenin available for this species. Regarding Arizona coral snake, *Micruroides euryxanthus* (AZ, NM), no fatalities ever reported but no antivenin for this species.

   ii. Bite results in minimal discomfort or necrosis. Effects *neurotoxic*. 50% envenomation rate, sx may take several hours to develop (30 min to 13 h range). *Sx*: N/V, weakness, dizziness, paresthesias, respiratory paralysis, diplopia, lid ptosis, salivation, etc. Onset of sx often *difficult to reverse* once present; definite bite of coral snake generally warrants 4–6 vials *antivenin*. Less often, fasciculations result in elevated CK and myoglobinuria; tx as w/ traumatic cause.

i. *Pregnancy and envenomation*

   i. Most likely the relatively small venom proteins cross placental barrier; early use of antivenin recommended.

   ii. *Management of anaphylaxis*: use ephedrine (25–50 mg IV) instead of epinephrine as the former acts as beta agonist helps prevent histamine release; less injurious to fetus than vasoconstrictive effect of epinephrine.

2. *Gila monster*

   a. *Range*: Sonora Desert (Mexico, S. Arizona). Similar to Mexican beaded lizard, but orange and black, not purple and black. Appear sluggish, but fast reflexes. Envenomation by capillary action as lizard grinds flesh (doesn't rapidly inject).

   b. Venom similar to crotalid + kallekrein, serotonin. Results in hypotension, respiratory arrest. Initially, pain, edema, local cyanosis. Pain may linger for several wks after event. GET IT OFF PT's BODY. (May require pliers, crowbar, knife, etc.) Irrigate wound, give tetanus, abx, supportive care, make sure no retained teeth.

E. Spiders:

1. *Black widow (Latrodectus mactans)*

   a. Female 2–2.5 cm long w/ characteristic red hourglass marking on ventral abdomen.

   b. *Range*: similar species worldwide in temperate/subtropics. In United States, most bites in South/SW states.

   c. *Habits*: defensive biters that build "cobweb" nests in corners of garages, gardens, and under logs/stones, etc. Guards oval white egg sac.

d. *Presentation*:
   i. Relatively little local inflammation, although initial bite may be painful.
   ii. Neurotoxic (multiple pathways including calcium flux) venom prone to induce muscle spasm of large muscle groups; effects may begin w/in 30 min.
   iii. HTN and autonomic/CNS dysfunction (fasciculations, ptosis, priapism, fever, bronchorrhea, respiratory muscle weakness) reported. Pregnant pts may experience contractions.
   iv. "Latrodectus facies" refers to characteristic swelling often mistaken for allergic reaction to medications.
   v. *Profound abdominal pain may mimic surgical abdomen.*
e. *Management*:
   i. *Local*: clean wound, apply ice, tetanus px.
   ii. *Pain/spasm*: narcotics, benzodiazepines.
   iii. Calcium infusion *not* recommended.
   iv. *HTN*: nitroprusside, nifedipine.
   v. Pain worst first 8–12 h, but sx may linger for days.
   vi. Admit symptomatic peds, pregnant pts, or if h/o HTN.
   vii. *Antivenin* (Merck, Sharp, Dohme):
      - Reserved for respiratory arrest, sz, hypertensive crises, and pregnancy.
      - Anaphylaxis, serum sickness risks.
      - Usual dose = 1–3 vials.

2. *Brown recluse (Loxosceles spp)*
   a. First clinical report TX, 1872. First death (ARF), TX, 1896. Five species in United States.
   b. 8–15 mm long. Violin-shaped mark on dorsal surface.
   c. May infest homes, preferring warm, undisturbed areas (i.e., garages, closets). Defensive biters.
   d. *Venom*: primarily a digestive juice w/ hemolytic and cytolytic enzymes including hyaluronidase and sphingomyelinase D (causes platelet aggregation, PMN chemotaxis, and cell membrane binding).
   e. *Presentation*:
      i. Initial bite may be painless or w/ sharp sting. Followed 6–8 h later by itching, aching w/ increasing ischemia (vasospastic). Local edema w/ surrounding erythema generally follows.
      ii. Severe cases develop bullae in center in 1–3 d, w/ underlying eschar. 2–5 wk later, eschar sloughs, leaving a muscle-sparing ulcer behind.
      iii. Systemic sx more common in peds, w/ hemolytic anemia, hemoglobinuria (usu. d 1–7). F/C/N/V, arthralgias, thrombocytopenia, DIC may occur. Rare ARF, death reported.
   f. *Management*:
      i. *Mild cutaneous dz*: cold compresses, elevation.
      ii. Debride necrotic areas.
      iii. Dapsone (inhibits PMNs) may be of benefit in first 48–72 h. 50–100 mg PO 2 times per day.
         - *Risks*: hypersensitivity, methemoglobinemia, hemolysis (if G6PD deficiency).
      iv. *Systemic sx*: admit if coagulopathy, hemolysis/hematuria, etc.
      v. Supportive wound care, IVF, abx, blood transfusion, etc. Dialysis has been required in rare cases.
      vi. *Severe tissue damage*: anecdotal reports of HBO benefit. Skin grafting sometimes necessary.
      vii. No antivenin shown to be of consistent benefit.

F. **Marine envenomation:**

1. *Coelenterates* (jellyfish/Portuguese man-o-war/coral)
    a. Sting via nematocytes, tiny specialized organs w/ venom sacs and barbs.
    b. Rinse w/ saltwater (not hypotonic fresh water, which will burst the fragile nematocysts, releasing venom).
    c. F/u tx w/ topical 5% acetic acid (vinegar), rubbing alcohol, or urine.
    d. Shaving affected area w/ cream/foam may help remove remaining nematocysts.
2. *Other*
    a. *Stingray*
        i. Cold irrigation. Remove spine/sheath. Constriction band. Suction first 15–30 min.
        ii. Soak in hot water (up to 113° F for 30–90 min) to address heat-labile venom.
        iii. Local anesthetics and narcotics prn.
        iv. Appropriate antibiotics include cefoxitin or clindamycin + gentamycin.
    b. *Catfish (Notorus* spp.) and *sea urchin* spines
        i. Spines may puncture skin w/ disproportionate pain and bleeding.
        ii. Immerse in hot water for heat-labile toxins and to reverse vasospasm.
        iii. Infiltration w/ alkalinized lidocaine may be of benefit.
        iv. Remove foreign bodies.
        v. For sea urchins, shaving pedicellariae may be useful.
        vi. Reports of benefit from application of catfish "slime" are anecdotal.
        vii. Consider prophylactic abx.

X. **EMERGENCY PROCEDURES**: see Chapter 26 on key steps in key operations.

CHAPTER 10

BURNS

I. **INITIAL CARE AND RESUSCITATION** (The following burns should be referred to a designated burn center if possible: 2nd- and 3rd-degree burns > 10% BSA; full-thickness burns > 5% BSA; any burn to face, hands, eyes, ears, or perineum that could result in cosmetic or functional disability; high-voltage electrical injury including lightning, inhalation injury, or assoc. trauma; chemical burns; burns in pts w/ major comorbidities [DM, COPD, etc.]. In addition to steps mentioned below, all significant burns merit NGT and Foley.)

A. **Airway, breathing, and other important considerations**

1. Always suspect inhalation injury; give 100% oxygen by mask.
2. Expose chest to assess breathing.
3. Consider early intubation, esp. if face/neck burns, or inhalation injury.

B. **Circulation:** fluid resuscitation (see below for calculation of TBSA)

1. BP may be difficult to assess in extremities; follow pulse, skin perfusion.
2. 2 peripheral IVs should be *sutured* at multiple points to the skin; as the pt will become edematous; this helps prevent lines from being dislodged.
3. While calculating fluid deficits, start RL at 500 cc/h (adult) or 250 cc/h (child > 5 yo).
   a. *Parkland formula* (for adults w/ burn BSA > 20%; peds/elderly BSA > 10%); developed by Dr. Charles Baxter:
      i. 4 cc/kg/24 h—initial guide, follow UOP, other clinical parameters.
      ii. *Can also be remembered as*:
         - *First 8 h*: LR 2 cc/kg/%TBSA
         - *Second 8 h*: LR 1 cc/kg/%TBSA
         - *Third 8 h*: LR 1 cc/kg/%TBSA
         - *Next 4 h*: 25% Albumin 0.1 cc/kg/%TBSA (may give 1/2 earlier if pt seems to need significantly more than would be estimated by Parkland formula)
      iii. *Note*: the Brooke formula recommends 2 cc/kg/24 h.
         - Second 24 h consider use of albumin.
   b. *Galveston formula* (designed for children):
      i. 5000 cc/m^2 burn + 2000 cc/TBSA m^2/24 h.
4. The Parkland, Brooke, and Galveston Formulas *all* use Ringer's lactate for the crystalloid, and *all* administer half the total fluid volume over the first 8 h *post-injury* (*not post-hospital arrival*), w/ the second half total fluid volume distributed over the ensuing 16 h. Follow clinical findings to avoid under- or overresuscitation. Also, in infants and children < 30 kg, recommend running a second line for maintenance fluid w/ D5LR to avoid hypoglycemia.
5. *Urine*:
   a. *UOP*: maintain ≥ 30 cc/h (30–50 ideal) (0.5 cc/kg/h) for adults or 1.0 cc/kg/h for children.
   b. *Alkalinization*: high-voltage burns, crush injuries w/ myoglobinuria/hemoglobinuria at risk of ATN. Not necessary to treat microscopic myoglobinuria, just grossly obvious cases. Consider use of mannitol a/o sodium bicarbonate for these pts (i.e., 2 amps sodium bicarbonate and 25 mg mannitol IV prn).
6. *Other adjuncts*: in the intensive care setting, pediatric pts may benefit from reducing the hypermetabolic demands on the heart by tx w/ beta blockade (i.e., propanolol).
7. Early use of albumin, or excessive fluids required should prompt placement of PA catheter.

C. **Nutrition and electrolytes**

1. *Energy expenditure*:
   a. *Nonintubated*: 629 – 11 (age) + 25 (wt in kgs) – 609 (if obese)
   b. *Intubated*: 1925 – 10 (age) + 292 (if trauma) + 5 (wt in kgs) + 281 (if male) + 851 (if > 20% TBSA burn)

2. Begin nutritional support postburn d 1.
3. Enteral feeds are preferred to parenteral nutrition.
4. Only stop tube feeds if residuals are > 150% of the hourly rate or 200 cc (whichever is more). Restart, then check again at 1 h, then 2 h, then q 4 h. Do not waste time w/ 1/2-strength formulas.
5. Adults w/ > 20% TBSA burns may benefit from anabolic medications such as oxandrolone.
6. Burn pts are essentially psychogenic drinkers—follow their sodium levels!

TABLE 10.1. Fluid Management for Serum Sodium Level

Serum Na*	Volume	Restricted Fluids*
≥ 136	No restriction	Water
133–135	1500 cc	Above plus juice, coffee, tea, soda, Jell-O, broth, watermelon, popsicles (Unrestricted: milk, Boost Plus, Deliver, Kindercal, Choice DM, ice cream)
130–132	1000 cc	Above plus milk, ice cream, Kindercal, Choice DM (Unrestricted: Boost Plus, Deliver)
< 130	500 cc	Same as above

*Note: Gatorade, Pedialyte, and ice are restricted fluids regardless of sodium level.

II. THERMAL BURNS

A. Initial pt considerations

1. Avoid hypothermia, remove all jewelry/constricting items; edema *will* follow major burns.
2. Perform standard trauma assessment as well as ABG, CXR, carboxyhemoglobin. Examine pulses, consider escharotomies (different incisions than fasciotomies) at bedside w/ IV sedation. Chest wall escharotomy on chest wall may be needed if ventilation impaired.

B. Immediate wound considerations

1. (Prehospital) Irrigate copiously w/ water and protect w/ clean dressing/sheet.
2. Gently clean, debride loose skin and blisters (blister fluid is proinflammatory and a good culture medium). In reliable pts, may leave intact blisters < 1 cm undisturbed.
3. Cover w/ topical antimicrobial (see section D. below on infection) and absorbent dressing.
4. *Accurately estimate burn size and depth* (4% TBSA error translates into 1 L error in 70-kg pt on the first day).
    a. *Wallace's rule of nines* (for 2nd-, 3rd-degree burns—in honor of A. B. Wallace, a Scottish plastic surgeon):
        i. *Adult*:
            - Head, 9%
            - Upper extremity, 9%
            - Neck, 1%
            - Anterior trunk, 18%
            - Posterior trunk, 18%
            - Lower extremity, 18%

        ii. *Child*:
            - Head/neck, 18%
            - Upper extremity, 9%
            - Anterior trunk, 18%
            - Posterior trunk, 18%
            - Lower extremity, 14%

        iii. *Note*: pt's palm (fingers included) is roughly 1% of BSA.

5. *Tetanus prophylaxis*: if burn > 10% BSA, give 0.5 cc tetanus toxoid. If tetanus immunization hx > 10 yr ago, or if received less than 3 total doses, or uncertain, also administer 250 U of tetanus immunoglobulin. Both Td and TIG are given IM. In short, treat all burn wounds like dirty wounds.

C. Scald injuries

1. Most common form of burn injury in pts < 5 yo.
2. Unlike other burns, which appear white or black (as well as dry and leathery), w/ full-thickness burns, 3rd-degree scald burns generally appear red (as well as dry and leathery).

D. Infection: leading cause of death in adequately resuscitated pts.

1. Mortality used to be from wound sepsis, but now pneumonia is main risk.
2. Generally do not consider a fever significant in a burn pt unless ≥ 39.5, as all pts will be hypermetabolic.
3. *Topical agents*: indicated immediately after debridement

TABLE 10.2. Topical Agents—Indicated Immediately After Debridement

Agent	Indications/Advantages	Caveats
Silver sulfadiazine (Silvadene)	Painless, nonstaining. Agent of choice except for face, ears, thick eschars, or skin grafts (causes sloughing)	Poor eschar penetration, mild reversible neutropenia
Silvadene + mycostatin (Silvamyco)	Extended coverage against fungi	Poor eschar penetration, mild reversible neutropenia
Mafenide acetate (Sulfamylon)	Good eschar penetration. Agent of choice for ears, thick eschars	Painful, metabolic alkalosis 2° carbonic anhydrase inhibitor. In some pts, allergy can cause a chondritis mimicking infection of auricle
Silver nitrate	Broad spectrum	Poor eschar penetration, electrolyte abnormalities
Sodium hypochlorite (Dakin's solution)	Broad spectrum	High doses impair wound healing
Neomycin	Useful for uncomplicated facial burns	Minimal
Bacitracin	Gram (+) coverage. Agent of choice for face	Minimal
Polymyxin B	Petroleum base moistens graft	Minimal
Polymyxin + mycostatin (Polymyco)	Good staph coverage—slightly better than bacitracin	Minimal
Bactroban	Good staph coverage—slightly better than bacitracin	Expensive

III. INHALATION INJURY

A. Generally do not cause direct thermal injury below level of vocal cords (exception = steam). Therefore, mechanism is from chemical injury. Majority of house burn fatalities are from anoxia, not thermal injury.

B. Injury may mature up to 48 h postexposure and is generally underappreciated initially.

C. Pulse oximetry not accurate. Obtain ABG and carboxyhemoglobin levels. If have high index of suspicion, treat w/ nonrebreather mask oxygen, and sit pt up at 45° to minimize airway edema.

1. *CO level of 50–60%* usu. fatal.
2. *CO level > 5%* abnormal except in smokers (> 10%).
3. *Tx until < 10%* (nonrebreather mask decreases half-life from 240 min to 40 min).
4. Suspect cyanide toxicity if persistent metabolic acidosis despite what should be adequate resuscitation.

a. If have pulmonary artery catheter, may also see increased SvO_2. (*Ddx*: sepsis, hepatic failure, AV shunt, nitroprusside toxicity.)

b. *Tx*: amyl nitrite, sodium nitrite, followed by sodium thiosulfate.

D. Bronchoscopy indicated to document dx, but can also be therapeutic (suctioning plugs, etc.). Xenon diffusion scan alterative means of dx.

E. **Nebulized heparin** (decrease cast formation) and acetylcysteine (loosen secretions, decrease oxygen toxicity) shown in one study to be of benefit along w/ bronchodilators and aggressive pulmonary toilet. [Desai, *J Burn Care Rehab*. 1998;19(3): 210–2.]

F. Avoid RSI for intubation (paralyzing pt w/ edematous airway high risk for losing airway). Instead, consider incremental use of morphine and Versed in 5-mg boluses until achieve desired sedation.

G. **Volumetric diffusive respiration:** of some benefit in retrospective analyses in documented cases inhalation injury.

H. **Oscillator:** most useful in neonates w/ surfactant deficiency.

IV. ELECTRICAL BURNS

A. **Low voltage** (< 1000 V)

B. **High voltage** (> 1000 V)

1. *Neurologic*: neurologic complications can develop early or late after trauma including encephalopathy, hemiplegia, aphasia, and brain stem dysfunction up to 9 mo after injury.
2. *Cardiac*: arrhythmias, particularly ventricular fibrillation can occur.
3. *Renal*: myoglobinuria can induce acute tubular necrosis. The earliest sign of impending problems is a distinctive "cranberry" color urine; once dark sediment is noted in the urine, more aggressive tx (beyond keeping UOP at 2 cc/kg/h) may be warranted. Mannitol and sodium bicarbonate may be given in a variety of methods. Some give a one-time dose of 25 mg mannitol and 1 bicarb ampule. Others recommend 25 mg IV of mannitol q 6 h and a 5% continuous bicarb infusion titrated to urine pH.
4. *Extremity*:
   a. Tetanic convulsions can lead to fxs/dislocations. Consider use of c-collar until injury can be ruled out.
   b. Fasciotomies (not just escharotomies) must be considered in any extremities w/ tense compartments, circumferential injury, rhabdomyolysis, or other evidence of muscle compromise. Unlike flame burns, damage to deep tissues is much greater than suggested by skin pathology, esp. around bone, which serves as a heat sink for electrical current.
5. *Abdomen*
   a. Intraabdominal injury, including bowel perforation, can occur.
6. *Other*
   a. Cataracts develop in almost 1/3 of pts after high-voltage injuries as a long-term complication.

C. **Lightning**

1. May cause *temporary* (unlike high-voltage electrical injury) paralysis (keraunoparalysis) a/o apnea.
2. Evaluate for blast effect (burst tympanic membranes).
3. Can cause arborizing, dendritic burn pattern over skin w/ (often) relatively spared internal tissues.

V. CHEMICAL BURNS

A. **General:** remove clothing, copiously irrigate w/ (minimum 15 L) water. Brush powders away before irrigation.

B. **Acids:** irrigate w/ water. Do not attempt to neutralize; tends to form eschars.

1. *Hydrofluoric/oxalic/phosphoric acids*: chelate calcium and magnesium, causing extensive, extremely painful local tissue destruction and potential arrhythmias. Copious irrigation w/ water followed by immediate application of calcium gluconate gel (2.5%); replacing the gel every 15 min until pain is relieved is appropriate. If significant pain persists after several cycles of gel change, intradermal calcium gluconate (10% at 0.5 cc/cm^2 involvement) may be of use. Alternately, intraarterial calcium gluconate may be tried. Failure to control the wound could lead to further extension of damage, including demineralization of underlying bone. Admission for telemetry monitoring (QT interval emphasis) is indicated, and 20 cc of calcium gluconate (10%) should be added to first liter of IV fluid. Frequent monitoring of calcium, magnesium, and potassium are indicated.

2. *Hydrochloric acid*: fumes can cause pneumonitis.
3. *Dichromate salts*: consider aggressive debridement (LD 50 is 50 mg/kg).
4. *Sulfosalicyclic/tannic/trichloroacetic acids*: systemic absorption can lead to hepato/renal toxicity.
5. *Formic acid*: can cause considerable electrolyte abnormalities, metabolic acidosis, renal failure, ARDS, and hemolysis. Hemodialysis may be required for large exposures. Wounds are characteristically greenish, deeper than are initially apparent, and are optimally managed by excision.

C. **Bases** (lime, bleach, sodium/potassium hydroxide): liquefactive necrosis invades more deeply than acid burns.
  1. Irrigate w/ water; may take longer than w/ acids.
  2. Cement (calcium oxide) leads to similar injury from hydroxyl ion. Irrigate (water/soap) until effluent has pH < 8.

D. **White phosphorus:** used in munitions and fertilizer. Spontaneously ignites upon contacting air. Immediate management includes covering w/ saline-soaked gauze (keep from air). Definite management includes copper sulfate (0.5%) irrigation and removal of particulate matter/foreign bodies.

E. **Hydrocarbons:** wounds are typically superficial and heal w/out extensive surgery, although ignition of the hydrocarbons would cause full-thickness injury. Neosporin or bacitracin are useful to help remove residual hydrocarbons. Systemic absorption, however, can result in respiratory embarrassment a/o hepatic toxicity.

VI. SURGICAL MANAGEMENT OF BURN WOUNDS

A. **Harvesting:**
  1. Dermatome harvest at 0.012" standard, consider 0.008" for elderly/very young. Clysis using LR w/ neosynephrine added (30 mg/L) minimizes blood loss.
     a. If wounds not ready for autograft, may temporarily cover w/ silver sulfadiazine or biologic dressing (allograft, pig xenograft) or synthetic (Biobrane® or Integra®).
  2. *Donor site may be managed w/*:
     a. Tegaderm, Xeroform, fine mesh gauze, or Aquacel (sodium carboxymethycellulose + ionic silver).
  3. *Postop*:
     a. Elevate extremities, generally take down dressings POD #5.

VII. RADIATION BURNS [Chambers JA, Purdue GF, *J Am Coll Surgeons*. Jan 2007;204(1):128–39.]

A. Acutely, treat ABCDEs. Decontaminate and debride wounds.

B. Estimate exposure based on hx, physical, radiation scanners/probes. Draw CBC (particularly important to check lymphocytes and granulocytes at baseline and 48 h). Draw *lymphocyte* culture (takes several days for results).

C. For whole body exposure (highly penetrating radiation such as gamma to > 1/3 of total bone marrow), anticipate acute radiation syndrome. Median survivable exposure 3–4.5 Gy. Hematologic syndrome (3+ Gy) often survivable w/ supportive medical care. GI syndrome (6–10 Gy) and neurovascular syndrome (15–30 Gy) not survivable w/ current technology. In pts w/ significant whole body exposure, avoid operations between d 3 and 60 postexposure or when wound is hyperemic.

D. For high-dose local tissue exposure, tissue necrosis results from a variety of factors, particularly obliterative arteritis. Determining the ultimate level of demarcation and viability is exceedingly difficult for several mo but may best correlate w/ initial level of bleb formation. Salvage of extremities w/ > 20 Gy local exposure has not been reported. Biologic dressings, physical therapy, and eventual flap coverage are most frequent interventions short of amputation.

VIII. FROSTBITE

A. Usu. occurs w/ temperature at or below 28°F (–2°C), resulting in freezing of tissue, intracellular ice crystal formation, a/o microvascular thrombosis.

B. Immediate tx includes removing all damp, cold clothing, immersion in warm (104°F, 40°C) saline (usu. 20–30 min), and prn analgesia. Aggressively tx hypothermia as well.

C. A conservative approach to wound debridement is appropriate as the level of necrosis may not be immediately apparent. Unless wet gangrene develops, there is no urgency for debridement or amputation. Triple-phase bone scan helps predict level of amputation.

IX. TOXIC EPIDERMAL NECROLYSIS

A. AKA Lyell's syndrome: diffuse erythema and bullous lesions in spectrum of dz predom. on face and trunk as well as mucous membranes and often (85%) conjunctiva.

1. *Nikolsky's sign*: lateral pressure to the epidermis → separation from underlying dermis. Commonly, 2–3 d nonspecific prodrome (malaise and flu-like), conjunctiva frequently developing lesions before skin.
2. *Classification*:
   a. *Extent*:
      i. *Bullous EM*: epidermal detachment < 10% of BSA w/ target lesions.
      ii. *Stevens-Johnson syndrome*: epidermal detachment < 10% BASA w/ widespread erythematous or purpuric macules or flat target lesions. Mortality ~ 5%.
      iii. *SJS-TEN*: epidermal detachment 10–30% BSA w/ widespread erythematous or purpuric macules or flat target lesions.
      iv. *TEN*: epidermal detachment > 30% BSA resulting in large areas of skin sloughing. Mortality 30–40% or higher depending on severity and care.
   b. *Distribution*:
      i. Some consider involvement of mucosa (conjunctiva, oropharnyx, tracheobronchial tree, genitalia, etc.) to be an exclusive feature of Stevens-Johnson syndrome, distinguishing it from TEN.

B. Dx: histopath → necrosis of basal keratinocytes, full-thickness necrosis, detachment superficial to basement membrane in absence of dermal inflammation. Differentiates from staphylococcal scalded skin syndrome (split is intraepidermal, not at junction of dermis and epidermis) NS pemphigoid lesions.

C. Likely immune-complex disorder → epidermal apoptosis. Weak risk factors include HIV, HLA-B27, and SLE. Usu. assoc. w/ following drugs: [sulfa drugs, chloramphenicol, Tegretol, phenytoin, NSAIDs—esp. piroxicam and tenoxicam] > [vancomycin, fluoroquinolones, allopurinol, aminopenicillins].

D. Tx mainstay = d/c instigating agent (consider plasmapheresis to remove medications), give supportive care during acute dz (3–6 wk). Manage wounds burns w/ topical abx (usu. NOT silver sulfadiazine, which has sulfa moiety) and biologic dressings prn. Ophthalmologic consultation to prevent conjunctival adhesions. Consider peridex mouthwax. Survivors often have significant scarring and functional sequelae.

CHAPTER 11

VASCULAR

I. ANATOMY

A. Supradiaphragmatic

1. Aorta gives off brachiocephalic trunk (innominate a.) to the right.
2. Common carotid is first branch off of both aorta and brachiocephalic trunk (innominate a.). Internal carotid has no extracranial branches. The branches of the external carotid are superior thyroid a., ascending pharyngeal a., lingual a., facial a., occipital a., posterior auricular a., maxillary a., and superficial temporal a. Consider mnemonic: **S**ome **A**stute **L**awyers **F**ind **O**ut **P**ost-**M**ortem **S**tudies.
3. After the common carotid, the innominate becomes the subclavian a. The first branches of the subclavian are the vertebral a.'s, which go cephalad while the interior mammary (int. thoracic) a. heads caudally.
4. Next, the thyrocervical trunk arises, giving off the inferior thyroid a., the lateral cervical a., and the suprascapular a. The last branch is the deep cervical a.
5. The subclavian a. becomes the axillary a. (important branch = thoracodorsal a.) once beyond lateral border of first rib.
6. The axillary a. becomes the brachial a. once beyond the lateral border of pectoralis major. See Chapter 26 on key steps in key operations for details on more distal upper extremity vasculature.
7. Bovine arch refers to common origin of left carotid and innominate a.'s.

B. Infradiaphragmatic

1. Aorta gives off phrenic arteries bilaterally once through hiatus.
2. Celiac axis is first major branch, giving off left gastric a., splenic a., and common hepatic a.
    a. *Left gastric a.* runs along the superior aspect of the lesser curvature of stomach, collateralizing w/ the right gastric a., which runs along the inferior aspect of the lesser curve.
    b. *Splenic a.* gives off dorsal and great pancreatic a.'s en route to spleen, then . . .
    c. *Common hepatic a.* divides into proper hepatic a. and gastroduodenal a. after giving off the right gastric a., which anastomoses w/ the left gastric a. in the lesser curvature of the stomach.
        i. Common hepatic divides into *right* and *left* hepatic a.'s. Typically the cystic a. comes off the right hepatic a.
        ii. *Gastroduodenal a.* gives off ant. and post. superior pancreaticoduodenal a.'s, which anastomose w/ their inferior counterparts stemming from the superior mesenteric a. (SMA) below. The gastroduodenal a. then turns left to become the right gastroepiploic a., running along the greater curve of the stomach, anastomosing w/ the left gastroepiploic, which has its origin w/ the distal splenic a.
3. *SMA is below celiac axis and yields 4 branches*:
    a. Inferior pancreaticoduodenal artery.
    b. Ileocolic artery.
    c. Right colic artery.
    d. Middle colic artery.
        i. Adrenal arteries take off the aorta near the SMA bilaterally.
        ii. Renal arteries are below the adrenal arteries.
4. Gonadal a.'s branch off between SMA and IMA.
5. *IMA yields 3 branches*:
    a. Left colic artery.
    b. Sigmoid artery.
    c. Superior rectal artery.
6. Aorta then branches into common iliacs.
7. Common iliacs divide into internal and external iliacs at L4, ~2 cm inferior to umbilicus.
    a. *Internal iliac* (hypogastric a.): can ligate unilaterally w/ impunity on 1 side only. Divides into large anterior (6 branches) and small posterior (3 branches) divisions. Important branch off

of anterior division is obturator a., which, through anastomosing w/ circumflex branches of profunda femoris, serves as collateral in external iliac or common femoral dz. Branches in pelvis including pudendal, uterine, gluteals, obturator, etc.

b. *External iliac*: gives off the inferior epigastric a. and deep circumflex a. before exiting the abdomen. The former forms the lateral side of Hesselbach's triangle and the latter travels around the anterior superior iliac spine, anastomosing w/ collateral vessels in the thigh. *Note*: ureter crosses external iliac, just distal to takeoff of internal iliacs (runs parallel to internal iliac a.).

C. **Infrainguinal**

1. Common femoral emerges from femoral canal (had been ext. iliac), giving off profunda femoris about 5 cm below inguinal ligament, then continuing on as superficial femoral.
2. Profunda femoris gives off obturator a., lateral femoral circumflex a., multiple perforators.
3. Superficial femoral a. emerges from adductor canal (Hunter's canal) as the popliteal a., which gives off superior geniculate arteries before trifurcating into the anterior tibial a. (most cephalad of the three—it leads anteriorly and penetrates interosseous membrane, and ultimately gives rise to the dorsalis pedis), posterior tibial a. (medial), and peroneal a. (lateral). Dorsalis pedis supplies metatarsals. Posterior tibial a. supplies sole of foot.

D. **Vessels that can be ligated w/ impunity**

1. *Arteries*: unilateral internal iliac (hypogastric); common hepatic artery (before takeoff of gastroduodenal; axillary; external carotid.
2. *Veins*
   a. Most veins can be sacrificed w/ relatively few consequences except for: IVC; portal v.; popliteal v.; bilateral jugular v.; right renal v.

E. **Important collateral pathways**

1. *Lower extremity*:
   a. "*Pathway of Winslow*:" subclavian → internal mammary → superior epigastric → inferior epigastric → external iliac → femoral.
      - Important collateral pathway in aortic occlusion.
   b. Internal iliac → obturator → medial circumflex → profunda femoris.
   c. Superficial circumflex iliac artery anastomoses w/ deep circumflex iliac a. and lateral femoral circumflex artery.
   d. Internal oblique → inferior gluteal a. → transverse branches of med/lat femoral circumflex a.
2. *Visceral*:
   a. Hepatic artery → gastroduodenal → ant/post sup pancreaticoduodenal → ant/post inf pancreaticoduodenal → SMA.
   b. *Colonic*: right branch of middle colic → marginal a. of Drummond → left colic a.
   c. *Sigmoid/rectal*: sigmoid and superior rectal a.'s come off of IMA (along w/ left colic), and anastomose w/ middle and inferior rectal (or hemorrhoidal) a.'s, which are supplied by hypogastric a.
3. *Cerebral*: ECA to cerebral circulation via ophthalmic collaterals/periorbital plexus; dural collaterals; leptomeningeal collaterals; persistent trigeminal a/o hypoglossal a.; collaterals from costocervical trunk.

II. PHYSIOLOGY AND VASCULAR SURGERY PRINCIPLES

A. **Arteries:** Endothelial lining regulate vascular tone, largely through NO^{--} vasodilatory (through cGMP, intracellular Ca^{++} release), antiinflammatory, and antithrombotic. eNOS expressed constitutively.

B. **Atherosclerosis and other vascular pathophysiology**

1. Endothelial injury → express adhesion molecules (i.e., VCAM-1), bind PMNs, which leads to expression of chemoattractant cytokines for monocytes. Monocytes become macrophages, which take up lipids, becoming foam cells. Meanwhile, B/T cells induce promotion and migration of smooth muscle cells. Plaques form w/ foam cell core and smooth muscle and connective tissue covering. Plaque rupture results in exposure of tissue factor w/ resultant thrombotic complications.
2. *Risk factors*:
   a. *Hypertension*: from mechanical stress, possibly also proinflammatory/pro-oxidant effects of angiotensin II.
   b. *Diabetes mellitus*:
      i. eNOS function and endothelial-driven vasodilation, vasoconstrictor endothelin-1.

ii. Platelet dysfunction w/ overexpression of GP IIb-IIIa.
iii. Bonding of advanced glycation end products to molecules stimulates inflammatory pathways.

c. *Dyslipidemia*:
i. Accelerates lipid deposition in arterial wall.

C. Physics and vascular surgery

1. *Law of LaPlace*: T (tension) = P × r/μ; P = pressure, r = radius, μ = wall thickness
   a. Predicts site of arterial rupture, also important in cecal perforation in bowel obstruction.
   b. P = Pressure = Force/Area.
2. *Poiseuille's law*:
   a. *Resistance*: $R = 8\eta L / \pi r^4$
      i. η = viscosity; L = length; r = radius of tube
   b. *Flow*: $Q = \pi \Delta P r^4 / 8 L = \Delta P / R$
   c. *Note*: in capillaries, the "fluidization of RBCs" and rouleaux formation also affect viscosity.
3. *Pascal's principle*: $F_1 / A_1 = F_2 / A_2$
4. *Continuity equation*: $Q = A_1 v_1 = A_2 v_2$
5. *Ohm's law*: V (potential difference between 2 points) = IR
   a. *Current*: $I = \Delta q / \Delta t$
   b. *Resistance*: $R = \rho\,(1/A)$
      i. *R in series*: $R_s = R_1 + R_2 + R_3 \ldots$
      ii. *R in parallel*: $1/R_p = 1/R_1 + 1/R_2 + 1/R_3 \ldots$
      iii. q = flow
      iv. ρ = flow constant
      v. A = cross-sectional area
6. *Joule's law*: $P = I^2 R$
7. *Capacitance*: $C = q / V$
8. *Bernoulli's principle*: "as the velocity of fluid increases, the pressure exerted by the fluid decreases"
   a. *Bernoulli's equation*: $P_1 + (1/2\rho v_1^2) = P_2 + (1/2\rho v_2^2)$
      i. ρ = density of fluid
9. *Reynold's number*: unitless value, < 2000 assoc. w/ laminar flow, > 3000 assoc. w/ turbulent flow
   a. $N_{Re} = \rho v_{av} D/\eta$
      i. ρ = density; v = velocity; D = diameter; η = coefficient of viscosity
10. Compliance = ΔV / ΔP
11. MAP = CO × TPR
    a. MAP ~ 1/3 (pulse pressure) + diastolic pressure
12. SVR = [(MAP – CVP)/CO] × 80
13. $CO = VO_2/(CaO_2) - (CVO_2) = HR \times SV$
14. Pressure differential proportional to $velocity_2 \times 4$

D. Principles of bypass

1. Need good inflow, good outflow, good conduit, appropriate pt.
2. Below the knee, do not use synthetic grafts.
3. Early failure (< 6 mo) is usu. technical. Failure less than 2 yr is usu. due to intimal hyperplasia. Late failure of vein grafts usu. from progressive atherosclerosis of inflow or outflow.
4. Infection means removal of graft w/ extraanatomic bypass (i.e., axbifem) or autologous vein graft in anatomic bed (i.e., neoaortoiliac system w/ femoral vein).
5. Don't treat anatomy, treat physiology.
6. Regarding anatomy, a diameter reduction of 50% means a cross-sectional area reduction of 75%—critical stenosis.
7. Arterial grafts have longest patency, followed by venous, then prosthetic.

8. *F/u*:
   a. *Graft failure*: perioperative (30 d) usu. technical or judgment error; midterm (up to 24 mo) usu. hyperplastic lesion in graft or anastomosis; late (> 24 mo).
   b. *Autologous*: degenerative stenosis or aneurysms primary problem.
   c. *Prosthetic grafts*: Anastomotic hyperplasia more common.
   d. *Surveillance*:
      i. *Infrainguinal vein graft*: U/S at 6 wk, then 3-mo intervals for 2 yr, then 6-mo intervals afterwards.
         - *Warning signs*: *reduction* in total graft flow velocity (i.e., < 40 cm/sec) and *elevation* of velocity at focal stenotic sites (i.e., velocity ratio > 3.5). Decreases in ABI > 0.15 in serial measurements also worrisome.
         - Focal defects can be approached w/ open surgery (patch angioplasty, resection, or jump graft) or percutaneous angioplasty (angioplasty less useful for long or anastomotic stenoses).

III. NONMESENTERIC ARTERIAL DISEASE

A. Carotid

1. *Dx*: duplex is excellent test, but least accurate in 60–70% stenosis range. Spectral analysis used to measure flow velocity; > 125 cm/sec is significant elevation. Check bilateral arm pressures. Obtain angiogram or MRA if abnormal symptoms present. *U/S*: to ECA is anteromedial to ICA and as triphasic flow, not continous flow as in the ICA (due to low pressure in CNS).
2. *Tx*:
   a. *Symptomatic (amaurosis fugax, CVA, TIA, etc.) tx guided by NASCET*: decreases 5-yr stroke risk from 26% to 9% w/ CEA if ICA is stenosed by 50% or more. In symptomatic pts, higher degrees of stenosis results in higher risk of stroke (unlike asymptomatic pts).
   b. *Asymptomatic tx guided by ACAS*: decreases 5-yr stroke risk from 11% to 5% w/ CEA if ICA is stenosed by 60% or more. Unlike symptomatic pts, those w/out sx do not have significantly higher risk of CVA w/ stenosis once beyond at/beyond 60–70%.
   c. *Carotid occlusion*: do not operate as recurrent CVA risk prohibitive. Antiplatelet therapy sufficient. If "stump syndrome" is present w/ amaurosis fugax or TIA, diagnose w/ external carotid endarterectomy may be of benefit.
   d. *Endarterectomy anatomy*:
      i. *ECA branches*: superior thyroid, lingual, facial, maxillary, superficial temporal, posterior auricular, occipital, and ascending pharyngeal.
      ii. *Important collateral paths*: the ECA provides important collaterals to the ICA circulation mainly through the ophthalmic, occipital, and I maxillary arteries.
      iii. *Nerves*:
         - *Vagus*: 90% posterior to carotid, 10% anterior, most commonly injured nerve (usu. causes hoarseness as gives off superior and recurrent laryngeal nerves).
         - *Hypoglossal*: loops in superior field, damage leads to ipsilateral tongue deviation.
         - *Ansa ("loop") cervicalis*: loops in midfield, can transect w/ impunity as only innervates strap muscles (sternothyroid, sternohyoid, omothyroid, omohyoid) w/ no significant function.
         - *Glossopharyngeal*: found high in superior field, damage results in dysphagia, gives off "Hering's nerve" to innervate carotid sinus.
         - *Facial*: marginal mandibular branch has motor function; damage results in inability to depress ipsilateral lip, may result in accidental lip biting.
   e. *Endarterectomy complications*:
      i. *Nerve damage*: see entry diii. above.
      ii. *Hyper-/hypotension*: results from denervation (i.e., neurapraxia) or increased stimulation (overlying plaque now gone) of carotid sinus. Treat HTN w/ nitroprusside, hypotension w/ dopamine. Generally self-limited 48–72 h.
      iii. *Hemorrhage*: stroke.
      iv. *CNS hypoperfusion*: stroke.
      v. *Restenosis*:
         - Up to 25–40% affected, only 10% significant flow velocity increase, 1–3% symptomatic over 5 yr.

- *< 2 yr*: secondary to intimal hyperplasia, comparatively benign natural hx.
- *> 2 yr*: atherosclerotic plaque more common.
- Operate if symptomatic and > 80% stenosis.

vi. If neuro deficit noted w/in first 6–24 h, prob. from thrombosis → take emergently back to OR.

- In OR, clamp ECA, CCA, check for backbleeding and pass Fogarty as appropriate (care should be taken not to pass the Fogarty too far or too aggressively as a carotid-cavernous fistula can result from injury to the ICA). After first 24 h, more likely pt has suffered reperfusion injury → CT head.

vii. *Cerebral hyperperfusion syndrome*: can occur up to 2 wk postop. Related to temporary loss of autoregulatory ability of intracranial circulation due to chronic vasodilation in vessels past the stenosis.

- Risk factors include a contralateral tight stenosis/occlusion, advanced age (> 70), ipsilateral tight stenosis.
- Manifested by headache, seizure, hemorrhagic stroke.
- Tx is aggressive blood pressure control titrated to relief of sx.

B. Lower extremity

1. *Acute arterial occlusion*

a. *6 Ps*: **P**ulselessness, **P**ain, **P**oikilothermia, **P**aralysis, **P**aresthesias, **P**allor.

b. If see foot drop, nonblanching skin, no capillary refill, no sensation, and no motor, do not revascularize (K^+, rhabdomyolysis can be fatal w/ reperfusion).

c. Anticoagulate (heparin inhibits propagation of thrombus via potentiation of antithrombin III, inactivating thrombin as well as activated factors IX–XII and plasmin, preventing conversion of fibrinogen to fibrin; it also promotes NO release), then thrombolysis or surgery:

i. Thrombolytics take several h to work, but may be appropriate if comorbidities, multiple levels of obstruction.

- *Indications*: if diffuse dz (i.e., multiple emboli), intact motor exam.
- *Types*:
  - *Tissue plasminogen activator* (TPA):
    - Urokinase
    - Streptokinase

ii. If do surgery, fix most proximal lesion first. Backbleeding is a poor predictor of success. Get intraop arteriography at completion. Have low threshold for fasciotomy. Watch carefully during reperfusion period for rhabdomyolysis, hyperkalemia, and renal failure.

2. *Chronic arterial occlusion*

a. *Px*: lower homocysteine (B_6, B_{12}, folate), improve HDL:LDL ratio, control HTN, antiplatelet tx, possible role of L-carnitine, naftidrofuryl, omega-3 fatty acids, arginine, etc.

b. *Medical tx*:

i. *Pentoxifylline* (Trental®):

- Uncertain mechanism, acts to decrease viscosity of blood by altering RBC rheology, 30% ↑ claudication distance.

ii. *Cilostazol* (Pletal®):

- A phosphodiesterase III inhibitor, unknown mechanism (vasodilator, platelet effects). 45–90% ↑ claudication distance.

iii. *Clopidogrel* (Plavix®):

- Blocks platelet ADP receptor, preventing fibrinogen binding and decreasing platelet adhesion/aggregation.

iv. *Acetylsalicylic acid* (aspirin):

- Blocks prostacycline synthetase, preventing formation of thromboxane A_2, a potent platelet aggregator.

c. *Intermittent claudication*: except for smokers and diabetics, most pts improve or remain the same. Risk of limb loss at 5 yr = 5%, 10 yr = 11%. Initial tx is exercise, smoking cessation, and rheologic agents. 10-yr limb loss risk drops to 2% w/ smoking cessation. Pentoxifylline helps claudication distance, but not rest pain. Nocturnal calf cramps common in general population, not assoc. w/ vascular dz.

d. *Limb threatening*: ulceration, gangrene, ischemic rest pain, metatarsalgia, dependent rubor (specificity increases if latter 3 increase w/ elevation of extremity). Rest pain means pain increases w/ elevation a/o decreases w/ dependency, generally over metatarsal heads; toe pain may mean gout or infection. Arterial ulcers form at distal areas of toes, foot. Venous insufficiency ulcers, in contrast, form at medial malleoli. Neurotrophic ulcers often between toes and over metatarsal heads (pressure points).

e. 90% have CAD, w/ significant 5- to 10-yr mortality (> 50%). 30% have > 50% internal carotid compromise.

f. *Dx*: Doppler, ankle-brachial indexes (ABIs) → 1–1.2 normal; 0.4–0.9 claudication; 0.0–0.4 rest pain/limb threat. Correlation poor in diabetics (get false negatives from Ca^{++} causing noncompressible vessels). Lower extremity formal ABIs w/ waveform analysis may be esp. useful w/ diabetics or ABI > 1.2. ABI is ratio of highest systolic pressure in either arm to systolic pressure in pedal vessels. Artificially elevated in diabetics frequently secondary to mural calcinosis in (particularly tibial, pedal) arteries. Toe pressures: 30 mm Hg nondiabetics, 50–55 mg Hg in diabetics should be down to level of transmetatarsal.

   i. In these pts esp., toe pressures are much more reflective of perfusion. 30–45 mm Hg good threshold for revascularization.

   ii. Pulse volume recordings can estimate burden of stenotic dz at various levels in LE.

   iii. W/ waveform analysis, waveforms become monophasic regardless if compressible or not. Inflow (above inguinal ligament) suggested by femoral artery waveform—upstroke prolonged to > 180 ms is c/w iliac dz. Toe pressures < 30 mm Hg (< 50 in diabetics) c/w severe ischemia, which will not heal tissue loss.

   iv. Normally, extremities have reversal of blood flow from resistance. Exercise dilates vessel, lessening this reversal. Additionally, an early change w/ atherosclerosis is loss of flow reversal (tri → biphasic).

g. *Manifestations*: claudication, arterial ulceration/painful/distal/pale, rest pain, dependent rubor, ulceration, gangrene. Differentiate from blue toe syndrome, esp. in asymptomatic pts, nonclaudicators. Typically see tissue loss only w/ multilevel dz; single-level dz more often just causes claudication.

h. *Tx*:

   i. *Inflow dz* (proximal to inguinal ligament):

      - *Aortoiliac occlusive dz*:

        - *Open*:

          - Aortofemoral bypass the standard w/ primary patency of 80–90% at 5 yr. Patency actually worse for younger pts, making them candidates for aortic endarterectomy in certain circumstances (aorta, proximal common iliac artery). Proximal anastomosis should be as close to renal arteries as possible as this area typically less calcified and less prone to degenerate.

          - Axillary-femoral bypass or fem-fem crossover have patencies of 60–65% and are reserved for pts unable to tolerate intraabdominal surgery.

          - *Endovascular guidelines*: note: recommendations are changing rapidly in favor of initial attempts at endovascular management. [Norgren L, et al., Inter-Society Consensus for the Management of Peripheral Arterial Disease (TASC II), *Eur J Vascendovasc Surg*. 2007;33:S1–7; Pentecost MJ, et al., Guidelines for peripheral percutaneous transluminal angioplasty of the abdominal aorta and lower extremity vessels, *Circulation*. 1994;89:511–31.]

      - *Aortoiliac (inflow) dz*:

        - TASC A and B lesions, endovascular intervention preferred; TASC C lesions best repaired using endovascular techniques in high-risk pts, but surgically in good-risk pts; TASC D lesions best repaired using open surgical techniques.

- *TASC A*:
  - Single stenosis < 3 cm in length in either CIA or EIA.
  - Endovascular the preferred tx.
- *TASC B*:
  - Single or multiple CIA stenosis 3–10 cm long; unilateral CIA occlusion; single short CIA occlusion; unilateral EIA occlusion not involving the origins of the internal iliac or CFA; endovascular approach is preferred.
- *TASC C*:
  - Bilateral CIA occlusions.
  - Bilateral EIA stenoses 3–10 cm long not extending into the CFA.
  - Unilateral EIA stenosis extending into the CFA.
  - Unilateral EIA occlusion that involves the origins of the internal iliac a/o CFA.
  - Heavily calcified unilateral EIA occlusion w/ or w/out involvement of origins of internal iliac a/o CFA.
  - Open surgical techniques in good-risk pts preferred; endovascular repair in high-risk pts.
- *TASC D*:
  - Infra-renal aorto-iliac occlusion.
  - Diffuse dz involving the aorta and both iliac arteries requiring tx.
  - Diffuse multiple stenoses involving the unilateral CIA, EIA, and CFA.
  - Unilateral occlusions of both CIA and EIA.
  - Bilateral occlusions of EIA.
  - Iliac stenoses in pts w/ AAA requiring tx and not amenable to endograft placement or other lesion requiring open aortic or iliac surgery.
  - Open surgical techniques preferred.

ii. *Outflow dz*:

- *Femoropopliteal dz.*
- *TASC classification*:
  - Type A lesions
    - *Single stenosis*: 10 cm in length.
    - *Single occlusion*: 5 cm in length.
  - Type B lesions
    - Multiple lesions (stenoses or occlusions), each 5 cm.
    - Single stenosis or occlusion 15 cm not involving the infra geniculate popliteal artery.
    - Single or multiple lesions in the absence of continuous tibial vessels to improve inflow for a distal bypass.
    - Heavily calcified occlusion 5 cm in length.
    - Single popliteal stenosis.
  - Type C lesions
    - Multiple stenoses or occlusions totaling > 15 cm w/ or w/out heavy calcification.
    - Recurrent stenoses or occlusions that need tx after 2 endovascular interventions.
  - Type D lesions
    - Chronic total occlusions of CFA or SFA (> 20 cm, involving the popliteal artery).
    - Chronic total occlusion of popliteal artery and proximal trifurcation vessels.
  - TASC A and B lesions endovascular approach is preferred. TASC C lesions in good-risk pts w/ good native conduit may be preferred. TASC D lesions are best managed w/ open surgical techniques.

- *Tibial dz*:
  - *Open*:
    - *Rank order of anastomotic preference is*: PT > AT > peroneal (not continuous w/ pedal arteries), if equal atherosclerotic burden.

C. **Aneurysms** (aneurysm = increase in diameter > 50% normal)

1. *Aortic*

a. *Epidemiology*: 3% men, 2.1% women; 13th leading cause of death in United States, most common peripheral arterial aneurysm. Assoc. w/ iliac (41%), femoral a/o popliteal aneurysms (15%), carotid stenosis/ectasia (if see carotid ectasia, do AAA U/S), and arterial ectasia. Normal diameter is 2.0 cm: 5.5 cm is indication for surgery (5.0 in females), as is increase in diameter > 0.5 cm/yr, or symptomatic aneurysms. 50% have CAD; 50% deaths due to CAD (5–15% postop MI).

b. *Presentation*: infrarenal (90%) >> juxtarenal > suprarenal. Usu. asymptomatic, but may manifest as abdominal, back, or groin pain, or thromboembolic sx. 20–25% present ruptured. If see midabdominal pain and shock, think ruptured AAA! Rupture risk (annual) assoc. w/ LaPlace's law (T = PR); < 5 cm 1%, 5 cm 3–15%, 6–7 cm 10–20%, 7–8 cm 20–40%, > 8 cm 30–50%. *Over 5 yr*: < 5 cm 20%, 5–7 cm 33%, > 7 cm 95%.

c. *Dx*: U/S good, but can't distinguish rupture (need CT); if unstable, straight to OR.

d. *Tx*:

i. *Open repair*:

- Generally avoid doing incidental appendectomy, cholecystectomy, or herniorrhaphy. If encounter cancer, fix aneurysm first, reperitonealize, then later address cancer.
- If make enterotomy, repair it, close the abdomen, and return later if possible.
- *Complications*:
  - *Ischemic colitis*: consider IMA reimplant if sluggish backbleed or diminished collaterals (don't do if brisk backbleeding—40 mm Hg backpressure adequate, or if occluded); biphasic Doppl signals on antimesenteric colon also suggests good flow. If see postop diarrhea (esp. bloody), get sigmoidoscopy; go to OR if necrosis is present. 2–4% of all AAA repair pts.
  - *Spinal ischemia*: 0.1% w/ infrarenal, 5–10% w/ suprarenal.
  - *Aortoenteric fistula*: best preventive maneuver is to interpose retroperitoneal tissue between graft and remainder of abdominal contents. GI bleeding is most common presentation warranting upper endoscopy. If no lesion (i.e., ulcer) seen on EGD to otherwise account for bleeding in pt w/ h/o AAA open repair, proceed to OR for repair. In stable pt, perform extraanatomic (i.e., axillo-fem w/ crossover or axillo-bifemoral) bypass. Next, open abdomen, clamp infrarenal aorta, remove graft, close GI defect, and oversew aortic stump. Unstable pts should be for immediate exploration of fistula; often simple suture repair of fistula at proximal suture line suffices, followed by repair of intestinal defect. Surgeon then has option for replacement of aortic section, augmented by wrapping tongue of omentum around gastrocolic ligament, underneath transverse mesocolon (w/ local infectious risks, but may less demanding for unstable pt in short term, and can soak graft in Rifampin or other abx, possibly w/ long-term PO abx such as second-generation cephalosporin or fluoroquinolone), or removal of graft.

ii. *Endograft*:

- As w/ all endovascular devices, anatomic criteria for endovascular repair are a moving target and change w/ newer technology.
- Studies show a perioperative mortality benefit EVAR vs open repair, but 2-yr survival is the same.
- *Requirements*: infrarenal neck 10–25 mm long, ≤ 26 mm diameter, angulation < 45–60° w/out excessive calcification. Common iliac artery landing zones at least 2 cm long w/ diameter < 16 mm, also w/out excessive calcification or thrombus.
- Possibly increased renal dysfunction (partially because requires contrast CT q 6 mo). Consider in older pts w/ good renal function. Currently > 70% infrarenal aneurysms repaired this way.
- Endograft leak (50% may have some type of leak, 25% w/in 1st yr; vast majority not clinically important).

- *Type I*: leak at proximal/distal aspect of device (type Ia and Ib, respectively). Often can be repaired w/ endovascular tx; must be repaired at the time of surgery if seen intraop.
- *Type II* (most common): leakage outside graft but inside native vessel from back-bleeding lumbar arteries, IMA, etc. Can embolize.
- *Type III*: mechanical problem w/ graft (i.e., modular disassociation).
- *Type IV*: leak from fabric porosity, usu. seals spontaneously.

- Aneurysm enlargement must be looked for on CT compared w/ baseline at time of graft placement (growth in size more important than presence of endoleak). Expect small decrease in size in first 6–12 mo, but no change is not uncommon. Growth in diameter > 0.25 cm in 6 mo warrants concern.

e. *Special circumstances*:

i. *"Mycotic" aneurysm*: *Staph* most common pathogen; *Salmonella* seen less commonly. Pts have abdominal pain, pulsatile mass, and *fever*. CT often reveals eccentric aneurysm that is thickened, w/ surrounding fluid. Tx w/ abx, debridement, and in situ grafting. "Mycotic" does not refer to infectious cause, but rather dates back to early (preantibiotic) days of "malignant endocarditis," which seeded systemic arterial tree w/ infectious emboli causing multiple aneurysms along path, resembling hyphae.

ii. *Inflammatory AAA*: 5% of cases; ↑ ESR; abdominal pain w/ ureteral obstruction/medial deviation. Get CT scan; use retroperitoneal approach to avoid duodenum. (Also use retroperitoneal approach for pts w/ horseshoe kidneys.)

2. *Visceral*

a. *Hepatic artery*: 20% of splanchnic aneurysms.

i. Rupture rate probably ~ 20%. Resection and repair warranted unless prohibitive operative risk.

b. *Splenic artery*: most common (60%).

i. Highest risk of rupture in gravid females (75% fetal loss, 50% maternal mortality).

ii. Ligation or embolization if > 2 cm, symptomatic, or in reproductive-age female.

iii. Splenectomy usu. not necessary, as short gastrics provide good collateral flow to spleen.

3. *Peripheral*

a. *True*

i. *Popliteal*:

- 1/2 bilateral.
- 1/3 assoc. w/ AAA (get abdominal U/S to evaluate aorta, iliac arteries).
- Risk is thrombosis/embolism, not rupture (40–50% limb loss over 5 yr if no tx).
- Exclude and bypass if > 2 cm.

ii. *Femoral*: most common true peripheral aneurysms, but low rupture and thromboembolic risk.

b. *Pseudoaneursyms*

i. Femoral most common. Iatrogenic. May be treated w/ local compression for ~ 1 h, but local injection of thrombin greatly accelerates closure (true for most peripheral pseudoaneurysms).

IV. VENOUS AND LYMPHATIC DISEASE

A. Deep venous thromboembolism (DVT)

1. *Impact and risk factors*:

a. *United States incidence* 1 per 1000 person/yr w/ mortality approaching 10% per case.

b. *Virchow's triad*: venous stasis, endothelial injury, hypercoagulable state.

c. *Risk factors*: trauma (esp. pelvic, spine), recent surgery, age > 65 yo, malignancy, exogenous estrogens, obesity, venous varicosities, family hx of thrombophilia.

d. *Thrombophilia*

i. Factor V Leiden (most common thrombophilia in Caucasians)

ii. Prothrombin 20210 (Factor II mutation)

iii. Protein C deficiency
iv. Protein S deficiency
v. Antithrombin IIII deficiency
vi. Hyperhomocysteinemia
vii. Antiphospholipid syndrome
viii. Lupus anticoagulant

2. *Presentation and pathology*:
   a. < 50% of pts have signs or sx initially.
   b. Most commonly begin in calf. (+) Homan's sign (pain w/ passive dorsiflexion of ankle) suggestive, although (–) test does not r/o DVT.
   c. Early findings may include pain a/o LE circumferential asymmetry. W/ large pelvic DVTs, may progress to *phlegmasia alba dolens*, or even *phlegmasia cerulea dolens*.
   d. *Sequelae*:
      i. 1/3 of calf DVTs embolize or propagate proximally.
      ii. Pulmonary emboli.
      iii. Chronic venous insufficiency.
3. *Dx*:
   a. Duplex study demonstrating noncompressible vein w/ no flow increase w/ distal compression is most commonly used modality. Pelvic or retroperitoneal DVT may be better assessed w/ magnetic resonance venography.
   b. Normal D-dimer level (marker for fibrin degradation by plasmin) essentially excludes dx; elevated level nonspecific in surgery pts (effects of trauma a/o surgery elevate level).
4. *Tx*:
   a. *Heparin*
      i. *Unfractionated*:
         - Begin w/ 80 U/kg bolus, then start 18 U/kg/h infusion for goal PTT of 60–80 sec as initiate warfarin (see section b. below); titrate as needed.
      ii. *Fractionated (low-molecular-wt) heparin*:
         - Given predictable response, no need to follow lab values.
         - Can use as bridge for warfarin or as stand-alone therapy (*agent of choice during pregnancy*, as warfarin teratogenic).
      iii. *Argatroban or hirudin if heparin-induced thrombocytopenia* (see Chapter 2 for choice of agent and dosing).
   b. *Warfarin*:
      i. Goal INR of 2.0–3.0 for 3 mo usu. indicated. Lifetime anticoagulation (or IVC filter, see c. below) likely indicated if recurrent DVTs or known thrombophilia.
   c. *IVC filter*: indicated if anticoagulation not appropriate (i.e., CNS hemorrhage) or if develop pulmonary embolism or propagation of iliofemoral thrombus while appropriately anticoagulated. < 5% PE rate. 5% long-term occlusion rate—tx w/ fluid resuscitation.
   d. *Other*: for significant pain or impending gangrene from *phlegmasia*, consideration may be given to thrombolysis or surgical thrombectomy followed by long-term anticoagulatoin.
5. *Prophylaxis*:
   a. Ambulation.
   b. Sequential compression devices.
   c. Unfractionated heparin 5000 U SQ 3 times per day.
   d. *Fractionated low-molecular-wt heparin*:
      i. Directly inhibits factors Xa, IIa.
      ii. More predictable response than unfractionated heparin, but additional cost limits its use to moderate- and high-risk pts.

B. **Venous insufficiency** (lower extremity)
   1. Twice as common in females. Secondary to valvular incompetence.

2. *Anatomy*:
   a. *Saphenofemoral*: reflux present in ~ 70% of pts w/ LE venous insufficiency.
   b. *Saphenopopliteal*: reflux present in ~ 15% of pts w/ LE venous insufficiency.
   c. *Perforators*:
      i. *Cockett* (posterior tibial): do not flow into GSV, but rather connect posterior arch vein to tibial vv. As a result, are unaffected by GSV stripping.
         - *Cockett I*: posterior to medial malleolus.
         - *Cockett II*: distal calf 2–4 cm posterior to tibia.
         - *Cockett III*: mid-calf 2–4 cm posterior to tibia.
      ii. Other perforators include lateral leg perforators and paratibial as well as Boyd perforators in proximal medial calf.
3. *Grading* (CEAP classification system: **c**linical severity, **e**tiology or cause, **a**natomy, **p**athophysiology):
   a. *Clinical severity*:
      i. *Class 0*: no clinical evidence of dz.
      ii. *Class 1*: telangectasias, "spider veins."
      iii. *Class 2*: varicose veins.
      iv. *Class 3*: edema, but no skin changes.
      v. *Class 4*: skin changes (lipodermatosclerosis, hyperpigmentation).
      vi. *Class 5*: class 4 skin changes + healed ulceration.
      vii. *Class 6*: class 4 skin changes + active ulceration.
4. *Dx*:
   a. On physical exam, pt often has swelling over legs/feet, relatively sparing toes (different than lymphedema).
   b. Physical exam adjuncts (now largely supplanted by radiography/ultrasonography).
      i. *Trendelenburg test*: elevate leg to drain veins, then apply pressure (hand or tourniquet) to saphenofemoral junction. Have pt stand and observe filling pattern.
         - Gradual calf filling occurs in normal anatomy w/ competent perforators.
         - Rapid (< 30 sec) calf filling occurs w/ incompetent perforators.
         - After observing calf, release pressure in thigh.
           - Rapid filling of thigh varices signifies saphenofemoral incompetence.
      ii. *Perthes test*: place tourniquet around upper leg, then have pt ambulate.
         - If varicosities disappear, signifies patent deep system w/ competent perforators.
         - If pt has pain w/ ambulation, signifies deep obstruction (pt relies on superficial veins for drainage).
   c. *Duplex U/S*: required for class 2–6 dz.
   d. *Plethysmography*: required (in addition to duplex U/S) for class 4–6 dz.
   e. *Venography*: required if evidence of deep system reflux/incompetence or obstruction.
5. *Tx*:
   a. *Class 1*: compression hose, injection sclerotherapy.
   b. *Class 2–6*:
      i. *Superficial incompetence only*:
         - Saphenous vein stripping (or ablation w/ RF or laser).
      ii. *Superficial* and *perforator incompetence*:
         - Saphenous vein stripping *and* subfascial endoscopic perforator surgery (SEPS).
      iii. *Deep reflux a/o obstruction*:
         - Valve reconstruction, transposition, or transplant; *or* PTA + stent; *or* bypass.

6. *Klippel-Trenaunay-Weber syndrome*: classic findings of limb hypertrophy, birthmark (port wine stain, or venous malformation), and varicose veins. In these pts, deep veins are frequently absent or otherwise anomalous; *saphenous vein stripping should be avoided.* Instead, more conservative measures such as support hose and stab avulsion are preferred.

C. Lymphatic insufficiency

1. *Etiology*:
   a. *Primary*: evident at birth (Milroy dz), puberty (lymphedema praecox—most common), or later in life (lymphedema tarda).
   b. *Secondary*: from surgery/radiation/tumor or infection (i.e., *Wuchereria bancrofti*).
2. *Dx*:
   a. On physical exam, swelling involves toes, w/ progressive involvement of more proximal structures.
   b. R/o other causes of edema/anasarca (cardiac, renal, hepatic, or venous insufficiency).
3. *Tx*:
   a. *Medical* (mainstay of tx):
      i. Address complicating medical complications (i.e., tx filarial infection w/ diethycarbamazine).
      ii. Wt loss, extremity elevation, compressive stockings, massage.
   b. *Surgical* (rarely utilized)
      i. *Physiologic*: lymphovenous shunts, lympholymphatic shunts, omental transposition.
      ii. *Excisional*:
         - *Charles procedure*: excision of skin, subcutaneous tissue, and fascia w/ skin graft coverage.
         - *Modified Homans procedure*: staged subcutaneous tissue excision under 1.5 cm thick skin flaps.
         - Arguably the surgical procedure of choice w/ the most consistent improvement.

V. MESENTERIC ISCHEMIA

A. Arterial

1. *Chronic* (CMI, intestinal angina):
   a. *Etiology*: most from atherosclerosis of mesenteric arteries, although vasculitides or compressive syndromes possible (i.e., median arcuate ligament syndrome from compression of celiac axis by part of diaphragm, esp. during full expiration).
   b. *Presentation*: generally elderly, *female* (3:1 over males) postprandial pain (w/in 10–30 min), develops into food avoidance. Wt loss, other GI complaints (diarrhea/constipation, flatulence, etc.) common. *As w/ acute dz, pain is classically out of proportion to physical findings.*
   c. *Dx*: duplex imaging may be useful for screening. Portal vein blood flow does *not* significantly ↑ w/ eating (abn). Arteriography gold standard, must show stenosis or occlusion of at least 2 of the major mesenteric vessels; 50% of cases involve all 3.
   d. *Tx*: if peritonitis → celiotomy. Attempt at revascularization should be made before resecting bowel if feasible. Prosthetic graft bypass to 1 or 2 vessels (SMA +/– celiac) standard unless contaminated abdomen (would require autogenous—i.e., reversed saphenous bypass vs femoral vein). Celiac a/o SMA endarterectomy also option for short stenoses; antegrade (supraceliac) is generally preferred over retrograde b/c of less atherosclerotic burden cephalad to celiac vessels and less risk of kinking (esp. w/ vein). Conversely, infrarenal aorta is easier to expose, and less potential for hemodynamic instability a/o distal embolization w/ clamping/unclamping. Endovascular stenting increasingly popular, esp. in elderly pts who are poor operative candidates, but patency is poor (50% primary patency at 1 yr; often serves as a bridge to definitive bypass). Divide median arcuate ligament along w/ bypass if this is offending structure (*note*: this is dx of exclusion). Predictors of success include female gender, postprandial pain, wt loss > 20 lb, no psych/drug abuse hx, arteriography w/ celiac axis compression w/ poststenotic dilatation a/o collateral flow.

2. *Acute mesenteric ischemia* (AMI):
   a. *Embolic*: ~ 50% of cases of AMI, majority from cardiac source (w/u CHF, MI, Afib, valve dz). Embolization of atheromatous plaques and iatrogenic insults generally result in smaller emboli that travel more distally, w/ more focal involvement (usu. middle/distal jejunum and ileum) than a proximal SMA lesion.
      i. *Presentation/dx*: abrupt onset acute abdominal pain, out of proportion to physical findings early on, +/– N/V/D. Progresses to frank peritonitis over time, often w/ sx of hypovolemia. Leukocytosis, hyperamylasemia, and later, increased lactate levels may be found. In the absence of perforation or bowel wall pneumatosis, plain films not helpful. U/S is operator- and properly prepared pt-dependent (i.e., pt should be NPO for at least 8 h prior to U/S to decrease bowel gas). Study of choice is abdominal CT angiogram (nonfilling of mesenteric vessel, bowel edema, and mesenteric stranding).
      ii. *Tx*:
         - Resuscitate, get EKG (check for Afib and MI), get invasive monitoring. Begin systemic anticoagulation and IV abx.
         - If peritonitis or unstable → resuscitate and celiotomy (bypass radiographic w/u—can do on-table angiography if necessary). Prep abdomen and both LE to knees. Make midline incision; assess viability of bowel. If amount of infarcted bowel is incompatible w/ life, close abdomen. Unless bowel is clearly necrotic, revascularize before resect. *Options*:
            - *SMA embolectomy*: open the vessel transversely if normal; longitudinally if atherosclerotic and a patch angioplasty is anticipated. Default should be longitudinal arteriotomy if uncertain.
            - *SMA bypass*: antegrade vs retrograde aorto-SMA vs retrograde ilio-SMA bypass. Prosthetic OK if no frank bowel necrosis or perforation.
   b. *Thrombotic*: accounts for ~ 25% of AMI. Usu. manifests during low-flow state from preocclusive lesion (see section 1. on CMI above). Presentation and dx are same as for embolic dz (see section 2a. above). Lesion more proximal than w/ embolic dz, usu. near SMA origin. Ischemic area usu. extends from ligament to Treitz to mid-transverse colon.
   c. *Nonocclusive*:
      i. *Etiology*: low perfusion despite patent vessels—CHF, hypotension/hypovolemia, digoxin, etc.
      ii. *Dx*: index of suspicion + "pruning" of mesenteric branch vessels typically seen on angiogram.
      iii. *Tx*: reverse etiology (increase perfusion w/ fluids, inotropes, etc., fluoroscopically guided papaverine or tolazoline may assist). Celiotomy if peritonitis. Bowel resection if nonviable.

B. **Venous thrombosis:** dx w/ abd CT—edematous bowel, venous thrombus. Assoc. w/ prothrombotic diatheses, intraabdominal inflammation (i.e., pancreatitis), postop state, and portal hypertension. Mild sx may be addressed w/ full heparinization alone. If have peritonitis, need celiotomy. Infarcted bowel (look at color, Doppler, Wood's lamp, etc.) should be resected, then reanticoagulate, planning for second-look celiotomy in 24 h. Should w/u predisposing conditions.

C. **Vasculitides and vasospastic disorders**

1. *Takayasu's*: chronic inflammatory dz primarily of aorta and large arteries, although subclavian, carotid, and renal arteries may also be affected. More common in females, and sometimes referred to as "pulseless dz" due to difficulty in palpating peripheral pulses in some pts. *Tx*: corticosteroids; cyclophosphamide may be used in refractory cases. Surgery rarely indicated for burned-out dz. Stenting and angioplasty → poor results.
2. *Buerger's dz* (thromboangiitis obliterans): poor response to medical and surgical tx. Only effective tx is cessation of smoking. *Dx*: young smokers (usu. male) w/ abnormal pressures and no risk factors for obstructive vasculopathies (hypercoagulable diathesis, etc.), essentially diagnostic w/out arteriogram. May present w/ nonhealing ulcers in fingers/toes. Arteriograms classically show normal vessels down to mid-leg/forearm w/ abrupt occlusions and "corkscrew" appearance of collateral vessels.
3. *Temporal arteritis* (giant cell arteritis): inflammatory disorder primarily of medium and large carotid artery branches. Classically, fever, HA, anemia, and high ESR + tender temporal artery +/– scalp pain and jaw/tongue claudication; severe cases may lead to blindness. Path dx via bx of temporal artery. Tx w/ prednisone usu. successful.

4. *Kawasaki's dz*: inflammatory dz of children; fever, cutaneous/mucosal, and vasculitis of small and medium blood vessels. Incidence is 10× higher in Asians. At risk for coronary aneurysms (~ 20–25%), which generally regress and are reduced in incidence w/ prompt medical tx. Peripheral ischemia reported. Tx 1st w/ ASA and IV IgG; steroids usu. avoided. PTCA, surgery rarely indicated.
5. *Complex regional pain syndrome* (formerly "causalgia" and "reflex sympathetic dystrophy"):
   a. Syndrome of pain and degenerative changes in extremity often in response to relatively minor trauma. Pathogenesis not fully understood.
   b. *Three stages*:
      i. *Acute*: hyperalgesic, painful, burning sensation, possible edema a/o hyperhidrosis.
      ii. *Dystrophic*: pain, edema w/ induration, relatively cool and cyanotic, often w/ brittle nails; muscle a/o bone wasting may begin.
      iii. *Atrophic*: atrophic skin and joint ankylosis accompanies spread of pain beyond initial area.
   c. *Dx*: clinical, augmented by symptomatic relief w/ sympathetic nerve block.
   d. *Tx*: acute stage may be self-limited. Dystrophic stage requires tx; both dx and tx may be achieved w/ lumbar sympathetic block. Other useful adjuncts include physical therapy and oral medications (i.e., gabapentin, amitriptyline, doxepin, etc.). Laparoscopic/open sympathectomy may be indicated. Spinal stimulation a/o intrathecal baclofen sometimes useful.
6. *Raynaud's dz*: vasospastic disorder triggered by cold exposure or emotional stress. Classically, white (pallor) → blue (cyanosis) → red (rubor) skin. Sometimes assoc. w/ connective tissue dz, occupational stress (i.e., vibration), diabetes mellitus. Tx includes avoidance of cold, tobacco/nicotine, beta antagonists, ergotamines, and oral contraceptives. Calcium channel blockers, Botox injections may be helpful.
7. *Polyarteritis nodosa* (PAN): inflammatory d/o of medium-sized arteries, w/ systemic sx such as fever. Etiology unknown, assoc. w/ hepatitis B. Skin changes may include predominantly lower extremity ischemic nodules a/o ulcerations, ischemia of digits, and nonblanching livido reticularis. Dx w/ bx of nodules/ulcer edges to include fat w/ blood vessels. Inflammatory vasculitic peripheral neuropathy may → mononeuritis multiplex, a significantly disabling condition. GI sx ~ 1/2 of cases, from postprandial discomfort to GI hemorrhage from mesenteric aneurysms or mesenteric infarction. About 1/2 respond to corticosteroids. Cyclophosphamide reserved for the remainder, or those w/ evidence of end-organ dz (renal, CNS, cardiac, etc.).

D. Miscellaneous extremity lesions, conditions, and dilemmas

1. *Subclavian effort thrombosis* (Paget-Schroetter syndrome)
   a. *Dx*: aching pain in the axilla in a high-risk pt (i.e., young male w/ repetitive exertion of shoulder muscles) w/ swelling and cyanosis should prompt UE venous duplex. (*Note*: neurogenic sx of thoracic outlet syndrome may also be present.) If abnormal, venography procures the dx.
   b. *Tx*: early catheter-directed thrombolysis results in better outcome than systemic anticoagulation. Recurrent episodes merits consideration for surgery for thoracic outlet syndrome (see Chapter 8 on thoracic and esophagus).
2. *Thoracic outlet syndrome*
   a. *Presentation*: compression of blood vessel(s) a/o nerve(s) as pass out of thoracic inlet to shoulder girdle. May present w/ paresthesias, weakness, swelling or coolness of extremity, pain, claudication. Anatomic lesions usu. due to congenital problems (bands, cervical rib) or repetitive trauma.
      i. *Neurogenic*: 85% of cases, most often due to compression in scalene triangle (anterior/middle scalene and first rib or cervical rib), although brachial plexus may be involved in costoclavicular space as well.
      ii. *Arterial*: classically assoc. w/ baseball players.
      iii. *Venous* (Paget-Schroetter syndrome): most often from congenital bands, although often seen in the dominant hand of young male throwing (i.e., pitchers, quarterbacks) athletes.
   b. *Dx*: hyperabduction maneuvers and positional changes in radial pulse somewhat unreliable.
      i. Maneuvers/clinical tests
         - *Adson test*: have pt slightly extend neck and turn head toward side of concern, take a deep breath and hold it for 10 sec. A positive test is when pulse diminishes, but this occurs in up to half of people w/out TOS.

- *Roos test* (elevated arm stress test/EAST): have pt sit w/ arms abducted 90°, w/ elbows flexed and forearms pointed toward ceiling, then open and close hands for 3 min. A positive test is reproduction of sx, w/ pt unable to complete 3 min of procedure. Some consider this most reliable screening test.
- *Wright test*: hyperabduction and external rotation of arm w/ head turned to opposite side; positive test is decrease in radial pulse or reproduction of sx.
- *Costoclavicular maneuver*: pull affected extremity down and backward to attempt to reproduce sx.
- Scalene muscle block (4 cc of 1% lidocaine into ant. scalene)–improvement of sx strongly predicts good operative result.

ii. Radiographic
- Initial screening w/ CXR, duplex worthwhile.
- Venography or arteriography is gold standard, depending on clinical picture.
  - Arteriography indicated if abn duplex, SBP difference of 20 mm Hg, or sx of emboli.

c. *Tx*:

i. Physical therapy is the mainstay of therapy for neurogenic TOS, w/ rib resection reserved for pts who have failed this modality (90% will have improvement w/ PT including stretching exercises and postural changes).

ii. Rib resection is required for arterial or venous TOS. Arterial or venous reconstruction may or may not be required depending on the patency and degree of vessel damage. Stents can be used but will crush if the entire rib is not removed. Usu. best NOT to place a stent in either arterial or venous TOS.

iii. *Operative*: rib can be resected via a transaxillay, supra- or infraclavicular approach depending on the surgeon's preference. Whatever the approach, the anterior (protect the phrenic nerve!) and middle scalene muscles should be divided and, if the pt has neurogenic TOS, some would argue that neurolysis should be performed (although this is controversial). The operative field should be palpated and any fibrous bands that might compress the neurovascular structures should be lysed.

3. *Popliteal artery entrapment syndrome* (PAES): from repetitive compression/trauma from medial head of gastrocnemius and popliteal artery leading to thrombus formation.
   a. *Dx*: MRI/MRA study of choice to study vessel above and below occlusion and the soft tissue anatomy of the popliteal fossa. There are five types of PAES (Types I-V) depending on the arterial relationship to the musculotendinous structures in the popliteal fossa. A sixth type ("functional" PAES) has also been described, which occurs w/ exercise in the absence of any demonstrable anatomic abnormality.
   b. *Tx*: depends on the type of popliteal entrapment and the patency of the artery. Arterial reconstruction or bypass; alternately division of medial head of gastrocnemius or popliteus muscle. Antiplatelet tx w/ ASA recommended.
4. *Fractures and dislocations assoc. w/ vascular problems*:
   a. *Distal humerus fx*: brachial artery; common cause of Sudeck's dystrophy.
   b. *Posterior knee dislocation*: popliteal artery.
   c. *Anterior hip dislocation*: femoral artery.
   d. *Chance fracture*: renal vessels.
5. *Arterial-venous access*
   a. *Indications*: ESRD. Nondiabetic: Cr > 6 mg/dL, GFR < 15 cc/min. Diabetic: Cr > 4 mg/dL, GFR < 25 cc/min. Quality of dialysis correlates w/ survival.
   b. Emergent need for dialysis (uremia, hyperkalemia, volume overload, acidosis) should be managed w/ temporary uncuffed catheter—not prosthetic AV graft; noncuffed catheters should usu. be removed after wks and any femoral catheter should be used no longer than a wk if possible. Avoid using subclavian vein. Cuffed hemodialysis catheters are used while waiting for AVF to mature.
   c. *W/u and priorities* (VA guidelines):

      i. Attempt upper extremities (nondominant, preferably) first. Palpate radial, ulnar, brachial aa's; perform Allen's test. Check patency/size of veins w/ elastic tourniquet.

      ii. Place distal fistulas before proximal ones to preserve options.

   iii. Preserve usable veins (esp. cephalic vein).
   iv. Attempt autologous fistulas first; will take 3–4 mo to mature, 70% primary patency at 1 yr.
   v. Prosthetic grafts ready for use almost immediately (< 1 m) but have only 40% primary patency at 1 yr.
   vi. Will often have to place central venous catheter (i.e., tunneled, cuffed catheter such as Permacath) for dialysis until fistula is mature. Should not be placed in subclavian vein as this places that outflow tract at risk (right internal jugular is first choice). Ideally, pts should have their fistula placed BEFORE requiring dialysis so that catheters are never required.

d. *Types*:
   i. *Native*:
      - *Radiocephalic* (Brescia-Cimino) *fistula*: site of preference, want at least 3 mm diameter of vein.
      - *Brachiocephalic fistula*: next choice after radiocephalic (more risk of arm swelling and steal syndrome).
      - *Basilic vein transposition*: highest risk of extremity swelling a/o steal syndrome.
   ii. *Prosthetic grafts*:
      - Forearm loop.
      - Upper arm loop.

e. *Complications*:
   i. *Steal syndrome*: preferential flow of arterial blood into venous outflow instead of perfusing distal artery.
   ii. *Dx*: manifests as hand pain, ischemic sx.
   iii. *Tx*:
      - Banding/plication of graft w/ clip/sutures, but high thrombosis rate.
      - Replacement of tapered graft not significant improvement in perfusion rate.
      - Distal revascularization and interval ligation (DRIL) procedure w/ vein or PTFE from brachial artery above graft to target below graft.
   iv. Neointimal hyperplasia in veins most common reason for stenosis/thrombosis and need for revision by interventional radiology or surgery (similar cost, outcomes for both).
   v. *Graft infection*: 10% incidence, usu. *S. epidermidis*. Refractory to abx, requires removal of graft. If *S. aureus* or *Pseudomonas*, must remove all graft. For *S. epidermidis* infections (more indolent), consider removing entire venous anastomosis w/ ligation. For arterial cuff, dissect to anastomosis clamp, leave 2–3 mm of cuff to which one can suture.
   vi. *Thrombosis*: consider endovascular/IR to open; otherwise, revise.

6. *Renovascular hypertension*

a. Most commonly seen at extremes of age w/ exaggerated diastolic hypertension (i.e., > 110 mm Hg).

b. *Physiology*:
   i. *Juxtaglomerular apparatus*: responds to decreased perfusion.
   ii. *Macula densa*: responds to hyponatremia.
   iii. *Renin*: converts angiotensiogen to angiotensin I. Angiotensin I is converted to angiotensin II by ACE, produced in the lungs.
   iv. *Angiotensin II*: potent vasoconstrictor, also induces the production of aldosterone.
   v. *Aldosterone*: stimulates resorption of Na (exchanging K) along w/ water, which passively follows.

c. *Dx*:
   i. Velocity > 200 cm/sec or ratio to aortic velocity > 3.5 suggest > 60% stenosis.
   ii. Renal vein renin ratio > 1.5:1 compared w/ contralateral side may be helpful if other side not stenosed (rare).

d. *Tx*:
   i. Not indicated in pts w/ mild hypertension (may not be cause of pt's HTN).
   ii. Consider if pt requires 3+ antihypertensives or if have renal insufficiency that may be improved as well.

iii. Most lesions can be managed by endovascular means.

7. *Dysphagia lusoria* [Valentine RJ, et al., *J Vasc Surg*. 1987;5(3):498–500.]
   a. Secondary to aberrant retroesophageal right subclavian artery.
   b. Variety of approaches (thoractomy, median sternotomy, etc.) have been used to resect and then reanastomose distal subclavian (i.e., to aortic arch); the right supraclavicular approach yields the lowest morbidity (subclavian to carotid transposition).
8. *Vascular surgery dilemmas*:
   a. AAA and concomitant intraabdominal malignancy (up to 4% of all AAA). Symptomatic or ruptured AAA trumps concerns w/ malignancy (treat the most life-threatening condition first).
      i. *Colon cancer*
         - If AAA asymptomatic and < 5 cm, resect cancer first, esp. if obstructing, bleeding, or perforated.
         - If AAA asymptomatic but > 5 cm and cancer asymptomatic, repair AAA first.
         - If AAA symptomatic or ruptured, repair first, then resect cancer at subsequent operation.
            - If cancer is obstructing, consider exteriorizing loop of colon after reperitonealizing AAA repair, keep pt on NGT suction, then mature ostomy the following day. Resect cancer at subsequent date.
   b. *Concomitant cholelithiasis and AAA*.
      i. Repair AAA first. Endovascular or open retroperitoneal approach facilitates subsequent laparoscopic cholecystectomy (compared w/ transperitoneal approach).
   c. *Aortoenteric fistula*:
      i. Most commonly occurs from erosion between proximal suture line of AAA graft w/ duodenum/proximal jejunum, although primary cases (unoperated AAAs) have been reported as have other parts of intestine.
      ii. Often presents w/ small "herald" bleed hours to wks before massive hemorrhage.
      iii. If suspect dx (and pt not hemodynamically unstable), procure upper endoscopy for confirmation.
         - If endoscopy negative, proceed to CT w/ oral and IV contrast to identify area(s) of possible inflammation. If CT negative, proceed to angiography (w/ lateral views).
      iv. *If dx secured or if pt unstable, proceed to operating room*:
         - Obtain proximal control of supraceliac aorta.
         - Mobilize affected bowel (i.e., Kocher maneuver) as necessary, then separate graft from bowel.
            - Maintain direct pressure over aortic defect.
         - Inject heparin in distal aortic segment to prevent stasis thrombosis.
         - Close bowel defect transversely if able.
         - If AAA has not previously been operated upon (rare) and bowel lesion is duodenal, many authors recommend standard graft repair followed by wrapping graft in omentum in absence of extensive local sepsis.
         - More commonly, fistula from aortic graft is encountered, which mandates removal of graft, oversewing aortic stump, and buttressing w/ local soft tissue (i.e., anterior spinal ligament, omentum, etc.).
            - Distal flow is achieved via extraanatomic bypass (i.e., axillobifemoral bypass). Aorta can also be reconstructed using femoral vein (NAIS) or cryopreserved aorta/vein, which avoids the issue of preventing aortic stump dehiscence and blowout.
         - *Note*: in hemodynamically stable pts w/ firm dx, one can perform extraanatomic bypass first, and then repair fistula or remove graft 1 to several days later.
9. *Vascular exposures*: see Chapter 26 on key steps for key operations.

CHAPTER 12

ONCOLOGY

I. GENERAL ONCOLOGY FACTS AND PRINCIPLES

A. General facts

1. Cancer mortality in USA: lung >> colorectal >> breast > prostate > pancreas > leukemia.
2. Cancer at 1- to 2-mm stage develops necrosis from outstripping blood supply, reaches a relative steady state (mo, yr) until angiogenesis provides more nourishment. Angiogenesis enhanced by fibroblast growth factor (FGF) and VEGF.
3. *Cell cycle*:
   a. G_1 (gap 1): prepares cell to enter S phase (most variable stage; will enter G_0 instead if not ready).
   b. *S* (synthesis): chromosomes replicate.
   c. G_2 (gap 2): prepares cell for entry into mitosis.
   d. *M* (mitosis): cellular elements divide into daughter cells (this stage most susceptible to radiation damage).

B. Genetics (gene → CA)

1. *p53*
   a. Regulates apoptosis by arresting cell cycle before G_1/S transition (facilitates repair vs apoptosis).
      i. Apoptosis mediated through class of proteases called caspases (10+ different types).
   b. Deletion or mutation results in damaged DNA replication.
   c. Likely most common genetic etiology for human neoplasms.
   d. *Li-Fraumeni syndrome*: sarcomas, breast CA, brain tumors, leukemia, adrenal CA, poss. uterine CA.
2. *Birc-5* (Survivin)
   a. Anti-apoptosis gene (bad for pts w/ cancer, good for pts w/ MI).
3. *C-myc*
   a. Small cell lung CA, neuroblastoma, Burkitt's lymphoma.
4. *K-ras*
   a. Proto-oncogene.
   b. Implicated in 90% pancreatic CA, 50% colon CA, some lung CA.
5. *Ret*
   a. Proto-oncogene.
   b. Assoc. w/ medullary thyroid CA (MEN II syndrome), Hirschsprung's dz.
6. *BRCA I, II*
   a. I = breast CA (50–80%), ovarian CA (40–65%).
   b. II = breast CA (35–80%), ovarian CA (10–20%), male breast CA.
7. *Adenomatous polyposis cancer* (APC)
   a. Tumor suppressor gene on chromosome 5q. Mutation assoc. w/ 80% of colorectal tumors.
   b. *Familial adenomatous polyposis (FAP) syndrome*: 100% get colon cancer if not taken out, almost universally AD.
      i. *Gardner's* (AD): GI polyposis, osteomas, epidermoid cysts, desmoid tumors.
      ii. *Turcot's* (AR): GI polyposis, CNS tumors (medulloblastoma, glioblastoma). Young presentation.
8. *Mismatch repair gene*
   a. *Hereditary nonpolyposis colon cancer* (HNPCC).
      i. *Lynch I, II*: defect in mismatch-repair gene, assoc. w/ microsatellite instability, right-sided colon cancer, and generally more favorable prognosis.

- *Lynch I*: no assoc. extracolonic malignancies.
- *Lynch II*: assoc. w/ malignancy in endometrium, ovaries, cholangiocarcinoma, stomach.
- *Muir-Torre*: Lynch (possibly other GI/GU malignancy) + cutaneous lesions (sebaceous adenoma/epithelioma/carcinoma, keratoacanthoma).

9. *Deleted in colorecal cancer (DCC) gene*
   a. Postulated to be tumor suppression gene on chromosome 18q.
   b. Possibly induces apoptosis in normal cells.
10. *COX-2 gene*
    a. Overexpressed in many colorectal tumors.
    b. Use of Cox-2 inhibitors may facilitate appropriate apoptosis and angiogenesis inhibition; reduce polyp burden in FAP pts (see section 7b. above).
11. *Hamartomatous* (no malignant potential) often confused w/ above, although no genetic locus identified
    a. *Peutz-Jeghers*: autosomal dominant, assoc. w/ STK11 gene mutation; mucosal hyperpig., mucocut. melanin spots. May develop extracolonic malignancies (GI, panc, breast/ov.).
    b. *Cronkhite-Canada*: GI polyps, nail dystrophy, alopecia, cutaneous hyperpigmentation. Nonfamilial, but up to 2/3 of pts have Japanese ancestry.
    c. *Cowden's*: autosomal dominant, assoc. w/ PTEN gene mutation. GI-tract hamartomas, breast CA, colon CA, uterine CA, lung CA, bladder CA, thyroid CA, circumoral papillomatosis, nodular gingival hyperplasia.

C. Genetics (CA → gene)

1. *Colon CA*: APC (esp. in FAP), COX-2, K-ras. p53, 18q (all are tumor suppressors except K-ras oncogene).
2. *Breast CA*: p53, bcl-2, c-myc, her 2 neu, BRCA I/II.
3. *Pancreas*: K-ras, INK4A, p53, SMAD4/DPC4, BRCA II.

D. Environmental factors

1. *Diet*: fatty diets lead to increased bile salts in gut, which is assoc. w/ colorectal CA.

E. Radiation therapy

a. *Indications*: see section II on specific malignancies.
b. *Arguments for neoadjuvant* (pre):
   i. Can downsize to make tumor more resectable.
   ii. Better oxygenation of tissues.
   iii. Less collateral tissue damage (usually).
c. *Arguments for adjuvant* (post):
   i. Can better stage tumor.
d. *Side effects*:
   i. Main complication is obliterative endarteritis, resulting in diminished blood flow. Tissue frequently becomes woody, less pliable, and often prone to malignant transformation (i.e., sarcoma, thyroid carcinoma, squamous cell carcinoma, etc.).
   ii. Radiation proctitis (may occur up to 1–2 yr later).
   iii. Tx w/ formalin, topical steroids.

F. Chemotherapeutic agents (see Table 12.1)

G. Common sites of metastasis

1. *Receiving metastases*:
   a. *Brain*: males—lung, colon, renal most common; females—breast, lung, colon, melanoma most common.
   b. *Lung*: breast, sarcoma.
   c. *Liver*: GI (esp. colorectal), pancreas.
      i. Liver has been shown to increase ICAM-1, VCAM-1, and selectin expression while decreasing iNOS expression during times of (even distant) inflammation, making the hepatic parenchyma more suitable for metastasis implantation and survival.
   d. *Bone*: breast (mixed osteoblastic/clastic), prostate (osteoclastic), follicular thyroid CA.
   e. *Ovaries*: stomach, colon.

TABLE 12.1. Chemotherapeutic Agents

Agent	Used For	Properties and *Side Effects/Toxicity
5-FU	Topical Systemic • Colon • Rectum	Antimetabolite (inhibits thymidylate synthase, important for pyrimidine/DNA synthesis) Radiosensitizer *Can cause *stomatitis* or *diarrhea*
Bevacizumab (Avastin)	Added to 5-FU tx for metastatic colorectal CA	Inhibits angiogenesis, binds VEGF *GI perforation, wound dehiscence reported *Hypertension
Cetuximab (Erbitux)	Added to irinotecan tx for metastatic colorectal CA	Monoclonal antibody against epidermal growth factor receptor Benefit seen for pts w/ nonmutant *Kras* only
Irinotecan	Colorectal CA	Inhibits topoisomerase I (DNA repair) *Can cause liver injury
Methotrexate		Antimetabolite (dihydrofolate reductase) • Decreases purine synthesis *Can cause dose-dependent *nephrotoxicity*
Leucovorin	Colon Rectum	Enhances 5-FU inhibition of thymidylate synthase *Can cause allergic reaction
Levimasole		*Can cause *arthralgia, myalgia, fever, neutropenia*
Cisplatinin	Esophagus Lung Head/neck Ovary/germ cell Bladder	*Can cause *nephrotoxicity* (Note: carboplatin better tolerated, less risk of nephrotoxicity)
Oxaliplatin		Adducts w/ DNA *Can cause peripheral neuropathy
Doxorubicin (Adriamycin)	Breast	Antibiotic • DNA basepair intercalation • Forms free radicals *Can cause *cardiomyopathy*
Bleomycin		Antibiotic *Can cause *pulmonary fibrosis*
Mitomycin C	Nigro protocol	Antibiotic *Can cause *hypercalcemia*
Cyclophosphamide	Breast	Alkylating agent • Causes DNA breaks *Can cause *hemorrhagic cystitis* (Note: ifosfamide can also cause HC)
Nitrogen mustard	Hodgkin's dz	Alkylating agent
Melphalan	Multiple myeloma, limb perfusion for melanoma	Alkylating agent
Chlorambucil	CLL	Alkylating agent

(Continues)

TABLE 12.1. Chemotherapeutic Agents *(Continued)*

Agent	Used For	Properties and *Side Effects/Toxicity
Vincristine/Vinblastine		Plant alkaloids—bind tubulin in metaphase *Can cause *myelosuppression* a/o *peripheral neuropathy*
Etoposide (VP-16)		Plant alkaloid—inhibits DNA topoisomerase II *Can cause neuropathy
Tamoxifen	Breast Desmoid tumors	**Endometrial cancer*, uterine sarcoma pulmonary embolism, stroke cataracts
Aromatase-inhibitors	Breast	Postmenopausal women

   f. *LN*: breast, papillary thyroid CA, liver, SCCA, melanoma
   g. *Adrenal*: lung, stomach, breast, melanoma, renal, prostate
   h. *Thyroid*: breast, kidney, colon, lung
2. *Sending metastases*:
   a. *Breast*: lung, bone, liver, brain, thyroid
   b. *Renal*: thyroid
   c. *Colon*: liver, lung, ovaries
   d. *Stomach*: liver
   e. *Melanoma*: liver, lung, GI tract, brain, skin
   f. *Prostate*: bone
   g. *Lung*: liver, adrenal, bone, brain
   h. *Pancreas*: liver
   i. *Sarcoma*: lung (for extremity sarcomas—retroperitoneal sarcomas usu. go to liver); sarcoma usu. does *not* spread via lymphatics

H. **Tumor markers** (**bold** represents primary usage)
1. *Carcinoembryonic antigen* (CEA): may be elevated w/ **colorectal** CA, melanoma, lymphoma, breast CA, lung CA, pancreatic CA, gastric CA, cervical CA, bladder CA, renal CA, thyroid CA, hepatic CA, ovarian CA, IBD, pancreatic dz, hepatopathy, and tobacco smoking.
2. *Alpha-fetoprotein* (AFP): may be elevated w/ **liver** CA or **germ cell** CA. Rarely elevated w/ cirrhosis, hepatitis, ataxia telangiectasia, Wiskott-Aldrich syndrome, and pregnancy.
3. *CA 125*: may be elevated w/ **ovarian** CA, uterine CA, cervical CA, pancreatic CA, liver CA, colon CA, breast CA, lung CA, GI tract CA, endometriosis, PID, pancreatitis, hepatopathy, pleuritis, menstruation, and pregnancy.
4. *CA 19-9*: cholangiocarcinoma, pancreatic adenocarcinoma.
5. *Lactate dehydrogenase* (LDH): extremely nonspecific, but used to follow testicular CA, Ewing's sarcoma, melanoma, NHL. Also elevated w/ CHF, hypothyroidism, anemia, and various lung and liver dz's.
6. *Prostate-specific antigen* (PSA): elevated w/ **prostate** CA, prostatitis, and BPH.
7. *Prostatic acid phosphatase*: elevated w/ **prostate** CA, testicular CA, leukemia, NHL, cirrhosis, PE, hyperparathyroidism, Gaucher's dz, and Paget's dz.
8. *Human chorionic gonadotropin* (hCG): elevated during pregnancy and may also be elevated w/ **choriocarcinoma** and cancers of **testis**, ovary, liver, stomach, pancreas, and lung. Marijuana may also elevate levels.
   a. *Neuron-specific enolase* (NSE): may be elevated w/ **neuroblastoma**, **small cell lung** CA, nephroblastoma (Wilm's tumor), melanoma, and cancers of thyroid, kidney, testis, and pancreas.

I. **Paraneoplastic syndromes**
1. *By source*
   a. Lung (*small cell*): ACTH, ADH
   b. Lung (*non-small cell*): PTH-like hormone

2. *By-product/result*
   a. *ACTH*: bronchial carcinoids, small-cell lung carcinoids >> gut/thymic carcinoids, endocrine pancreatic neoplasms, pancreatic cystadenomas, thyroid medullary carcinoma, pheochromocytoma
   b. *CRH*: thyroid medullary CA, prostate CA
   c. *Hypercalcemia*: breast, lung, kidney, multiple myeloma, parathyroid CA, renal cell, SCCA
   d. *SIADH*: small cell CA of lung >> prostate, adrenal, esophagus, pancreas, colon, head/neck, carcinoids, mesotheliomas
   e. *Hypoglycemia*: insulinoma, hepatoma, adrenocortical, mesothelioma, fibrosarcoma, neurofibrosarcoma
   f. *Tumor lysis syndrome* (hyperuricemia, hyperkalemia, hyperphosphatemia, hypocalcemia): lymphoma, leukemia, rarely small cell lung CA, metastatic breast CA, metastatic medulloblastoma

J. **Multiple Endocrine Neoplasm (MEN):** see Table 12.2.

TABLE 12.2. Multiple Endocrine Neoplasia (MEN) Syndromes

	MEN I	MEN IIa	MEN IIb
Acronym	Wermer's Syndrome	Sipple's Syndrome	Sizemore's Syndrome
Associated tumors	**P**arathyroid (90%) (4-gland hyperplasia) **P**ancreas (80%) (gastrin > insulinoma) **P**ituitary Adenoma (55%) (prolactin >> GH > ACTH)	**P**arathyroid (20–60%) (4-gland hyperplasia) *Medullary thyroid CA* (100%) *Pheochromocytoma* (20–40%)	*Medullary thyroid CA* (100%) *Pheochromocytoma* (20–40%) Neuromas (lips, tongue, oral mucosa, GI tract)
Other findings	Adrenal adenomas (30%) Thyroid nodules (10%)	RET 2 A, B lesion	Often marfanoid habitus. RET 2 A, B lesion Worse prognosis than other MEN syndromes
Manage	More aggressive pancreatic resection than for sporadic tumors often indicated	Prophylactic thyroidectomy for by age 5 Consider annual screening for calcium, calcitonin, catecholamines	Prophylactic thyroidectomy by age 1 Consider annual screening for calcium, calcitonin, catecholamines

II. SPECIFIC CANCERS ORGANIZED BY ORGAN (ALPHABETICALLY)*

A. Anal

1. *Risk factors*: immunosuppression, anal receptive intercourse, and (for squamous cell cancers) HPV (subtypes 6, 11, 16, 18) infection.
2. *Subtype by location*:
   a. *Anal canal cancers* (proximal to anal verge): $^2/_3$ of all anal cancers, more common in women. Locally aggressive, w/ $^1/_2$ locally advanced at dx, $^1/_3$ to $^1/_2$ w/ mesenteric LN spread.
   b. *Anal margin cancers* (distal to anal verge, including 5-cm radius of perianal skin): more common in homosexual males. Relatively favorable prognosis; rarely metastasize (usu. to superficial inguinal LN—15% of cases overall).
3. *Subtype by histology*:
   a. *SCCA*: 80% of anal cancer. Includes basaloid, mucoepidermoid, and cloacogenic.
   b. *Adenocarcinoma*: exceptionally rare; poor prognosis. Optimal tx likely surgery + chemo + XRT.
   c. *Melanoma*: poor prognosis. Typically tx w/ WLE (1–2) cm if able to spare sphincter mechanism; otherwise APR indicated. See section O. below on skin cancers for more information.

*Staging information from Edge SB, et al., *AJCC Cancer Staging Handbook*, 7th ed. New York: Springer Inc.; 2010.

4. *W/u*:
   a. Complete H&P, w/ focus on anal sphincter function. CXR, abdomen/pelvis CT scan, proctoscopy endorectal U/S appropriate. Clinically (+) inguinal LN should be investigated w/ FNA.
5. *Tx*:
   a. *Anal canal cancers*:
      i. Tumors < 5 cm (T1, T2) that do not invade sphincter → WLE.
      ii. All others → Nigro protocol of chemoradiation (*note*: below regimen assoc. w/ high incidence of complications in AIDS pts; alternatives may be appropriate). 85% 5-yr survival.
         - *Day 1*: Mitomycin C IV bolus (or bleomycin or cisplatin).
         - *Days 1–4*: 5-FU continuous IV infusion.
         - *Days 1–35*: XRT 5 d/wk for 45–55 Gy. Boosts to anus a/o inguinal basins allowed.
         - *Days 29–32*: 5-FU continuous IV infusion.
         - *Exceptions*: surgery still indicated for:
           - Salvage for persistence or recurrence after Nigro tx → APR.
           - Significant local sx (rectovesical fistula, perineal sepsis, incontinence, etc.) → APR.
           - Recurrent LN dz after XRT → inguinal LN dissection.
           - Obstructing lesions → temporary fecal diversion.
   b. *Anal margin cancers*:
      i. Tumors < 5 cm (T1, T2) that do not invade sphincter → WLE (80% 5-yr survival).
         - XRT alone yields similar survival, but w/ higher incidence of complications.
      ii. Tumors > 5 cm (T3) or w/ LN (+).
         - APR w/ inguinal XRT (inguinal LN dissection if residual/recurrent LN).
6. *Premalignant lesions*
   a. Paget's dz (intraepithelial adenocarcinoma).
   b. Bowen's dz (intraepithelial squamous cell carcinoma).
   c. Both manifest as perianal eczematoid plaque; r/o synchronous invasive colorectal CA w/ endoscopy. Local excision is preferred tx (although topical agents such as 5-FU may be effective), along w/ "anal mapping" bx's of remaining perianal skin (sample 4 quadrants of verge, margin, and dentate line).

TABLE 12.3. AJCC TNM Classification for Anal Carcinoma

Primary Tumor (T)	Regional Lymph Nodes (N)–Clinical and Pathological	Distant Metastasis (M)
Tis – Carcinoma *in situ*	N1 – Metastasis in perirectal LN(s)	M1 – Distant metastasis
T1 – < 2 cm in greatest dimension	N2 – Metastasis in unilateral internal iliac a/o inguinal LN(s)	
T2 – > 2 but not > 5 cm in greatest dimension	N3 – Metastasis in perirectal and inguinal lymph nodes a/o bilateral interal iliac a/o inguinal LN(s)	
T3 – > 5 cm in greatest dimension		
T4 – Any size tumor that invades adjacent organ(s)		

TABLE 12.4. AJCC Staging for Anal Carcinoma (2009 Version)

Stage	TNM	Survival (Squamous)	Survival (Nonsquamous)
0	TisN0M0		
I	T1N0M0	71.4	59.1
II	T2N0M0 T3N0M0	63.5	52.9
IIIa	T1N1M0 T2N1M0 T3N1M0 T4N0M0	48.1	37.7
IIIb	T4N1M0 Any T, N2, M0 Any T, N3, M0	43.2	24.4
IV	Any T, Any N, M1	20.9	7.4

B. Breast

1. *Genetics*:
   a. Majority of breast CA are sporadic (90–95%), not familial.
   b. *Risk factors*: early menarche, late menopause, hormone replacement therapy, late childbirth.
   c. *BRCA I*; chromosome 17q, tumor suppressor gene. Lifetime risk breast CA 50–85%. Risk of ovarian CA 40–65%. Assoc. w/ medullary breast CA.
   d. *BRCA II*; chromosome 13, autosomal dominant. Lifetime risk breast CA ~ 35–80%. Lifetime risk ovarian CA 10–20%. Increased risk male breast CA.
   e. *Syndromes*: Li-Fraumeni assoc. w/ p53 mutation; sarcoma, brain, leukemia, adrenocortical CA. Cowden syndrome assoc. w/ PTEN; uterus, lung, bladder, thyroid, colon, GI polyps. RBI w/ bilateral retinoblastoma, soft tissue sarcoma.
2. *Screening*: USPTF 2009 recommendations: biennial mammogram starting at age 50; however, ACS and NCCN still recommend annual screening at age 40 (in cases of 1st-degree relatives w/ breast CA, recommend 10 yr before age of cancer dx). Clinical breast exam by physician at least every 3 yr in 20s–30s, then annually therafter. Breast self-exam may be suggested in the 20s, but evidence of significant benefit compared to other screening modalities is lacking.
3. *LCIS*: a marker of increased risk for breast CA, most frequently found in white females; 80–90% premenopausal. Risk of developing cancer = 21% over 17 yr (~ 1%/yr), usu. favorable histology. Of those who develop invasive dz, 2/3 ductal. Can observe as high risk (most common), chemoprevention (tamoxifen), or prophylactic B mastectomy. NSABP Cancer Prevention Trial showed tamoxifen for 5 yr → 56% ↓ risk invasive cancer. *F/u*: PEx and MMG (or MRI) q 6–12 mo × 5 yr, then annually.
4. *DCIS*: 20–25% of breast CA. Presents as microcalcifications or mass. Prognosis excellent, tx w/ total mastectomy or lumpectomy and radiation.
   a. DCIS w/ widespread dz (2+ quadrants) requires total mastectomy w/out LN dissection. 1–2% (+) LN. For more limited dz and those w/ (–) margins (primary or re-excised), either total mastectomy or breast conserving therapy. If apparent pure DCIS tx'd w/ mastectomy or tail of breast (could compromise future SLNBx), consider doing SLNBx. If < 0.5 cm, unicentric, low-grade of solid, cribriform, or papillary subtype, can do excision + RT; TM w/out LN dissection; or excision alone + observation. Margins > 10 mm are negative; less than 1 mm inadequate.
   b. Long-term survival w/ mastectomy = excision and whole breast irradiation. Whole breast irradiation added to margin-free resection ↓ recurrence, but no ↑ in survival. XRT indicated after local excision for DCIS > 0.5-cm diameter.
   c. *Early Breast CA Trial overview*: 5 yr of tamoxifen → 52% ↓ annual recurrence in pts w/ ER (+) or receptor-unknown tumors. NSABP B-24 = tamoxifen of benefit for DCIS after breast conservation tx and XRT (5% absolute ↓ recurrence and 37% relative risk ↓), esp. good for ER (+) dz.
   d. *F/u*: PEx q 6 mo for 5 yr and then annually, and annual mammography.

TABLE 12.5. DCIS Grading (Van Nuys Prognostic Index)

Score	1	2	3
Size (mm)	< 15	16–40	> 41
Margins (mm)	> 10	1–9	< 1
Pathology	Non-high grade, no necrosis	Non-high grade, w/ necrosis	High grade +/– necrosis

TABLE 12.6. DCIS Treatment

VNPI (total)	Intervention
3–4	• Excise to 1-inch margins
5–7	• Excise/reexcise to 1-inch margins • XRT if < 1-cm margin or no reexcision
8–9 (can't get 1-cm margin)	• Mastectomy • +/– SLNBx • No XRT necessary after mastectomy

5. *Breast CA staging and prognosis*
   a. *Stage I, II breast CA*: partial mastectomy + XRT vs total *and* SLNBx.
      i. *Breast conservation contraindicated if*: pt doesn't want it, (+) margins (if positive after re-excision mastectomy indicated), diffuse malignant calcifications, 1st/2nd-trimester pregnancy, pregnant, widespread dz, inadequate radiation, or hx of prior XRT in the area. Breast-conserving tx relative contraindications: connective tissue dz in skin (lupus, scleroderma), tumor > 5 cm, focally positive pathologic margins. In women 70 yo or older w/ clinically negative LN and ER (+) cancer, can pursue breast-conserving therapy plus tamoxifen or aromatase inhibitor w/out irradiation. [Intergroup CALCGB/RTOG/ECOG Study.]
      ii. *Initial w/u*: hx, physical, CBC, LFTs, CXR, B diagnostic mammography, bx results for estrogen/progesterone receptors, HER2/neu expression.
         - If bone or abdominal sx or elevated alkaline phosphatase, obtain bone scan a/o abdominal CT/MRI as appropriate (some will get CT of c/a/p if > 1 cm).
         - For clinical stage I/II cancer, assess axillary LN status; perform SLNBx and complete axillary dissection if SLNBx +. For level I and level II dissections, at least 10 LNs are required for accurate staging. Only dissect level III if gross dz in I or II.
            - Still, consider as optional if esp. favorable tumors, if adjuvant therapy is unlikely to help pt, elderly pts, and those w/ serious comorbidities (BINV-B).
         - In literature regarding tx of neoplasms w/ "favorable histology," this refers to tubular (almost always HER2/neu non-overexpressed, ER [+]), colloid. Medullary risk of metastasis is equal to other high-grade carcinomas; do not treat as favorable histology.
         - *SLNBx*: must have clinically negative axilla, or negative core or FNA bx of suspicious nodes. If cannot indentify sentinel LN or if is (+) for metastasis, a full axillary LN dissection indicated or axillary RT is given. Internal mammary node excision is optional if sentinel nodes identified in internal mammary chain.
   b. *Stage III and inflammatory BRCA*
      i. "Inoperable" locally advanced.
         - *Tx*: anthracycline-based + taxane neoadjuvant chemotx indicated. Follow w/ total mastectomy and axillary LN dissection or lumpectomy and axillary dissection and adjuvant XRT *and* postop hormonal therapy. Some have advocated option of chemo/XRT alone. If inoperable, palliative XRT may be considered along w/ hormonal tx if hormone receptor (+) or unknown.
   c. *Stage IV* (metastatic or recurrent)
      i. Eval w/ H&P, CBC, LFT, CXR, bone scan, x-rays of abn areas of bone scan, +/– CT/MRI of chest and abdomen, bx of any possible site of recurrence. PET is optional.
      ii. *Tx*:

- *Local recurrence only.* (*Note*: consider all for chemo/endocrine tx.)
  - If previous mastectomy, then resect local recurrence if able to get clear margins and give XRT if prior irradiation doesn't preclude. If unresectable, consider XRT if no limiting prior irradiation.
  - If previous breast-conserving therapy, perform total mastectomy.
- *Systemic recurrence* (all get chemo/endocrine tx unless toxicity significantly impairs quality of life).
- *Bone metastasis*: bisphosphonate, calcium citrate, vitamin D if expect survival > 3 mo, and Cr < 3.

6. *F/u for breast CA*:
   a. Regular physical exam and MGM. If breast-conserving tx used, then first MGM is 6 mo after surgery. LFTs, tumor markers, and routine bone scans not utilized.
   b. If on tamoxifen, get annual pelvic exams and expedited exams for vaginal spotting.
   c. If on aromatase inhibitors, monitor bone health w/ DEXA scan or other modalities.
7. *Chemotherapy for breast CA*
   a. Neoadjuvant chemotherapy should be considered for large clinical stage IIa, IIb, T3N1M0 (stage III) tumors that meet all criteria for breast-conserving therapy except for tumor size (i.e., > 5 cm or disproportionately large compared w/ breast size); also inflammatory breast CA, and those w/ fixation to skin/muscle. Consider percutaneously placed clips to guide postchemotherapy excision. NSABP B-18 trial showed neoadjuvant tx results in higher rates of breast conservation.
      i. Neoadjuvant tx w/ trastuzumab in addition to paclitaxel followed by FEC chemotherapy is indicated for overexpression of HER2/*neu* (more than doubles complete response rate).
      ii. If pursue neoadjuvant chemotherapy, consider pretreatment SLNBx. If negative, can omit axillary dissection at time of local surgery. If positive, perform level I/II axillary dissection w/ local surgery. Can also do SLNBx at time of definitive surgery.
   b. *Adjuvant chemotx*: FU, doxorubicin, cyclophosphamide (FAC/CAF); or CEF (epirubicin, FU, doxorubicin).
      i. If adjuvant chemotherapy indicated, complete this before XRT, esp. if involves methotrexate (may be concurrent w/ other CMF—cyclophosphamide, 5-FU).
      ii. Tumors < 0.5 cm w/out (+) LN, chemotx not indicated, although tamoxifen can be used prophylactically for additional tumors, esp. if ER (+).
      iii. Invasive lobular or ductal tumors 0.6 to 1.0 cm and no LN, but unfavorable features (angiolymphatic invasion, high nuclear grade, high histological grade, HER-2 overexpression, or hormone receptor-negative status) may be considered for chemotx.
      iv. If (+) LN or tumors > 1 cm should receive chemotherapy. If LN (–), hormone (–) tumors > 1 cm, give chemotherapy. If LN (–), hormone receptor (+) tumors 1–3 cm in diameter, give endocrine and chemotherapy. Any pt that is hormone receptor (+), add endocrine (if pt is postmenopausal, give aromatase-inhibitor w/ or following taxmofen; if premenopausal, just tamoxifen as aromatase-inhibitors ineffective if ovarian function). In general, tamoxifen should be given after chemotherapy, as tamoxifen is effective regardless of ovarian function.
         - *Estrogen tx side effects*:
           - *Both*: hot flashes, night sweats, vaginal dryness.
           - *Tamoxifen*: uterine/endometrial CA, DVT.
           - *Aromatase inhibitor*: musculoskeletal sx, osteoporosis, fractures.
         - *ATAC Trial*: anastrozole superior to tamoxifen *or* combination of both in adjuvant endocrine tx of postmenopausal women w/ hormone receptor (+) cancer regarding recurrence, not survival.
      v. If invasive cancer is ER or PR (+) should be considered for adjuvant endocrine tx (regardless of age, LN status, or if adjuvant chemotx appropriate unless LN (–) and less than 0.5 cm or if 0.6–1.0 cm and have favorable prognostic features).
      vi. *In other words . . .* chemotx (more effective in premenopausal pts) is given to all pts w/ lesions > 1 cm unless they are postmenopausal and ER (+). Tamoxifen/aromatase inhibitors are given to anybody who is ER (+) w/ tumor > 1 cm a/o (+) LN.

8. *Radiation for breast CA*
   a. *Indicated if*:
      i. Tumor size > 5 cm.
      ii. 4 or more (+) LNs.
      iii. Stage I or II dz managed w/ breast conservation surgery or advanced DCIS tx'd w/ WLE.
      iv. Locally advanced/inflammatory breast CA refractory to neoadjuvant chemotherapy.
   b. Usu. 50 Gy w/ local 10- to 15-Gy boost, starting 2–4 wk postop, and lasting ~ 6 wk, 5 d/wk.
9. *Less common situations*
   a. *Breast CA during pregnancy*:
      i. Compared w/ nongravid pts, larger tumor size at dx, less differentiated, less frequently ER/PR (+). ~ 30% HER-2/neu (+). Usu. (+) axillary lymph nodes.
      ii. *Staging*:
         - *Clinically T1, T2, node-negative*: CXR w/ shielding, B diagnostic MMG w/ shielding, LFT, BUN/Cr, CBC w/ differential.
         - *Clinically T3, or node-positive*: also get liver U/S, +/– MIR of thoracic/lumbar spine.
         - If indicated, SLNBx w/ radionuclide is considered safe during pregnancy, but blue dye is not recommended.
         - *Chemotx*: contraindicated during first trimester or after 35th wk, but otherwise is not assoc. w/ increased risk of fetal malformation; fetal monitoring prior to each cycle is appropriate, however. FAC is regimen of choice (5-FU, doxorubicin, cyclophosphamide).
            - Taxanes/endocrine tx and XRT not recommended for use during pregnancy. Trastuzumab assoc. w/ oligohydramnios and not recommended during pregnancy.
   b. *Breast CA in men*: 1% of all breast CA, usu. invasive ductal, assoc. w/ BRCA II.
10. *Less common pathology*
   a. *Paget's dz*: defined by neoplastic cells in epidermis of NAC, usu. manifests as local eczema, excoriation, ulceration, bleeding, a/o pruritis of NAC.
      i. 80% have other site of malignancy in breast (invasive CA or DCIS).
      ii. *Evaluation*: H&P, NAC bx, bilateral diagnostic MMG. If no lesion on MMG, get breast MRI.
      iii. *Tx*:
         - Traditionally, total mastectomy w/ ax dissection.
         - Alternatively, breast-conserving surgery of any assoc. CA + resection of NAC followed by breast XRT. Address axilla as indicated for invasive tumor if additional malignancy found; if no detectable additional malignancy, axillary dissection not indicated.
         - If assoc. DCIS or other assoc. malignancy tx'd w/ breast conservation, consider hormone tx.
   b. *Phyllodes tumor* (cystosarcoma phyllodes)
      i. Encompass a spectrum of dz from benign to malignant.
      ii. Most important risk factor for recurrence is ability to achieve margin-free resection. Recurrences usu. local, although rarely cavitary or solid metastases may occur in lung.
      iii. Indistinguishable from fibroadenomas on MMG and U/S. FNA and core-needle unable to consistently distinguish, either.
      iv. Given above, excisional bx w/ 1-cm margins is indicated in large or enlarging fibroadenoma, particularly in pts w/ Li-Fraumeni syndrome (increased risk). Axillary LN dissection unnecessary unless clinically positive. XRT not uniformly recommended. Adjuvant chemo/endocrine tx not indicated.
   c. *Inflammatory breast CA*: may be confused w/ breast abscess or other infectious etiology: breast imaging and skin bx mandatory. Initial management is generally chemotherapy+/– XRT followed by MRM (and XRT if not given previously).
   d. *Variants of invasive ductal carcinoma*
      i. *Medullary*: anaplastic, undifferentiated epithelial component w/ lymphocytic infiltrate. Assoc. w/ BRCA I (test for this gene). Favorable prognosis.

ii. *Mucinous* (colloid): well-differentiated cells surrounded by mucin. Relatively favorable prognosis. Small tumors may not warrant SLN/AND.

iii. *Tubular*: infiltrating tubular structures w/ open central space, usu. small, w/ excellent prognosis. Small tumors may not warrant SLN/AND.

iv. *Adenoid cystic*: favorable prognosis; small tumors may not warrant SLN/AND.

e. *Papilloma*: most common cause of ductal system bleeding; tx = subareolar excision.

TABLE 12.7. AJCC TNM Classification for Breast Carcinoma

Primary Tumor (T)	Regional Lymph Nodes (N)–Clinical and Pathological	Distant Metastasis (M)
Tx – Primary tumor can't be assessed	Nx – Regional LNs can't be assessed	Mx – Presence of distant mets can't be assessed
T0 – No evidence of primary tumor	N0 – No regional LN mets	M0 – No distant mets
Tis – Carcinoma *in situ*	N1 – Mets to 1–3 movable ipsilateral axillary LNs or internal mammary detected by SLN bx N1mi – micrometastases – > 0.2 mm and < 2.0 mm	M1 – Distant mets
T1 – ≤ 2 cm in greatest dimension	N2 – Mets to 4–9 ipsilateral axillary LNs clinically fixed or matted OR ipsilateral internal mammary in absence of axillary dz	
T2 – > 2 but ≤ 5 cm	N3 – Mets to > 10 axillary LNs *or* ipsilateral internal mammary LNs in presence of axillary dz *or* ipsilateral supraclavicular LNs	
T3 – > 5 cm		
T4 – Direct extension to chest wall or skin; includes inflammatory carcinoma		

TABLE 12.8. AJCC Staging for Breast Carcinoma (2009 Version)

Stage	TNM	5-Year Survival
0	TisN0M0	92.7
I	T1N0M0 T0-1N1mi	87.8
IIa	T0N1M0 T1N1M0 T2N0M0	81.4
IIb	T2N1M0 T3N0M0	74.0
IIIa	T0N2M0 T1N2M0 T2N2M0 T3N12M0	66.7
IIIb	T4, Any N, M0	41.0
IIIc	Any T, N3, M0	49.3
IV	Any T, Any N, M1	14.8

11. *Sentinel lymph node*
    a. *Indications*
        i. Early, nonmulticentric invasive breast CA (< 4.5 cm), clinically node (–), *w/out* neoadjuvant chemo/XRT.
        ii. *Certain cases of DCIS*: > 2.5 cm, comedo, multifocal/multicentric, high grade.
    b. *Contraindications*
        i. Palpable axillary LAD.
        ii. Tumors > 5 cm (multiple drainage routes probable).
        iii. Previous axillary surgery or neoadjuvant chemotx or XRT.
        iv. Large bx cavity (> 6 cm); cavity drainage may be different than tumor drainage.
    c. *Technique*
        i. Inject subareolar (generally the highest sensitivity) or peritumoral.
        ii. Blue dye (isosulfan blue, methylene blue, vital blue dye). Methylene blue assoc. w/ rare cases of anaphylaxis; also skin necrosis if inject too superficially. Inject 5 min preop if lateral to nipple, or 10–15 min preop if medial to nipple.
        iii. Technetium-99m. Inject 30 min to 24 h preop.
12. *Axillary dissection*
    a. Assists w/ staging and local control, but not survival.
    b. Perform level I, II axillary dissection for stage I, II cancer if SLN not performed. The Auchincloss modification of Patey's MRM has been the standard for several decades, and does not resect pectoralis minor or level III nodes unless those nodes are clinically involved.
13. *Breast reconstruction*
    a. By federal law, is covered by health insurance after mastectomy.
    b. May be immediate or delayed. Candidates for immediate reconstruction are generally low stage (I, II).
    c. Reconstruction delay is typically to permit XRT, which can adversely affect the reconstruction, particularly if prosthetic/implant is used (if implant is used, it must be covered by muscle if XRT employed).
    d. Choice of autologous (latissimus, TRAM, etc.) vs prosthetic reconstruction depends on variety of factors, such as pt habitus, comorbidities, and need for adjuvant therapy.

C. Carcinoid

1. *General*: arise from enterochromaffin cells (neural crest origin), and variably secrete vasoactive substances (5-HT/serotonin, histamine, dopamine, substance P, prostaglandins, etc.).
2. *Appendiceal* (40%)
    a. Appendectomy sufficient for tumors < 1.5 cm in diameter w/out evidence of spread.
    b. Right hemicolectomy indicated if tumor > 1.5 cm in diameter or gross evidence of spread to lymph nodes, mesoappendix, etc.
3. *Rectal* (15%)
    a. Diameter < 1 cm → local excision.
    b. Diameter 1–2 cm → wide local excision; if invade muscularis propria → LAR or APR.
    c. Diameter > 2 cm → regional excision; majority succumb to systemic dz and thus sphincter-sparing is generally advocated.
4. *Pulmonary* (11%): as blood flow bypasses liver, more likely to manifest w/ carcinoid syndrome.
5. *Small intestine* (27%)
    a. Wide resection indicated; 70% metastatic to lymph nodes.
    b. 40% assoc. w/ second GI malignancy.
6. *Metastatic*
    a. *Medical tx*:
        i. Octreotide (note, operations on pts w/ metastatic carcinoid can induce *carcinoid crisis*, which is managed w/ IV octreotide drip)

ii. Loperamide, diphenoxylate

iii. Albuterol

iv. H_2 blockers

v. Cyproheptadine (serotonin receptor antagonist)

D. Colorectal

1. Decreased w/ fiber, calcium, omega-fatty acids possibly. Increased risk w/ fatty diets, possibly due to effects of additional bile salts in gut. 94% spontaneous, 5% HNPCC, 1% FAP.
   a. *Genetics*: loss of APC, DCC, p53, K-ras most common
   b. *Syndromes*:
      i. *Familial adenomatous polyposis* (FAP)
         - Loss of APC gene on chromosome 5q. Autosomal dominant, 20% spontaneous. 100% CRCa by age 40. Dx requires > 100 polyps, and vast majority of pts will have many more.
         - Begin surveillance in puberty w/ flex-sig. Recommend total colectomy by age 20.
         - Assoc. w/ small intestinal (duodenal/ampullary) tumors as well; need routine EGD.
         - *Gardner's syndrome*: FAP + desmoid tumors (treat w/ sulindac, taxmoxifen, or resection) +/– osteomas (classically in mandible).
         - *Turcot's syndrome*: FAP + brain tumors.
      ii. *Lynch syndrome* (hereditary nonpolyposis colon CA [HNPCC])
         - 5% of population, autosomal dominant, assoc. w/ DNA mismatch repair genes, right colon cancers, and metachronous cancers.
         - *Amsterdam criteria*: at least 3 1st-degree relatives over 2 generations, w/ at least 1 before 50 yo.
         - *Bethesda criteria*: similar in principle to Amsterdam criteria but less stringent.
         - Lynch I—no assoc. extra-colonic malignancies.
         - Lynch II—assoc. w/ ovarian, endometrial, cholangiocarcinoma, a/o gastric CA.
         - Surveillance colonoscopy at 25 yo or 10 yr before age of earliest CRCA in family.
         - Operation should be subtotal colectomy (and TAH/BSO if no longer able or desires fertility).
      iii. *Polyps*
         - *Hyperplastic*: most common colonic polyp, but no concerns for malignant transformation as w/ adenomatous polyps.
         - *Hamartomas*: ectopic nonneoplastic tissue, assoc. w/ below:
           - *Peutz-Jeghers*—in addition to GI hamartomas, have perioral hyperpigmented lesions, overall increased risk in GI cancer (not from hamartomas, though—usu. duodenal or colonic) as well as breast, biliary, possibly reproductive.
           - *Cronkhite-Canada*—hamartomas + nail/hair atrophy/alopecia + hypopigmentation.
           - *Juvenile polyposis*—polyps w/ no increased malignant potential, but pts do have increased overall risk of other neoplasia(s). Recommend routine colonic surveillance and total colectomy if cancer arises.
           - *Adenomatous*—malignant potential, more so if villous than tubular; remove endoscopically.
             - If carcinoma *in situ* present, no further intervention other than surveillance colonoscopy.
             - If carcinoma invades muscularis mucosa, 8.5–20% (+) LN. *Options*:
               - Do standard cancer procedure.
               - If pedunculated (nonsessile), well-differentiated, no vascular/lymphatic invasion, and has clear margin on stalk for > 5 mm, can offer close surveillance colonoscopy.

- If tubular adenoma, < 1 cm, usu. f/u colonoscopy in 5–10 yr. If villous, > 1 cm, or 3–10 adenomas removed, then repeat colonoscopy in 3 yr.
    - If sessile, villous, and can't be entirely removed via endoscopy, perform segmental resection. If > ~ 7 cm, generally need celiotomy. If lower, can attempt transrectal resection.
    - If have invasive carcinoma w/ < 2-mm margin, or lymphovascular invasion, or poorly differentitated, then colectomy indicated.

2. Rectal 43%, sigmoid 25%, ascending 18%, transverse 9%, descending 5% (c/c → 83% polyps in left colon, but only 61% of cancer w/ 55% total in rectum).
3. *Right-sided tumors*—less common, tend to grow larger before producing sx, generally present w/ bleeding/anemia, but SBO, biliopancreatic-like sx (RUQ pain, nausea) can occur.
4. *Left-sided tumors*—more common, can present like diverticulitis, fistula.
5. Rectal CA most commonly presents w/ hematochezia, but tenesmus, rectal pain, urgency, or mucous discharge can occur as well as fistula-in-ano.
    a. Assess if sphincters can be spared w/ U/S (TRUS or EUS) or MRI.
    b. May be able to spare (i.e., LAR) if proximal to last 3–5 cm of rectum (10 from anal verge). Neoadjuvant radiation +/– chemo may downsize tumor to allow easier resection; ~ 5000 cGy over 6 wk w/ 5-FU during first and last wks reduces depth of wall invasion and lessens LN involvement in ~ 70%.
6. Regardless of location, all CRCA can present w/ change in bowel movements. Colonoscopic eval is gold standard. Obstructive CA generally merits segmental colectomy w/ end colostomy. Bleeding or obstructive CA get metastatic w/u; includes LFTs (if LFT abnormal, get liver CT or MRI) and CEA. Preop, get baseline CEA; will need to follow every 4 mo postop to survey for recurrence or metastasis. Also get preop CT if tumor is in rectum or if > 4 cm (higher risk for invasion into adjacent structures).
7. Chemotherapy consider for stage II or III tumors—FOLFOX; add Avastin if stage IV.
8. *Radiation therapy*: effective in rectal tumors (w/in 12 cm from anal verge) in decreasing local recurrence and prolonging dz-free survival. Pts w/ locally advanced rectal CA (≥ T3) should get neoadjuvant chemoradiation prior to surigical resection.
    a. *Advantage to postop XRT*: good perfusion provides high oxygen tension, which facilitates radiation injury by free radical damage.
    b. *Disadvantages to postop XRT instead of preop*: increased small bowel in XRT field and creation of a relatively hypoxic field. Further, postop XRT in pts post-LAR is sphincter dysfunction and fecal incontinence.

TABLE 12.9. AJCC TNM Classification for Colorectal Carcinoma

Primary Tumor (T)	Regional Lymph Nodes (N)	Distant Metastasis (M)
T1 – Invades submucosa	N0 – No LN mets	M0 – No distant mets
T2 – Invades muscularis propria	N1a – Mets in 1 LN N1b – Mets in 2–3 LNs N1c – Tumor in subserosa, mesentery or nonperitonealized pericolic tissues w/out LN mets	M1a – Distant mets present
T3 – Invades subserosa, but no further than nonperitonealized paracolic fat	N2a – Mets in 4–6 LNs N2b – Mets in ≥ 7 LNs	
T4 – Invades peritoneal cavity or contiguous organs		

TABLE 12.10. AJCC Staging for Colorectal Cancer (2009 Version)

Stage	TNM	5-Year Survival	5-Year Survival
0	TisN0M0	Colon	Rectal
I	T1N0M0 T2N0M0	74.0	74.1
IIa	T3N0M0	66.5	64.5
IIb	T4aN0M0	58.6	51.6
IIc	T4bN0M0	37.3	32.3
IIIa	T1–T2N1/N1cM0 T1N2aM0	73.1	74.0
IIIb	T3–T4aN1/N1cM0 T2–3N2aM0 T1–T2N2bM0	46.3	45.0
IIIc	T4aN2aM0 T3–4aN2bM0 T4bN1–N2M0	28.0	33.4
IV	Any T, Any N, M1a–b	5.7	6.0

TABLE 12.11. Colorectal Tx Based on Stage

Stage	Definition	Tx Based on Stage
I	T1 or T2	Surgery (see Table 12.12 for appropriate procedure)
II	Invasive to local area or continguous structures, but no (+) LN. T3 or T4	Surgery + FOLFOX
III	LN (+)	Surgery +FOLFOX
IV	Metastatic	FOLFOX +/– Avastin; surgery for obstruction/symptomatic lesions

TABLE 12.12. Colorectal Surgical Tx Based on Location

Location	Procedure
Ascending	Right hemicolectomy (distal 4–6 cm of TI to transverse colon supplied by right branch of middle colic a.)
Transverse	Extended right hemicolectomy. Divide right and middle colic aa's at their origin, then remove colon supplied by them
Splenic flexure	Segmental colectomy
Descending	Left hemicolectomy (from splenic flexure to rectosigmoid junction)
Sigmoid	Segmental colectomy

(Continues)

TABLE 12.12. Colorectal Surgical Tx Based on Location *(Continued)*

Location	Procedure
Prox 1/3–2/3 of rectum (5–6 cm above dentate line, or ~10 cm above anal verge)	LAR: removal of sigmoid colon *and* proximal rectum w/ anastomosis in pelvis below the peritoneal reflection
Mid-rectum	LAR or APR: excision of rectum and anus w/ permanent closure of perineum and creation of end colostomy. Must do APR if involves anal sphincters, rectovaginal septum
Lower rectum	APR or transanal excision. Latter feasible if tumor is mobile, < 4 cm in diam, are T1–2, N0 on U/S or MRI, well or mod differentiated, involve < 40% of rectal wall, and are located w/in 6 cm of anal verge

**Note*: Some advocate the "no-touch technique" for intraoperative handling of specimen: First close off venous outflow and obliterate the lumen of cancerous segment before resecting/touching specimen. This has not proven to improve outcome in any measure.

E. Desmoid tumor (aggressive fibromatosis)

1. Occurs sporadically (esp. upper extremity/shoulder, abdominal wall) or assoc. w/ hereditary disorders such as FAP (esp. intraabdominal/mesenteric). Extraabdominal desmoids more common in females of reproductive age, likely due to stimulatory effects of estrogen. Although some desmoids may regress spontaneously, the majority continue to grow and compress or invade surrounding structures.
2. Present w/ enlarging mass, often w/ compressive sx.
3. *Dx*:
   a. MRI demonstrates homogenous masses, isointense w/ muscle on T1-weighted images and decreased signal intensity compared to fat on T2-weighted images.
   b. Bx reveals spindle cells and may appear similar to a low-grade sarcoma except for *lack* of mitotic activity in fibroblasts and *high* degree of differentiation.
4. *Tx*:
   a. Complete surgical extirpation (negative-margins) is foundation of effective tx. Frequent recurrence (30–80%; mesenteric desmoids worse than extraabdominal) is a frustrating aspect of management.
   b. Radiation tx most commonly employed in incompletely excised tumors, but also as a palliative adjunct for unresectable dz.
   c. Medical management usu. reserved for unresectable tumors, although minimally; symptomatic, small intraabdominal tumors may be initially observed w/ medical tx. Most commonly, NSAIDs (i.e., sulindac) a/o anti-estrogen (i.e., tamoxifen) are used w/ about 1/2 of pts responding. Less frequently, cytotoxic drugs such as doxorubicin or carboplatin are prescribed.

F. Esophagus

1. *Epidemiology/etiology*: fastest-growing cancer in United States (4% of CA), but 9th most common CA worldwide.
   a. SCC traditionally more common than adenocarcinoma, but the latter has been increasing much faster in incidence in the United States (70% new dx's in United States).
   b. *Risk factors for SCC*: highest endemicity in N. China, Iran, Russia, India, and S. Africa. In the United States, blacks more affected than whites, Hispanics. Excessive intake of nitrates/nitrosamines, alcohol, tobacco (smoking), and deficiencies in vitamins A, C, B_2, as well as achalasia, esophageal strictures/webs, prior radiation, tylosis assoc. w/ esophageal SCC.
   c. Primary risk factor for esophageal adenocarcinoma is Barrett's esophagus (malignant transformation rate 1–2% per yr).
2. *Staging and w/u*:
   a. CT chest and abdomen (some advocate PET scan; good to eval for metastatic dz).
   b. Endoscopic U/S (best means to determine depth of invasion and local LN; provide tissue dx).
   c. Bronchoscopy for upper 2/3 lesions (r/o fistula).
   d. CT head a/o bone scan if sx are suggestive; cervical LAD should be biopsied.

e. Consider bronchoscopy, thoracoscopy, a/o laparoscopy to determine if metastatic dz present.

3. *Tx*:

a. *Contraindications*: distant mets, enlarged mediastinal or celiac (not paraesophageal) LN, esophagobronchial fistula. Most upper $^1/_3$ cancers are nonresectable.

b. *Neoadjuvant therapy*: cisplatinum + 5-FU concomitant w/ XRT of 4500 rad may be of benefit for ≥ T2 tumors.

c. *Surgery*: Optimize nutrition (i.e., TPN).

i. Celiotomy, should first check for metastatic dz—most commonly will be to liver or celiac nodes. If (+), then only resect if other palliative interventions are not feasible.

ii. *Subtotal esophagectomy*: distal tumors (i.e., at GE junction) appropriately managed w/ Ivor-Lewis (or Tanner-Lewis modification). Need right thoracotomy (mobilize esophagus, anastomose stomach to esophagus in chest). If proximal esophageal margin (+) for cancer, perform total esophagectomy w/ cervical anastomosis. 10-cm margins are desirable in esophageal tumors as they tend to spread horizontally.

iii. *Total esophagectomy*: proximal (cervical, upper esophageal) neoplasms are more appropriately managed this way. Esophageal mobilization may be approached in 2 ways:

- Mobilize esophagus via right thoracotomy and bring conduit substernally or through posterior mediastinum to neck.
- Transhiatal esophagectomy, avoiding thoractomy. Disadvantage of this is less thorough periesophageal lymphadenectomy, risk of injuring blood vessels or tracheobronchial tree.
- *Note*: cervical anastomosis leaks more frequently than intrathoracic anastomosis (12% vs 5%), but mortality w/ cervical leak is far less than than w/ intrathoracic leak (2% vs 50%).

iv. *Conduit*: stomach preferred (easy to mobilize, good blood supply; preserve right gastroepiploic; important to do pyloromyotomy/plasty to avoid stasis), followed by colon. Free jejunal grafts rarely utilized.

d. *Adjuvant therapy*: XRT only recommended if (+) margins or residual dz. No proven advantage w/ adjuvant chemotx.

e. *Palliative tx*:

i. *Dilation* (caveat = perforation risk).

ii. *Laser*: reported use in Japan for cure in superficial, *in situ* lesions as well as for palliation.

iii. *Self-expanding stents* (oral or operative insertion)—facilitate pureed diet.

iv. *Chemoradiation palliation*: SCCA more responsive than adenoca, and upper $^1/_2$ lesions have less morbidity (esp. N/V).

4. *Prognosis*: if able to perform R0 resection, anticipate 15–20% 5-yr survival. However, less than 60% of pts w/ locoregional dz can be fully resected.

G. **Gastric** (adenocarcinoma: GIST and lymphoma are discussed in separate sections)

1. *Epidemiology/etiology*: overall decreasing in United States although cardia/GE junction CA increasing. *Wide geographic variation*: Japan, Costa Rica, Korea >> United States, W. Europe. In United States, non-Caucasian (African Americans, Native Americans, Hispanic) males at increased risk gastritis, EBV, h/o operation for benign peptic ulcers. *H. pylori* risk factor for distal cancers and MALT, but could be protective against proximal CA. HNPCC is genetic risk factor.

2. *Pathology*: 95% in United States = adenocarcinoma. GIST, lymphoma, carcinoid, SCCA in remainder. Most often found on lesser curve. 10% *linitis plastica* (malignancy spreads beyond gross mass) w/ esp. poor prognosis.

a. *Lauren classification*:

i. *Intestinal*: from mucosal glands, usu. more distal, and in older pts, often assoc. w/ *H. pylori*, atrophic gastritis.

ii. *Diffuse*: from lamina propria, more invasive (transmural, across submosa, and in lymphatics—more frequent peritoneal mets), usu. more proximal and in younger pts.

3. *Dx*:

a. *Clinical*: generally presents w/ abdominal pain, wt loss. Anemia common. Advanced dz may manifest w/ dysphagia (prox. tumor) or gastric outlet obstruction (distal tumor).

i. *Eponymic signs of metastasis include*: supraclavicular (usu. left) lymphadenopathy—*Virchow's node*; periumbilical met/mass—*Sister Mary Joseph's nodule*; ovarian drop met—*Krukenberg tumor*; prerectal drop met—*Blumer's shelf.*

ii. *Acanthosis nigricans*: velvety, hyperpigmented, hyperkeratotic skin changes, usu. of axilla and groin classically assoc. w/ internal malignancy. Gastric CA is the most common malignancy found w/ this, although in some series lung CA is seen as frequently; many other cancers (i.e., pancreatic, endometrial, etc.) have reportedly been assoc. w/ acanthosis nigricans, as have nonmalignant conditions (i.e., metabolic syndrome). "Tripe palms" refers to similar changes in the palms.

b. *Advanced*: EGD w/ bx is cornerstone. EUS useful to eval. depth and LN status (~ 75% accurate). CT scan to determine if unresectable (visceral metastases, malignant ascites). Diagnostic laparoscopy more sensitive regarding resectability, esp. when combined w/ peritoneal washings.

4. *Staging*: AJCC/UICC more widely used than Japanese system (see Table 12.13 and Table 12.14).

5. *Tx*:

a. *Surgery*

i. *Partial/total gastrectomy w/ gross margin of 6 cm is mainstay*; decide surgery by region involved.

- *GE junction*: most common. Often very advanced. Siewert classification, 3 types:
  - *Type I*: originate in distal esophagus; assoc. w/ Barrett's esophagus. Need gastric pull-up to neck or Ivor-Lewis esophagogastrectomy.
  - *Type II*: adenocarcinoma of gastric cardia; w/in 2 cm of squamocolumnar junction. Total or proximal subtotal gastrectomy. Former has advantage of less esophagitis w/ plus Roux-en-Y reconstruction, and LNs along lesser curve are more easily removed.
  - *Type III*: subcardial infiltrating GE junction; tx same as type II.
- *Midbody*: 15–30% of cases. To achieve adequate margin, total gastrectomy usu. indicated.
- *Distal*: ~ 35%. Total vs distal subtotal gastrectomy have similar survival, w/ latter having better quality of life and should be performed if able to achieve adequate margins.

ii. *Endoscopic mucosal resection* (EMR)

- More frequently performed in Japan than in United States. Appropriate candidates have T1 tumors (confined to mucosa), which are well differentiated and polypoid or fungating or w/ elevated borders (Borrmann type I, IIa/b). Serial pathology sections should be performed after excision. If invades into submucosa but not beyond, pylorus-preserving gastrectomy may be appropriate.

iii. *Lymphadenectomy classification* (not part of AJCC, but commonly described)

- Japanese reports of improved survival in extended lympadenectomy, esp. in stage II/III dz, and authors recommend level of LN resection 1 level higher than involved nodes. Translates into a D2 resection for most cases, and certain centers in the United States have approached levels of success near those in Japan w/ no increased morbidity over D1 resections; most centers in United States and Europe though have experienced increased M&M w/ D2 vs D1 resections, so not uniformly recommended except for select specialist centers.
- *D1*: removal of all LN w/in 3 cm of primary tumor (perigastric).
- *D2*: D1 + removal of all hepatic, splenic, celiac, and left gastric LNs.
- *D3*: total gastrectomy + omentectomy + splenectomy + distal pancreatectomy + porta hepatic + periaortic lymphadenectomy.

iv. *Reconstruction options*:

- *Subtotal gastrectomy*: BI, BII (ante- or retrocolic), or Roux-en-Y gastrojejunostomy (ante- or retrocolic). Roux-en-Y easier than BI w/ less risk of anastomotic tension, and less risk of bile reflux than w/ BII (w/ Roux limb > 40 cm).
- *Total gastrectomy*: of Roux-en-Y esophagojejunostomy, pouch, or jejunal interposition, the first is usu. the easiest to perform w/ the least morbidity.
- Lawrence-Hunt (jejunal) pouch.

TABLE 12.13. AJCC/UICC TMN Classification for Gastric Cancer

Primary Tumor (T)	Regional Lymph Nodes (N)	Distant Metastasis (M)
Tx – Unknown	Nx – Unknown	Mx – Unknown
T0 – No tumor	N0 – No LN mets	M0 – No mets
Tis – *In situ*, no invasion of lamina propria	N1 – 1–2 (+) LNs	M1 – Distant mets
T1a – Invades lamina propria T1b – Invades submucosa	N2 – 3–6 (+) LNs	
T2 – Invades muscularis propria	N3a – 7–15 (+) LNs N3b – 16 (+) LNs	
T3 – Penetrates subserosa		
T4a – Invades serosa, but not adjacent structures T4b – Invades adjacent structures		

*Additional descriptors for gastric cancer:
Histologic Grade (G): Gx = unknown; G1 = well-differentiated; G2 = mod differentiated; G3 = poorly differentiated; G4 = undifferentiated.
Residual Tumor (R): Rx = unknown; R0 = no residual tumor; R1 = microscopic residual tumor; R2 = macroscopic residual tumor.

TABLE 12.14. AJCC/UICC Staging for Gastric Carcinoma

Stage	TNM	5-Year Survival
0	TisN0M0	
Ia	T1N0M0	70.8
Ib	T2N0M0 T1N1M0	57.4
IIa	T1N2M0 T2N1M0 T3N0M0	45.5
IIb	T1N3M0 T2N2M0 T3N1M0 T4aN0M0	32.8
IIIa	T2N3M0 T3N2M0 T4aN1M0	19.8
IIIb	T3N3M0 T4aN2M0 T4bN0–1M0	14.0
IIIc	T4aN3M0 T4bN2–3M0	9.2
IV	Any T, Any N, M1	4.0

b. *Neoadjuvant therapy*: MAGIC trial: periop use of ECF (epirubicin/cisplatin/5-FU) [Chua YJ, et al., *Ann Surg Onc*. 2007;14(10):2687–90.]. Improved 5-yr overall survival compared to surgery alone for = T2 tumors. Similarly, combination chemoradiotherapy w/ XRT shows some benefit in ongoing studies.

c. *Palliative options*: chemotx, XRT, resection, or endoscopic laser ablation/dilation/stenting may be appropriate alone or in various combinations.

H. Gastrointestinal stromal tumors (GIST)

1. A form of soft-tissue sarcoma, assoc. w/ mutation of c-KIT/CD117 (tyrosine kinase receptor protein).
   a. Not all are CD117 (+), however.
   b. Rarely spread by lymphatics, much more commonly to liver or elsewhere in abdomen.
   c. *Location*: stomach > small intestine > colon.
2. *Dx*: w/u should include CT or MRI of abdomen, CXR or CT chest, possibly EUS. Bx depends on index of suspicion or plans for neoadjuvant tx to facilitate surgery. As tumor is friable, care should be taken to not violate tissues unnecessarily.
3. *Staging*: TNM + mitotic rate; size and mitotic rate most important for determining likelihood or recurrence.
4. *Tx*:
   a. *Neoadjuvant therapy*: reserved for tumors that appear only marginally resectable (read about c-KIT tyrosine kinase inhibitors, below); optimal response require up to 6 mo.
   b. *Surgery*: mainstay of tx.
   c. *Adjuvant therapy*: Gleevec (imatinib mesylate) is an inhibitor of c-KIT (as well as platelet-derived growth factor and Bcr-Abl receptor) tyrosine kinases; 50% response rate. FDA-approved for pts at high risk of recurrence (≥ 5 cm, high mitotic rate, small bowel origin), unresectable a/o metastatic tumors. Sunitinib malate (Sutent) is FDA approved for GIST tumors resistant to imatinib.
5. *Prognosis*: historically, overall 50% 5-yr survival; however, limited data on survival after initiation of imatinib therapy.

I. Hepatobiliary

1. *Hepatocellular carcinoma*
   a. *Etiology*: worldwide, most common lethal malignancy in men. Incidence rising rapidly in United States due to epidemic hepatitis C (up to 1/3 develop chronic dz, of which up to 1/3 develop cirrhosis, of which experience up to 2% chance/yr of developing HCC). Other risk factors include toxins (aflatoxin, polyvinyl chloride, etc.).
   b. *Dx*: frequently presents w/ jaundice and nonspecific constitutional sx. Alpha-fetoprotein (AFP) elevated in ~ 75%. Bx appropriate for any solid hepatic lesion w/ elevated AFP (> normal but < 400 ng/mL if hepatitis B surface antigen [–], or > 4000 if hepatitis B surface antigen [+]).
   c. *Staging*:
      i. T1 = solitary tumor, no vascular invasion.
      ii. T2 = single or multiple tumors, none > 5 cm, none w/ vascular invasion.
      iii. T3 = multiple tumors > 5 cm, or any involving branch of portal/hepatic vein.
      iv. T4 = direct invasion of any organ other than gallbladder.
      v. N, M status based simply on presence/absence of LN/distant spread.
      vi. Multiple histologic types, of which fibrolamellar has the best prognosis, and is less frequently assoc. w/ cirrhosis.
   d. *Tx*:
      i. *Surgical*:
         - *Resection*: method of choice for peripheral lesions in Child's A cirrhotics.
           - Hepatic reserve physiology largely determines resectability. See Chapter 16 on hepatobilary and pancreas for details of evaluation of liver function such as indocyanine green and MEGX. Preop portal vein embolization of planned resection area may be of benefit to induce hypertrophy of remaining hepatic parenchyma, and thus postop hepatic function.
         - *Transplant*: method of choice if Child's B or C, and if single tumor < 5 cm or up to 3 tumors, none of which are > 3 cm in diameter, and no evidence of extrahepatic spread.
      ii. *Other*:
         - Ablation
           - *Radiofrequency* (RFA): of limited success if near large vessel due to "heat sink" phenomenon.
         - Embolization
         - Arterial infusion

e. *Postop*:

i. *Prognosis*: overall 5-yr survival is ~ 35% after resection, and up to 75% after transplantation.

ii. *Surveillance*: liver CT/MRI along w/ AFP levels (if initially elevated) should be followed frequently for 2 yr, then annually if normal.

2. *Cholangiocarcinoma* ("Klatskin tumor" refers to neoplasm at bifurcation of extrahepatic bile duct)

a. Risk factors include choledocholithiasis, hepatolithiasis, choledochal cysts, nitrosamines, hepatic flukes (i.e., *Fasciola* spp.), ulcerative colitis, HNPCC, and sclerosing cholangitis.

b. *W/u*:

i. CT and ERCP generally obtained. Like pancreatic adenocarcinoma, CEA and CA 19-9 may be elevated.

ii. *Usu. unresectable. Criteria for unresectability include*: (+) LN outside hepatic pedicle; distant metastasis; bilateral extension into secondary hepatic ducts; bilateral extension into hepatic parenchyma; combination of vascular involvement w/ contralateral ductal spread.

c. *Surgery*:

i. *Lower third* (distal): pancreaticoduodenectomy (Whipple).

ii. *Middle third*: local excision (remove GB and CBD from hepatic duct to pancreas) and LN dissection. Reconstruct w/ hepaticojejunostomy.

iii. *Upper third* (proximal): bile duct resection beginning distally, including GB and LN in porta hepatis, possibly along w/ caudate lobe (controversial). Reconstruct w/ hepaticojejunostomy.

d. *Adjuvant tx*: XRT +/– 5-FU may be of some benefit; limited data.

3. *Gallbladder carcinoma*

a. *Risk factors* include cholelithiasis, gallbladder polyps (solitary polyp > 1 cm greater risk than multiple or smaller polyps), porcelain gallbladder (mucosal calcification higher risk than uniform, transmural calcification), and typhoid carrier state.

b. *Management*:

i. *Surgery*:

- Regardless of operation performed, bile spillage significantly worsens outcome. As bile spillage is also increased in gallbladder cancer operations, *strong consideration should be given to open cholecystectomy in all suspected cases of gallbladder cancer.*
- Known gallbladder carcinoma should undergo staging laparoscopy, as ~ $^1/_2$ have metastatic dz.
- If does not penetrate muscularis (T1), cholecystectomy is adequate.
- If invades muscularis or deeper (stage ≥ T2), lymphadectomy (portal, periductal, right celiac, posterior pancreaticoduodenal) should be added to liver parenchyma excision (IVb/V), typically w/ 2+ cm margins beyond palpated or imaged tumor. Some recommend consideration of port site excision as well.

ii. *Adjuvant tx*: chemotx (5-FU) + XRT recommended for all, except T1, N0 pts.

J. Lung

1. *Lung cancer* = number 1 cause of cancer death in United States; tobacco smoking = number 1 risk factor.

a. *Histological types*: adenocarcinoma (50%), squamous cell (30%), small cell (20%), large cell (10%).

2. *Lung cancer management*:

a. *Non-small cell* (NSCLC—adenocarcinoma, squamous cell, large cell, bronchoalveolar, etc.):

i. *Presentation/dx*: freq. presents w/ cough and constitutional sx such as wt loss or fatigue; SCCA may also cause hypercalcemia. Imaging should include CT of chest/liver/adrenals. *Tissue dx*: percutaneous, broncoscopic, or thoracoscopic means (FNA, brushings, etc.). Mediastinoscopy standard for mediastinal LN; should be considered for central T1 tumors and all T2 or T3 tumors. 40% of pts present w/ metastatic dz.

ii. *Tx*: surgical resection (lobectomy +/– mediastinal lymphadectomy) gold standard for curative tx of stage I and II cancers. Prohibitive operative risk pts may be offered XRT for stage I and II dz; RFA is other option for small (i.e., < 3 cm) peripheral lesions. Adjuvant chemotx

TABLE 12.15. AJCC TNM Classification for Lung Cancer

Primary Tumor (T)	Regional Lymph Nodes (N)	Distant Metastasis (M)
Tx – Primary tumor cannot be assessed *or*, tumor proven by malignant cells in sputum or bronchial washings, but not seen by imaging or bronchoscopy	Nx – Regional LNs cannot be assessed	Mx – Presence of distant met(s) cannot be established
T0 – No evidence of primary tumor	N0 – No regional LN mets	M0 – No distant met(s)
Tis – Carcinoma *in situ*	N1 – Mets to ipsilateral peribronchial *a/o* ipsilateral hilar LNs, and intrapulmonary nodes involved by direct extension of the primary tumor (ipsilateral parynchymal spread only)	M1a – Tumor nodule in contralateral lobe w/ pleural nodules or malignant pleural or pericardial effusion M1b – Distant mets
T1 – ≤ 3 cm in greatest dimension, surrounded by lung/pleura, w/out bronchoscopic evidence of invasion more proximal than lobar bronchus	N2 – Mets to ipsilateral mediastinal *a/o* subcarinal LNs	
T2 – 3–7 cm in greatest dimension *or* invading visceral pleura *or* involving main bronchus ≥ 2 cm distal to carina *or* assoc. w/ atelectasis or obstructive pneumonitis that extends to the hilar region but doesn't involve whole lung T2a – 3–5 cm T2b – 5–7 cm	N3 – Mets to contralateral mediastinal, *or* contralateral hilar, *or* any scalene or supraclavicular LNs	
T3 – > 7 cm OR any size that directly invades chest wall (including superior sulcus), diaphragm, mediastinal pleura, parietal pericardium; *OR* in main bronchus < 2 cm distal from carina; *OR* associated atelectasis or obstructive pneumonitis of entire lung		
T4 – Invades vital structures of heart, great vessels, trachea, recurrent laryngeal n. esophagus, vertebral body, carina, satellite tumor nodules in different ipsilateral lobe		

TABLE 12.16. AJCC Staging for Lung Carcinoma

Stage	TNM	Median Survival (Months)
0	TisN0M0	
Ia	T1N0M0	115
Ib	T2aN0M0	76
IIa	T2bN0M0 T1N1M0 T2aN1M0	47

(Continues)

TABLE 12.16. AJCC Staging for Lung Carcinoma *(Continued)*

Stage	TNM	Median Survival (Months)
IIb	T2bN1M0 T3N0M0	24
IIIa	T1N2M0 T2a–bN2M0 T3N1–2M0 T4N0–1M0	17
IIIb	T1N3M0 T2N3M0 T3N3M0 T4N2–3M0	10
IV	Any T, Any N, M1	7

(i.e., cisplatin) standard for T2+ or N1+ dz. T3 and stage III tumor management is individualized, but usu. involves neoadjuvant chemotherapy. *Surgery is not recommended as primary tx for N2–3 or M1 dz,* although resection of a solitary brain metastasis may favorably impact survival.

b. *Small cell lung cancer* (SCLC):

i. *Presentation/dx*: similar for NSCLC (above), except that frequently manifest paraneoplastic syndrome(s) such as Eaton-Lambert (proximal LE asthenia), Cushing's syndrome, and SIADH. In addition to w/u listed for NSCLC, obtain MRI of head and bone scan, +/– bone marrow bx. 2/3 of pts present w/ metastases, and the majority of the remainder have locally unresectable dz.

ii. *Tx*:

- SCLC is exceptionally chemo-sensitive; all pts are given chemotx +/– XRT may be added for relatively local/limited dz.
- Surgical resection is indicated for less than 5% of pts w/ SCLC (rarely limited to T1/T2 and N0).

3. *Prognosis*: overall, 15% 5-yr survival. However, stage I non-small cell w/ appropriate tx has > 70–90% 10-yr survival; only 10% of pts are dx'd this early, however. Some have advocated screening high-risk pts w/ chest CT to identify these cancers early, thus improving survival.

K. Lymphoma

1. *Hodgkin lymphoma*

a. *Presentation*:

i. A = *asymptomatic*, B = *symptomatic* (fever, night sweats, pain, pruritus).

ii. *Staging*:

- I = 1 area or 2 contiguous areas on same side of diaphragm.
- II = 2 noncontiguous areas on same side of diaphragm.
- III = both sides of diaphragm involved.
- IV = liver, marrow, lung, or other nonlymphoid tissue except spleen.
  - Staging celiotomy rarely indicated w/ high-resolution CT scanners, but still may be indicated for stage Ia or IIa (may avoid chemotx if can prove not more advanced). Contraindicated if have B sx, if XRT not an option, or if have (+) marrow, mediastinal LAD, or other extranodal dz.
    - 2 liver bx's. Splenectomy. Lymphadenectomy of suspicious LNs, as well as LN bx of splenic hilum, porta hepatic, celiac trunk, para-aortic/caval/iliac. Clip areas of suspicious LNs. In females, ovaripexy to assist w/ XRT management.

b. *Dx*: dependent on tissue (intact LN); Reed-Sternberg cells diagnostic.

c. *Tx*: CHOP chemotx (**c**yclophosphamide, **h**ydroxydaunomycin [doxorubicin], **O**ncovin [vincristine], and **p**rednisone) + rituximab standard. Assoc. w/ infertility, esp. young males. XRT may be given instead if stage Ia, IIa.

2. *Non-Hodgkin lymphoma*
   a. Presentation same as above, need tissue dx.
   b. Worse prognosis than Hodgkin. Usu. systemic at dx.
   c. *Tx*: XRT and MOAP chemotx (vincristine, cyclophosphamide, prednisone, adriamycin).
3. *Gastric lymphoma*
   a. Most common site of primary lymphoma in GI tract.
   b. *Dx*:
      i. Endoscopy w/ bx's and EUS appropriate for initial dx. Subsequent evaluation should include: *H. pylori* histologic and serologic testing; CT of chest and abdomen; bx of bone marrow and any identified LAD appropriate to assess extent of dz.
      ii. Dx appropriate if lymphoma appears to be sole or primary locus of dz. ~ 2% of all lymphomas, ~ 15% of all gastric malignancies. Most commonly B-cell lymphoma > MALT > other.
   c. *Tx*:
      i. Early MALT (**m**ucosa-**a**ssociated **l**ymphoid **t**umors—now termed extranodal marginal zone lymphomas of MALT type) and potentially early diffuse large B-cell lymphoma should be treated for *H. pylori*, which may induce remission (effective in $^2/_3$ of localized MALT lymphomas). F/u serial endoscopy mandatory.
         - Positive nodal status, transmural extension, and certain genetic markers (as well as *H. pylori*-negative MALT cases) likely to fail this management; XRT usu. tx'd w/ chemotx used for antibiotic-resistant MALT tumors (surgery reserved for failure of XRT and chemo).
      ii. B-cell gastric lymphoma appropriately tx w/ chemotherapy (CHOP + rituximab) +/– XRT w/ > 80% dz-free 5-yr survival rate for early stage dz. Main risk of chemotx is perforation (~ 5%). XRT useful for tumors less than 3 cm in size, markedly less so if > 6 cm.
      iii. Uncommonly, surgery may be pursued for localized dz in some institutions, or recommended for cases resistant to chemotherapy; surgical resection, even w/ positive margins, can be of benefit in such select cases.
4. *Intestinal lymphoma*
   a. Second most common site of GI lymphoma. In adults, represents up to 25% of all small bowel malignancies and is the most common small bowel malignancy in children under 10 yo. Frequently mimics celiac or tropical sprue as malabsorptive dz (also increased incidence in pt w/ celiac dz as well as AIDS), but also causes bleeding, obstruction, or perforation. Generally located in lymphoid-rich ileum.
   b. *Dx*: histological—Kiel classification subtypes into low-, intermediate-, and high-grade lesions.
   c. *Tx*:
      i. As w/ small bowel adenocarcinoma (most common small bowel malignancy; tx w/ resection, which if is in duodenum right of SMA means Whipple), resection of bowel and lymph-containing mesentery is indicated. Duodenal lymphoma may require pancreaticoduodenectomy. Obtain frozen section to confirm clear margins; tumor widely infiltrates submucosa.
      ii. Unlike small bowel adenocarcinoma, adjunctive chemotx such as CHOP (particularly for intermediate- and high-grade dz) and XRT is often indicated.
5. *Thyroid lymphoma*
   a. Rare. Typically presents as rapidly growing goitrous mass +/– fever, dysphagia, a/o dysphonia. Increased risk after Hashimoto's thyroiditis. Non-Hodgkin B-cell most common subtype, followed by MALT tumors.
   b. *Dx*: U/S, FNA, CT of head/neck, chest, abdomen.
   c. *Tx*:
      i. Chemotx w/ CHOP alone yields good survival rates for B-cell tumors.
      ii. Surgery (near-total or total thyroidectomy) may provide some additional survival benefit to CHOP, but assoc. w/ significantly higher (than resection for carcinoma) complication rates due to edema, anatomic distortion. Not consistently recommended.
      iii. MALT tumors of thyroid often may be treated w/ XRT alone.

L. Occult primary

1. Represents up to 10% of all malignant dx's. Most commonly involves liver, lungs, lymph nodes, a/o bone. Primary site ultimately found in < ⅓ of cases.
2. *3 broad categories*: (1) adenocarcinoma and other nonsquamous carcinoma (majority of cases); (2) squamous cell carcinoma; (3) neuroendocrine tumors.
   a. *W/u may be aided by*:
      i. *PET/CT*
      ii. *Immunohistochemical stains*: cytokeratins (CK7, CK20)—patterns of (+) and (–) status helpful for evaluating carcinomas such as lung/breast/endometrium/ovary/urothelium/thyroid/pancreas/colon.
      iii. *Other*:
         - *Axillary lymphatic adenocarcinoma in female*: often from breast CA. Consider breast imaging, including MRI.
         - *Supraclavicular SCCA*: likely from head/neck source; obtain head/neck CT, panendoscopy (nasopharyngoscopy, bronchoscopy, direct laryngoscopy, esophagoscopy).
         - *Mediastinal lymphatic adenocarcinoma*: possible germ cell tumor; get β-hCG, AFP, LDH levels.
         - *Bone scan as indicated by sx.*
         - *Adenocarcinoma or poorly differentiated carcinoma in men*, particularly in retroperitoneum: also consider testicular U/S, PSA, CA-125, β-hCG, AFP, LDH.
         - *Neuroendocrine tumors*: octreotide scan may be of benefit.
3. *Tx*: based on presumptive primary. Regional lymphadenectomy and XRT generally appropriate for adenocarcinoma or squamous cell carcinomas. Chemotherapy appropriate for histologic type may result in significant response in 10–50% of pts. Overall median survival little more than 6 mo.

M. Pancreas

1. *Pancreatic adenocarcinoma*
   a. *Epidemiology/etiology*:
      i. Main risk factors are male gender, age over 60 yo, and cigarette smoking.
      ii. Almost always has mutation of codon 12 of K-ras oncogene, but p53 tumor suppressor gene also mutated in up to 75% of cases. p16 and BRCA mutation linked to some cases as well.
      iii. Familial cases assoc. w/ HNPCC (see section D. above on colorectal cancer), familial (*BRCA II* mutation) breast CA, ataxia-telangiectasia, familial atypical multiple mole melanoma syndrome, and Peutz-Jeghers syndrome.
   b. *Dx*: classically presents w/ wt loss and painless jaundice. Helical CT scan is generally modality of choice for making dx. If CT doesn't demonstrate mass, ERCP/EUS can be useful (even if classic "double duct" sign of CBD and pancreatic duct stricture is absent), particularly if brushings are obtained. However, tissue dx is not required before pursuing surgery for pancreatic head mass.
   c. *Staging*
      i. Considered unresectable if involves SMA, celiac axis, or invades posteriorly on preop CT. Distant metastasis (including para-aortic or celiac LNs) is a contraindication for surgery. Involvement of portal vein or SMV means borderline resectability to most surgeons, but this is controversial, as is direct invasion of adrenal, kidney, or colon. Many surgeons will proceed w/ laparoscopy (to look for peritoneal implants, etc.) if CT doesn't demonstrate evidence of unresectability or metastasis, and then open for pancreatic resection if still no evidence of spread.
   d. *Tx*:
      i. *Neoadjuvant*: consider in tumors that appear to be nonmetastatic, but locally advanced to make them potentially resectable. Pursuing neoadjuvant tx is one of the few indications for obtaining tissue bx before intervening.
      ii. *Surgical*
         - *Curative* (pancreaticoduodenectomy ["Whipple" operation]); appropriate for < 20% of pts. "Pylorus-preserving" Whipple has not been proven to improve postop gastric

emptying. Nor has extensive lymphadenectomy beyond peripancreatic LNs been proven to improve survival in the United States.

- *Palliative*
  - *Biliary bypass*: hepaticojejunostomy. Preop stenting only recommended if evidence of cholangitis or severely symptomatic (i.e., pruritic) and surgery is not imminent.
  - *Duodenal bypass*: only about 1/4 of pts will develop duodenal obstruction, thus gastrojejunostomy is usu. reserved for pts w/ no evidence of distant metastasis who are therefore more likely to survive long enough to become symptomatic from obstruction.

iii. *Adjuvant*:
- *Chemotx*: gemcitabine agent of choice for metastatic dz. May have some role as adjuvant tx.
- *Radiation*: when given w/ 5-FU, *may* be of benefit in some cases (not proven).

e. *Prognosis*: after resection, median survival just over 15 mo (5-yr survival 20%). If metastasis, 3–6 mo.

2. *Intraductal papillary mucinous neoplasms*
   a. First described in 1980s.
   b. Usu. present in 7th–9th decade of life, slightly more often in men, and are usu. in the pancreatic head.
   c. Subtypes include main-duct, branch-duct, or combined IPMNs. Increased risk of malignancy w/ main-duct IPMN. Commonly mucin will be found at the ampulla of Vater.
   d. Small, branch-duct IPMNS w/out solid component can be managed conservatively; otherwise, tx is pancreas resection.
3. *Mucinous cystic neoplasm*
   a. Lesions w/ increasing malignant potential w/ age, formerly referred to as cystadenoma or cystadenocarcinoma.
   b. Typically occur in 5th–6th decade of life, more commonly in women, and tend to be located in body or tail of pancreas.
   c. Unlike IPMNs (above), these do *not* communicate w/ duct. Characteristically have thick wall w/ ovarian stroma.
   d. Tx is most often w/ distal pancreatectomy.
4. *Serous cystic neoplasm*
   a. Account for 1/4 of cystic neoplasms of the pancreas, and are seen more commonly in pts w/ von Hippel-Lindau dz.
   b. Differentiate from mucinous variety by aspiration of contents for mucin (if find mucin, consider malignant or premalignant).
      i. Also, on CT, serous cystic neoplasms characteristically have a much thinner wall than mucinous cystic neoplasms; they also often demonstrate a "sunburst" pattern of calcification w/in a central scar on CT.
      ii. These tumors may have honeycomb appearance w/ thin septa dividing tumor into microcysts.
      iii. These tumors have clear demarcation between cyst and pancreatic parenchyma (unlike MCN).
      iv. These tumors do not communicate w/ pancreatic duct.
   c. Almost always benign (< 1 per 10,000 contain a malignancy). WHO refers to more common benign variant as *serous cystadenoma* and the rare malignant type *serous cystadenocarcinoma.*
   d. More common in females (2:1) and assoc. w/ von Hippel-Lindau dz; usu. present in 7th decade.
   e. *Tx*: resection is curative, and is primarily performed to avoid sx assoc. w/ mass effect of large tumors, as malignancy is exceedingly rare.
5. *Insulinoma*
   a. *Pathology*: most common pancreatic endocrine tumor, followed by gastrinoma.
      i. Majority sporadic, solitary, benign (85%), less than 2 cm, and equally distributed throughout pancreas.
      ii. > 3 cm or angioinvasive more likely malignant. Mets most often in surrounding lymphatics and liver. Multiple tumors suspect for MEN I.

b. *Dx*:

i. *Whipple's triad suggestive*: sx of hypoglycemia w/ rest or exercise, glucose < 45 during sx, and relief of sx w/ glucose administration.

ii. *Hypoglycemia w/ insulin*: glucose ratio > 0.4 indicative.

iii. *To r/o factitious dz*: check for elevated C-peptide, proinsulin (not seen if factitious). Can also screen for anti-insulin antibodies and sulfonylureas to r/o factitious hypoglycemia.

iv. Nesidioblastosis may have identical presentation, but usu. presents early in life (often in infancy), and is not assoc. w/ any mass.

c. *Localization*:

i. Gold standard = intraop 10 MHz U/S and palpation; 96–100% successful.

ii. Spiral CT and gadolinium MRI are primarily to r/o hepatic mets; only 45% successful in locating primary, and neither good if < 1 cm. U/S and somatostatin receptor scintigraphy also have been used, but results are no better. Rarely, calcium gluconate injection and selective venous sampling used 88–100% (sensitive).

d. *Tx*:

i. *Medical*: diet change and diazoxide generally not effective.

ii. *Surgical*: tx = enucleation. Some give IV secretin afterwards to identify ductal leak.

- Subtotal pancreatectomy (enucleation of tumor if in head and distal pancreatectomy) indicated for MEN I pts and familial pts who often have multifocal dz. Subtotal resection also indicated for nesidioblastosis.

6. *Gastrinoma* (Zollinger-Ellison syndrome)

a. 2nd most common islet cell tumor (after insulinoma), most common pancreatic tumor in MEN syndrome, and most common symptomatic malignant endocrine pancreatic neoplasm. 75% sporadic, 25% MEN I syndrome. Malignancy not based on pathology, but behavior. Initially reported rates of 60–90% malignancy have decreased in recent years to ~ 1/3 of cases (except in MEN I cases—85% LN mets, prognostic significance of LN mets uncertain, however). Large (> 3 cm), sporadic tumors most prone to hepatic mets.

b. Usu. presents as abdominal pain, w/ 2/3 having diarrhea, and 15% w/ diarrhea alone. N/V not uncommon. GI bleeding in 10%.

i. Diarrhea stops or significantly decreases w/ NGT aspiration, an important distinguishing feature (i.e., from carcinoid or VIPomas).

ii. May present as persistent, virulent peptic ulcer (esp. if persist after tx for *H. pylori* or H_2 blockade) or GERD w/ severe esophagitis.

iii. Also consider dx if pt has other indicators of MEN I (hypercalcemia, elevated PTH, pituitary tumor).

c. *Dx must include hypergastrinemia in presence of increased gastric acid secretion.*

i. Fasting gastrin level usu. not above 100 pg/cc in normal pts, but occasionally non-ZES pts will have levels up to 1000 pg/cc; > 1000 pg/cc is essentially diagnostic in pts w/ acid secretion. Significant hypergastrinemia (enough to cause ZES) rarely may also be caused by certain ovarian tumors.

ii. Basal acid output (BAO) normally < 5 mEq/h. ZES produces a BAO of > 15 mEq/h, or a ratio of BAO to maximum AO > 0.6. Usu., gastric pH < 2.5 for in ZES.

iii. *If unsure of dx, may administer secretin provocation test*: check fasting gastrin level, then give 2 CU/kg IV of secretin, then recheck gastrin at 2, 5, 10, and 20 min; paradoxical increase in gastrin > 200 pg/mL is 87% sensitive (most false negative results from *H. pylori*) and 100% specific.

iv. *Differential dx for hypergastrinemia*:

- *Excess stimulation*
  - ZES, antral G-cell hyperplasia (+/– pheochromocytoma), pyloric obstruction
- *Insufficient gastrin inhibition*
  - Atrophic gastritis
  - Pernicious anemia
  - Gastric carcinoma

- Vitiligo
- H_2 blockers, PPI
- Antral-exclusion operations (also, retained antrum in duodenal stump after Billroth II)
- Vagotomy

- *Decreased metabolic processing of gastrin*
  - Chronic renal failure
  - Small bowel resection (usu. transient)
- *Miscellaneous*
  - Rheumatoid arthritis

d. *Localization*:

i. > 50% in duodenum (45–60% of all, 60–80% in MEN I), 60–90% in gastrinoma triangle (junction of D2 and D3, junction of cystic duct and CBD, junction of head and neck of pancreas). Rarely in renal capsule, ovarian malignancies.

ii. ^{111}In-octreotide scintigraphy most useful test. CT scan and arteriogram each miss 50%; venous sampling not helpful.

e. Preop prep should include NGT, PPI (titrate to gastric acid output to < 5 mEq/h).

f. Palliative care includes tumor debulking, PPI, somatostatin; consider total gastrectomy.

7. *Glucagonoma*

a. Assoc. w/ "migratory necrolytic erythema" (related to amino acid deficiency), wt loss, diabetes, VTE. Almost always malignant w/ 70% having metastatic dz, and only 30% cure rate; octreotide can be used for palliation of sx.

b. *Dx*: confirmed w/ elevated glucagon level, which can be provoked w/ secretin. Normal upper limit is 150–190 pg/cc.

c. Localization typically achieved via enhanced CT, MRI, or angiography. Most often in body or tail.

d. Preop prep should included TPN w/ amino acid supplementation, octreotide prn sx.

e. *Tx*: surgical excision of primary (and mets, if any).

f. ~ 30% of cases assoc. w/ postop thrombotic complications; consider use of periop anticoagulants.

8. *VIPoma*

a. *"Werner-Morrison syndrome," or WDHA syndrome*: watery (secretory) diarrhea, hypokalemia, achlorhydria.

i. Diarrhea is secretory (not related to intake), high volume (dx unlikely if < 700 cc/d) and persists w/ NGT aspiration and H_2 blockers (unlike most cases of gastrinoma), but is consistent feature along w/ hypokalemia. Other features more variable, and may also include cutaneous flushing, hypercalcemia, a/o hyperglycemia.

ii. ~ 1/2 metastatic at dx.

b. Dx confirmed w/ elevated VIP and diarrhea (consider gastrinoma, carcinoid, or infectious source if VIP normal). Upper limit of normal is 200 pg/cc.

c. Localization via enhanced CT, MRI, or angiography. Up to 10% intrathoracic; consider chest CT if initial studies (–).

d. Preop prep should include octreotide to assist w/ fluid management.

e. *Tx*: distal pancreatectomy is sufficient for most; if no tumor found, also examine other retroperitoneal tissues such as adrenals. Debulking of tissue is indicated even if metastatic, and octreotide can be used for palliation as well.

9. *PPoma*

a. Equal distribution in pancreas.

b. No assoc. clinical syndromes.

c. Tx = surgical resection.

10. *Somatostatinoma*

a. Gallstones, steatorrhea, pancreatitis, diabetes mellitus are present w/ variable consistency (i.e., 10% have hypo-, not hyperglycemia). Rarely assoc. w/ neurofibromatosis. 70–90% malignant.

b. Localization may be procured via CT, MRI, angiography, a/o somatostatin-receptor scintigraphy. Most situated in pancreatic tail and generally large enough to localize w/out difficulty.

c. *Tx*: surgical resection (distal pancreatectomy, not enucleation). Debulking of mets (usu. hepatic) indicated. Simultaneous cholecystectomy is indicated even if gallbladder w/out stones as cholelithiasis eventually develops in the majority of cases.

N. Sarcoma—soft tissue (for GIST tumor, see section H. above)

1. *Rare cancers* (0.6% of malignancies in United States) arising from mesenchyma.
2. *Distribution*: Location (~ 1/2 in extremities) 33% lower extremity; 16% viscera; 15% retroperitoneal/intraabdominal; 14% upper extremity; 10% trunk; 12% other. Histopathology 20–25% liposarcoma; 19% leiomyosarcoma; 18% malignant fibrous histocytoma (MFH) (*Note*: *many sources rank MFH as most common type*); 10% fibrosarcoma; 7% synovial; 4% malignant peripheral nerve tumor (MPNT); 22% other.
3. *Behavior*:
   a. *Locally*: locally compress structures, expanding from w/in pseudocapsule.
   b. *Metastatic*:
      i. Almost always spread hematogenously; *exceptions*: clear cell (only 30% hematogenous), fibrohistiocytoma, synovial, epithelioid (15% LN; consider SLNBx).
      ii. Lung usu. involved in metastasis (*exception* = GI sarcomas → liver).
4. *Risk factors*:
   a. *Environmental* (possible): radiation, trauma, pesticides/herbicides, infectious agents.
   b. *Genetic*: Li-Fraumeni syndrome, neurofibromatosis, familial adenomatous polyposis.
5. *Dx and grading*:
   a. *Bx*: bear in mind future potential definitive procedures when orienting bx. Core-needle bx more likely than FNA to give definitive pathology. Open bx in the extremity can be performed w/ pneumatic tourniquet after exsanguination of the limb. Small incision directly over lesion, oriented along Langer's lines or axis of limb. < 5 cm: *excisional bx*. > 5 cm: *incisional bx*. Frozen and permanent pathology are indicated. Meticulous hemostasis is important to diminish risk of seeding from postop hematoma.
   b. *Radiographic*: MRI is the standard for dx, staging, and surveillance. CXR/CT are important adjuncts for detecting pulmonary metastases. Low grade → CXR and MRI of tumor. High grade → chest CT and MRI of tumor.
      i. T1 ≤ 5 cm in greatest dimension.
      ii. T1a tumor above superficial fascia.
      iii. T1b tumor invading or deep to superficial fascia.
      iv. T2 > 5 cm in greatest dimension.
      v. T2a tumor above superficial fascia.
      vi. T3b tumor invading or deep to superficial fascia.
      vii. N1 regional lymph node metastasis. (*Note*: sarcoma is unique in that N1 dz as well as M1 dz constitutes stage IV.)
      viii. M1 distant metastasis.
   c. FNCLCC Histologic Grading System
      i. Based on 3 parameters and scored as follows:
         - Differentiation (1–3)
         - Mitotic activity (1–3)
         - Extent of necrosis (0–2)
      ii. Scores are summed to designate a grade:
         - Grade 1: 2 or 3
         - Grade 2: 4 or 5
         - Grade 3: 6–8

TABLE 12.17. AJCC Staging for Soft-Tissue Sarcoma

Stage	TNM	Grade
I	T1a/b–T2a/b N0M0	G1, GX
IIa	T1a–b N0M0	G2–G3
IIb	T2a–bN0M0	G2
III	T2a–bN0M0	G3
	T any N1M0	G any
IV	T any N0M1	G any

6. *Tx*:
   a. *Extremity/trunk*: < 5 cm → excision w/ negative margins (attempt 1- to 2-cm gross margin). > 5 cm, *low grade* → excision and postop external beam radiation (EBRT), 50 Gy. > 5 cm, *high grade* → excision w/ periop brachytherapy (BRT) or postop EBRT. > 10 cm, *high grade* → consider preop EBRT tx; complete excision and BRT or EBRT—appropriate chemo: antracyclin a/o ifosfamide.
      i. Currently, ~ 90% of pts are able to undergo limb-sparing surgery, not amputations.
      ii. Compartment resection does not improve survival.
      iii. Reconstruct vessels in thigh. Sacrifice sensory nerves, but not motor if possible.
      iv. In shoulder, popliteal region do amputation or limb salvage + XRT.
      v. In hand/feet, do local amputation.
      vi. *Viscera*: bowel resection. If incomplete, give postop EBRT-morbid.
      vii. *Retroperitoneal/intraabdominal*: bx not indicated for suspicious retroperitoneal mass unless suspect lymphoma or germ-cell tumor, contemplate neoadjuvant tx, dx if suspect unresectable dz, or suspect metastases from another primary. Instead, go directly to excision of mass.
   b. *Metastatic dz*: consider metastasectomy on case-by-case basis.
   c. *Adjuvant tx*:
      i. *Radiotherapy*: preop generally advantageous over postop (smaller field, may reduce intraop seeding, may facilitate dissection). Chief disadvantage is impairment of wound healing (wait 3–6 wk post-XRT to operate); if give XRT postop, also wait 3–6 wk. Usual XRT dose = 50 Gy. If anticipate close margins, consider brachy tx. Consider postop XRT if margins < 1 cm, but should be standard for resectable high-grade sarcoma.
      ii. *Chemotherapy*: doxorubicin, anthracycline, ifosfamide, etc., appears to benefit pts w/ large, high-grade tumors.
7. *Surveillance*:
   a. F/u w/ physical exams, regional imaging, and CXRs or chest CTs.
   b. Resect or amputate local recurrence (56% 5-yr survival).
   c. Chemo may be of some benefit for disseminated dz (ifosfamide, adriamycin).
8. *Prognosis*:
   a. 56% 5-yr survival overall.
   b. Grade most important (> 5–6 mitoses in 30 HPF is *high grade*); extremities better than retroperitoneum. Margins only important for local recurrence. In primary extremity dz overall *low grade* dz → 90% 10-yr survival, *high grade* dz → 55% 10-yr survival.

O. Skin cancers

1. *Melanoma*
   a. 3% of skin cancers, 67% skin cancer mortality. Assoc. w/ mutations in p16 (INK4a), CDK4, and B-RAF.
   b. *Management*:

TABLE 12.18. AJCC TNM Classification for Melanoma

Primary Tumor (T)	Regional Lymph Nodes (N)	Distant Metastasis (M)
Tx – No evidence of primary or unknown primary	Nx – Minimal requirements to assess regional nodes cannot be met	Mx – Minimal requirements to assess the presence of distant mets cannot be met
T0 – Atypical melanocytic hyperplasia (Clark I), not a malignant lesion	N0 – No regional LN involvement	M0 – No known distal mets
Tis – Melanoma *in situ*	N1 – Metastasis limited to 1 LN N1a – Clinically occult/ microscopic N1b – Clinically evident/ macroscopic	M1 – Distant metastasis M1a – To skin, subcutaneous tissue, or distant LN M1b – To lung M1c – To other viscera or any distant metastasis w/ elevated LDH
T1 – < 1 mm thick T1a – No ulceration and mitosis < 1/mm^2 T1b – W/ ulceration or mitoses ≥ 1/ mm^2	N2 – Metastasis in 2–3 regional LNs *or* intralymphatic regional metastasis w/out LN metastasis N2a – Microscopic only N2b – Macroscopic (clinically evident) N2c – Satellite or in-transit metastasis, but no LN metastasis	
T2 – 1.01–2 mm thick T2a – No ulceration T2b – W/ ulceration	N3 – Metastasis in 4+ regional LNs, *or* matted LNs, *or* in-transit metastasis/satellite metastasis plus regional LN metastasis	
T3 – 2.01–4 mm thick T3a – No ulceration T3b – W/ ulceration		
T4 – > 4 mm thick T4a – No ulceration T4b – W/ ulceration		

TABLE 12.19. AJCC Staging and Management for Melanoma

Stage	TNM	Management	5-Year Survival
Ia	T1aN0M0	0.5-cm margin if *in situ*; otherwise 1-cm margin	> 90%
Ib–II	T1b–T4bN0M0	1- to 2-cm margin (2 cm if > 2 mm thick) + SLNBx	70%
III	Any T ≥ N1M0	WLE, regional lymphadenectomy	60%
IV	Any T, any N, M1	WLE; regional lymphadenectomy; selective metastasectomy	10–15%

i. *W/u*:
   - If palpable LN in region, consider FNA; if inguinal LAD, consider pelvic CT.
   - If evidence of regional spread, consider CXR and LDH, PET scan.
   - If CNS sx, consider head CT/MRI.

ii. *Wide local excision*:
   - *In situ*: 0.5-cm margins. (*Note*: *in situ* dz is the only level of melanoma appropriate for Mohs.)
   - *Depth < 1 mm*: 1-cm margins.
   - *Depth 1.01–2 mm*: 1- to 2-cm margins.
   - *Depth 2.01–4 mm*: 2-cm margins.
   - *Depth > 4 mm*: 2-cm margins (some advocate 3-cm if able).

iii. *Lymph nodes*:
   - *Indications for SLNBx*: stage Ib, II. (Primary cutaneous melanoma w/ Breslow thickness > 1 mm; lesions < 1 mm w/ invasion of reticular dermis to Clark's level IV; poor prognostic indicators [ulceration, regression, lymphovascular space invasion]).
   - *Indication for regional lymph node dissection*: regional LN metastasis (established by FNA or SLNBx).
     - Unlike many other cancers (e.g., breast), regional lymphadenectomy may prolong survival in addition to decreasing rate of local recurrence. Adequate numbers of LN for dissection: groin = 10; axilla (level I–III), neck = 15.
     - *Iliac/obturator LN dissection*: indicated if Cloquet's node (+), if pelvic CT or PET (+), or (more controversial) if 3+ superficial groin LN (+).

iv. *Aduvant tx*:
   - *Immunotherapy*:
     - *IL-2*: FDA approved for metastatic dz since 1998; long-term response in only 6%, though.
     - *IFN-α2b*: FDA approved for stage IIb–III dz. May increase dz-free survival in limited subsets of pts; probably appropriate for pts w/ local dz > 4 mm thick or w/ (+) regional LN metastasis.
   - *Chemotx*: dacarbazine, temozolomide most frequently used in clinical trials for metastatic dz.
   - *Radiation*: consider for stage III pts w/ 4+ LN, particularly in head/neck or if recurrent dz.

v. *Special circumstances*:
   - *Ear*: generally requires resection of underlying cartilage and reconstruction.
   - *Face*: lymphatic drainage frequently involves parotid; operative surgeon should be prepared for parotidectomy.
   - *Trunk*: Sappey's line imperfectly predicts the lymph node drainage. Lymphoscintigraphy should be used to demonstrate drainage pattern.
   - *Subungual*: requires amputation of distal phalanx along w/ sufficient dorsal skin to achieve recommended margins; volar skin used to fashion flap. 40% 5-yr survival.
   - *Anus*: very poor prognosis. Excision to clear margins is recommended if able to preserve sphincters; otherwise, APR is performed, but the extra morbidity w/ this operation does not improve overall survival.
   - *Distant metastasis*: resection of isolated distant metastasis is often appropriate; consider HILP/infusion w/ melphalin for in-transit mets.

vi. *F/u*:
   - Complete hx and physical q 6 mo for several years, then annually.
   - CXR, LDH, LFT q 6 mo, depending on circumstances, may be appropriate.

2. *Squamous cell carcinoma* (SCCA)
   a. *Risk factors* include immunosuppression and UVA exposure. Somewhat unique to SCCA (not seen in BCCA, below), is risk of tumor in areas of chronic inflammation (i.e., Marjolin's ulcer).
   b. *Prognosis*:
      i. If < 2 cm in diameter, 5% local recurrence, 7% distant spread.
      ii. If > 2 cm in diameter, recurrence doubles, distant spread triples.

c. *Tx*:

i. *Precursor lesions* (actinic keratosis, etc.): cryotherapy, topical 5-FU, curettage, dermabrasion, CO_2 laser, etc., may be utilized.

ii. For SCCA, surgical resection preferred, generally w/ 4-mm margins appropriate for tumors < 2 cm in diameter. For tumors > 2 cm in diameter, 10-mm margins may be more appropriate.

iii. Mohs surgery or XRT may be appropriate around critical structures such as eye, nose, ear, and mouth.

iv. Regional lymph node involvement merits lymphadenectomy.

v. Adjuvant XRT if > 1 LN (+), (+) margins, which cannot be resected further, or perineural tumor involvement.

3. *Basal cell carcinoma* (BCCA)

a. *Risk factors* similar to those for SCCA. Pts w/ Gorlin syndrome (autosomal dominant: multiple BCCAs, odontogenic keratocysts, and palmar/plantar pitting) and nevus sebaceous of Jadassohn also at increased risk.

b. *Most common skin cancer w/ several variants*:

i. Nodular—most common form.

ii. Aggressive variants include morpheaform, infiltrative, and sclerosing—more likely to recur.

c. *Tx*: same as for squamous cell carcinoma. 10-mm margins should be considered for aggressive variants, regardless of size.

4. *Merkel cell carcinoma*

a. Aggressive neuroendocrine tumor from pressure receptors; 1/4 to 1/3 locally recur, and the same proportion have either regional lymph node spread a/o distant metastasis. Classically encountered on the face of older white males.

b. Histopathologically difficult to distinguish from small cell lung cancer. Get screening CXR to evaluate for the latter; staining for cytokeratin-20 also helps differentiate from small cell lung cancer.

c. *Tx*:

i. WLE w/ 2- to 3-cm margins (or Mohs surgery) recommended.

ii. SLNBx should be performed unless clinically positive dz prompts lymphadectomy instead.

iii. XRT recommended by many if either (+) LN (in addition to lymphadectomy) or if no SLNBx done.

5. *Kaposi's sarcoma*

a. Spindle-cell malignancy assoc. w/ human herpes virus 8, primarily in immunosuppressed persons, although a variety of clinical and epidemiological forms exist. Most commonly encountered in the skin (almost invariably) or GI tract.

b. *Tx*: excision (rarely performed), XRT, cryotherapy, or local injection of chemotherapeutic agent. Therapy is generally considered palliative (i.e., for GI hemorrhage).

P. Thymoma: see Chapter 8 on thoracic and esophagus.

TABLE 12.20. Therapy of Common Malignancies in Alphabetical Order*

Cancer	Surgery and Margins	Chemotx	Radiation	Comments
Breast	Stage I, II—BCT *or* MRM Stage III, IV—usu. MRM *10-mm margins ideally.	• None if < 1 cm • > 1 cm, node (–)—unless post-menopausal and ER (+) • (+) LN • Tamoxifen/AI if: > 1 cm & ER (+) or (+) LN	• If BCT used • After MRM if: T > 5 cm or > 4 LNs (+) *or* (+) margins	• SLNBx if: invasive carcinoma *or* severe DCIS (latter, DVF—see text)
Colorectal: Anus, squamous	Consider WLE if < 5 cm, no sphincter invasion APR for failure of Nigro protocol	Nigro protocol—first-line therapy	Nigro protocol—first-line therapy	

(Continues)

TABLE 12.20. Therapy of Common Malignancies in Alphabetical Order* (*Continued*)

Cancer	Surgery and Margins	Chemotx	Radiation	Comments
Colorectal: Colon, adeno	Hemicolectomy Sigmoidectomy	If > T3 5-FU + LCV	Postop if posterior extension T4 dz	Avastin may be added to 5-FU if M1
Colorectal: Rectum, adeno	Low anterior resection Abdominoperineal resection *2-cm margin good goal; 0.5 cm acceptable	If > T2 5F-U + LCV	• Preop for sphincter-sparing • Postop if T3	Avastin may be added to 5-FU if M1
Esophageal, adeno	Distal tumors: transhiatal Proximal tumors: transthoracic 10-cm margins	Neoadjuvant cisplatin + 5U	Neoadjuvant	
Gastric, adeno	Proximal: total gastrectomy w/ Roux-en-Y Mid-body: totalgastrectomy Distal: distal subtotal gastrectomy w/ 5- to 6-cm margin *All involve resecting 2 cm of duodenum and +/– omentectomy. LN dissection variable.	peri-operative ECF for ≥ T3	DFV	
GIST tumors	Segmental resection	Gleevec for high risk, recurrent or metastatic dz	NCE	
Hepatobiliary: cholangio	Lower third: pancreaticoduodenectomy Middle third: local excision and LN dissection Upper third: resect bile duct +/– caudate	NCE	C/V	
Hepatobiliary: gallbladder	Stage I: cholecystectomy Stage II/III: extended cholecystectomy— regional LN dissection, IVb/V liver resection Stage IV: palliative	NCE	NCE	
Hepatobiliary: hepatocellular	Peripheral tumor, Child's A → resect Child's B or higher → transplant ideally for local dz	NCE	NCE	• RFA • Emboliz. • Cryo • PEI
Intestine/duodenal: adeno	Pancreaticoduodenectomy vs segmental resection; 5- to 10-cm margin	NCE	NCE	
Lymphoma, NHL	Surgery not primary tx except in intestinal	Rituximab + CHOP	DVF	
Pancreas, adeno	Whipple	C/V	NCE	
Sarcoma	Resection	NCE	Adjuvant for high-grade tumors or > 5–10 cm	

(Continues)

TABLE 12.20. Therapy of Common Malignancies in Alphabetical Order* (*Continued*)

Cancer	Surgery and Margins	Chemotx	Radiation	Comments
Skin: melanoma	*In situ* → 0.5 mm WLE < 1 mm → 1 cm WLE 1–4 mm → 2 cm WLE > 4 mm → > 2 cm WLE	IFN → or IL-2 for metastatic dz	NCE	SLNBx for ≥ 1-mm depth
Skin: basal cell, squamous cell	< 2 cm, non-recur. → 0.4 cm > 2 cm, recur., aggress. → 1+ cm	Instead of excision: • 5-FU • Local IFN • Photodynamic • Systemic	DVF (may be used instead of surgery for small tumors; or adjuvant for positive margins)	Consider SLNBx
Skin: Merkel cell	WLE (i.e., 3 cm), SLNBx	NCE	C/V	

*Information in this table is extremely generalized and abbreviated, not necessarily reflecting variations common in clinical situations. Refer to text in chapter for more complete details. NCE = not commonly employed, C/V = controversial/variable, DVF = depends on various factors.

CHAPTER 13

ENDOCRINE

I. THYROID (BENIGN AND NEOPLASIA)

A. Embryology and anatomy

1. *Embryology*: descends from foramen cecum at base of tongue (branchial pouches I and II). Joins ultimobranchial bodies IV and V.
2. *Vascular*:
   a. Inferior thyroid artery arises from thyrocervical trunk, runs close to recurrent laryngeal, and also feeds parathyroids.
   b. Superior thyroid is first branch of external carotid. In minority of persons, an ima thyroidea arises from aortic arch.
   c. Superior, middle, and inferior thyroid veins drain into internal jugular.
3. *Nerves*:
   a. Internal branch of sup. laryngeal nerve provides sensation to larynx.
   b. External branch of sup. laryngeal nerve gives motor supply to tense larynx.
   c. Recurrent laryngeal inn. all other muscles of larynx.

B. Physiology

1. *Thyroid-stimulating hormone* (TSH) secreted by anterior pituitary, stimulates thyroid growth, uptake and organification of iodine, and releases of T_3 and T_4 from thyroglobulin.
   a. TSH release prompted by ↑ hypothalamic thyrotropin-releasing hormone (TRH) a/o ↓ T_3.
   b. Catecholamines and ß-hCG also stimulate thyroid function.
   c. TSH ↓ by (–) from ↑ T_3 and T_4. Glucocorticoids, prolonged starvation also ↓ thyroid function.
   d. *Wolff-Chaikoff effect*: transient ↑ in iodine organification followed by ↓ thyroid activity in response to large doses of iodine.
2. *Follicular cells*:
   a. Predominant thyroid cell type. Traps iodine by complexing w/ tyrosine to form monoiodotyrosine (MIT) or diiodotyrosine (DIT), stored intracellularly to thyroglobulin.
   b. MIT coupled to DIT results in thyroid hormone T_3 (triodothyronine). DIT coupled to another DIT results in thyroid hormone T_4 (thyroxine). Usu., ~ 2 wk worth of the hormones are bound to thyroglobulin intracellularly.
   c. *In periphery*:
      i. T_3 ↑↑ biologically active than T_4, binding directly to nuclear receptors.
      ii. Majority of peripheral T_3 derived from T_4 in plasma, liver > brain, brown fat.
         - Conversion ↓ by certain drugs (corticosteroids, propranolol, PTU) and clinical states (sepsis, brain death?) → clinical hypothyroidism.
      iii. Half-life of T_3 ~ 10 h. Half-life of T_4 ~ 7 d. Body usu. has > 1 wk worth of biologically active hormone in periphery.
      iv. Thyroxine-binding globulin (TBG) transports ~ 80% of thyroid hormones. Hormones unable to act on cells while bound.
         - During pregnancy (hyperestrogenemia), TBG levels ↑, leading to ↑ plasma *bound* T_4. As *free* T_4 is unchanged, pt remains clinically euthyroid.
3. *Pharmacology*:
   a. *Thioamides*: inhibit organification of iodine and oxidation to MIT/DIT. *Risks*: agranulocytosis (< 1%), hepatic dysfunction, rash, and arthralgias.
      i. *Methimazole* (Tapazole)
         - *Advantage*: once-daily dosing.

- *Disadvantage*: crosses placenta, contraindicated in pregnancy.

ii. *Propylthiouracil* (PTU):

- *Advantage*: additional action of inhibiting peripheral conversion of T_4 to T_3; useful for more rapid control of hyperthyroid sx vs methimazole.

b. *Lugol's solution*: high concentration of inorganic iodine. Helps control vascularity of thyroid, preparing Graves' pts for surgery.

c. *Corticosteroids*: ↓ peripheral conversion of T_4 to T_3 (like PTU and beta antagonists).

d. *Beta antagonists*: ↓ end-organ manifestations of thyrotoxicosis (HTN, tachycardia, tremor). Additionally, propanolol ↓ peripheral conversion of T_4 to T_3 (like PTU and corticosteroids).

4. *Laboratory assessment of follicular physiology*:

a. *TSH*: most sensitive assay of thyroid function, gen. reflecting pathology before sx.

b. *Total T_4*: affected by levels of serum protein, which bind much of the T_4.

c. *Free T_4 index*: serum free T_4 difficult to measure directly, so the index is calculated using the levels of total T_4 (above) and the T_3 resin uptake test (below).

d. *T_3 resin uptake test* (indirectly measures free T_4): low levels of available (measured) T_3 indicate low levels of free T_4 (means lots of binding sites were unoccupied by T_4, thus available to bind T_3). Conversely, high levels of measured (free, available) T_3 indicate large levels of T_4 (occupying binding sites, making the T_3 free to be measured).

e. *Radioactive iodine uptake* (RAIU): used to distinguish hyperthyroidism (low TSH and increased RAIU) from subacute thyroiditis (low TSH and low RAIU).

f. *Thyroid autoantibodies*

i. *Thyroid antimicrosomal antibodies*: Hashimoto's dz, Graves' dz.

ii. *Antibodies to TSH receptor*: Graves' dz.

iii. *Thyroglobulin antibodies*: assoc. w/ Hashimoto's dz.

g. *Thyroglobulin*: synthesized by follicular cells. Useful for surveillance in pts after thyroid ablation for cancer.

5. *C cells*:

a. Neural crest cells that migrate into superolateral areas of thyroid during development.

b. Produce calcitonin, which inhibits osteoclast liberation of calcium from bone (effect = decrease calcium level, though effects often not clinically significant). Calcitonin release stimulated by hypercalcemia, alcohol, a/o pentagastrin.

c. May transform into medullary thyroid carcinoma. Elevated risk MEN IIa, IIb. Serum marker = calcitonin, not thyroglobulin.

C. Benign disease

1. *Graves' dz*: indications for surgery → contraindication to RAI (pregnant, child) or question of CA.

a. *Presentation*: hyperthyroid sx such as tachycardia, weakness, and tremors may be present along w/, classically, proptosis.

b. *Dx*: circulating TSH low or absent, serum T_4 a/o T_3 elevated, along w/ FTI. Suggestive stigmata such as diffuse goiter and exophthalmos in addition to these serum tests are sufficient to make the dx. Thyroid radioactive iodine uptake will be elevated as well (45–90% localization to gland), and pts also often have high titers of thyroid antibodies.

c. *Tx*:

i. *Antithyroid meds*: best for pts who are young, pregnant, or lactating.

ii. *Radioactive iodine*: for older pts w/out above concerns, pts w/ toxic multinodular goiter.

iii. *Surgery* (subtotal thyroidectomy): for children/young adults w/ severe dz or those who want rapid response; also if unable to exclude cancer, or for tx of endemic goiter or hyperfunctioning adenoma.

2. *Goiter*: "Endemic form" from iodine deficiency, in 12% of world's population, rare in United States. 3–4% of United States population has goiter, usu. nonendemic, most often from multinodular goiter.

a. Perform careful physical exam and check TSH, T_4 levels.

b. FNA bx should be procured on single, dominant, or particularly large nodules.

i. 20% of "indeterminate" are actually malignant, whereas "benign" readings have only 1–2% false negative rate.

ii. If h/o neck irradiation, forego FNA; 40% will have malignancy, w/ less than half in the most suspicious nodule. For the same reason, forego FNA if family hx of thyroid cancer. Substernal goiters should not be assayed w/ FNA.

c. *Tx*:

i. *Medical*:

- TSH suppression w/ thyroxine does not predictably decrease goiter size, may actually induce hyperthyroidism. Only considered for young pts (less risk of arrythmias and osteoporosis) w/ small goiters who desire nonoperative management.
- Radioactive iodine more effective than TSH suppression, but may induce hyperthyroidism in ~ 5% of pts. Hypothyroidism in ~ 1/4 of pts after tx. Resistance to tx because goiters largely nonfunctional thyroid tissue. Pts w/ respiratory embarrassment may experience actual worsening of sx w/ radioactive iodine tx. Best candidates are those who are too ill from other problems to be good surgical candidates; exception is the pt w/ substernal goiter, which should always be addressed surgically because of airway concerns.

ii. *Surgical*:

- For enlarging/large, symptomatic (respiratory compromise, dysphagia, SVC obstruction), or substernal goiters. Also indicated if radiographic studies demonstrate tracheal displacement or compression, or if FNA results in malignancy concerns, or if pt has cosmetic concerns.
- Total or subtotal thyroidectomy may be pursued, depending on size, symmetry, pt's desire regarding supplemental exogenous thyroxine vs risk of recurrence. Cervical approach is almost always adequate, although median sternotomy useful for substernal goiters.

3. *Thyroiditis*

a. *Hashimoto's* (chronic lymphocytic; autoimmune): most common cause of hypothyroidism, although euthyroid state or even thyrotoxicosis may be transiently present. 15× common in women. Thyroid usu. symmetrically enlarged, may be tender. *Histopath*: demonstrates oxyphilic changes (Askanazy cells), and lymphocytic infiltrate. *Dx*: ↑ serum thyroid Ab titers. ↑ incidence of malignant lymphoma. No tx necessary if euthyroid and no goiter. If symmetrically enlarged (non-nodular) and no compressive sx, suppressive medications OK. Surgery (subtotal thyroidectomy) indicated for compressive sx; to r/o malignancy; cosmesis.

b. *Suppurative*: the rarest form of thyroiditis, most often due to *Streptococcus/Staphylococcus* and generally follows URI in children. Commonly presents w/ fever, dysphagia, neck pain. *Tx*: surgical drainage. Recurrent cases should be evaluated w/ barium swallow to r/o piriform sinus fistula.

c. *Riedel's* (struma): hard thyroid w/ fibrosis extending into surrounding soft tissues (may be assoc. w/ other sclerosing conditions such as sclerosing cholangitis and retroperitoneal fibrosis). Bx to r/o anaplastic carcinoma. Usu. hypothyroid. Surgery (division/resection of isthmus to partial thyroidectomy) frequently indicated to decompress trachea a/o esophagus.

d. *Subacute* (deQuervain's; granulomatous): usu. in relatively young (20–40 yo) women, sometimes assoc. w/ recent viral illness. Most have fever, palpitation, asthenia, malaise, wt loss, and usu. (but not always) thyroid swelling and head/neck pain. May mimic Graves' dz. *Labs*: ↑ ESR and serum gamma-globulin w/ ↓ RAIU, but normal; elevated thyroid hormone levels. Often resolves spontaneously; relief poss. accelerated w/ ASA a/o corticosteroids.

D. Neoplastic disease

1. *General*:

a. Best prognostic indicator for mortality age > 40–50 yo. *Other concerning factors*: very young age (< 15 yo), fam h/o thyroid CA or MEN II syndrome (other familial hx syndromes such as FAP, Gardner's, or Cowden's, increase risk as well), hx of head/neck irradiation, large (> 4 cm) nodule, or U/S findings of irregular border or microcalcifications.

b. W/u should include neck U/S w/ FNA.

c. Invasive thyroid carcinoma of any size usu. tx'd w/ total/near-total thyroidectomy to maximize dz-free survival.

d. *Complications* (rates for experienced endocrine surgeons):
   i. *Recurrent laryngeal nerve damage* (persistent): ~ 3% after total, ~ 2% after subtotal thyroidectomy.
   ii. *Hypoparathyroidism*: ~ 2.5% after total, < 0.5% after subtotal thyroidectomy.
   iii. *Hypothyroidism*: note, performing "only" a lobectomy may still result in hypothyroidism; pts should be counseled on this preop.

2. *Papillary*:
   a. 80% of thyroid cancers, gen. best prognosis. Type most assoc. w/ h/o head/neck irradiation.
   b. *Pathology*: concentric calcifications in psammoma bodies. Often multicentric. Mets usu. via lymphatics.
   c. *Tx*:
      i. Total thyroidectomy is generally tx of choice. Modified radical neck dissection (and level VI/central neck dissection as thyroid cancer usu. spreads here first) if clinically (+) nodes.
      ii. Lobectomy + isthmusectomy may be done in *absence* of the following: size ≥ 1 cm; fam h/o of thyroid CA; personal h/o of head/neck irradiation; clinically or histologically (+) lymph nodes; (+) margins; grossly multifocal dz; aggressive variant of papillary cancer (i.e., columnar cell, tall cell, oxyphilic, insular, or poorly differentiated).
3. *Follicular*:
   a. Unlike other thyroid neoplasms, malignancy cannot be determined w/ FNA; 80% of "follicular neoplasms" from FNA turn out to be benign.
   b. Unlike other thyroid neoplasms, metastasizes primarily hematogenously, not via lymphatics. Usu. metastasizes to bone.
   c. *Tx*: If FNA dx of follicular neoplasm and no evidence of metastasis at the time of operation, performing a thyroid lobectomy and waiting for final path is reasonable (if pt willing to undergo poss. 2nd operation). Completion thyroid done if path = malignancy.
4. *Hürthle cell* (oxyphilic cell carcinoma):
   a. Usu. considered a follicular variant, (note: a rare papillary variant occurs as well) but more commonly spreads to LN, concentrates iodine less well, and slightly worse prognosis than standard follicular carcinoma.
   b. *Tx*: similar for follicular carcinoma.
5. *Medullary*:
   a. From Clara, or "C," cells, (predominantly upper pole) secrete calcitonin (less commonly, also ACTH). 80% sporadic, but may be familial, or assoc. w/ MEN II (latter 2 both assoc. w/ RET proto-oncogene). May have flushing, diarrhea (similar to carcinoid syndrome) a/o Cushing's syndrome. Metastasizes to LNs (stage IV if outside level VI), bone, lung, and liver.
   b. *Preop*:
      i. Calcium or pentagastrin stimulation can sometimes detect occult tumor.
      ii. Baseline serum markers of calcitonin; CEA should be drawn.
      iii. For RET proto-oncogene (+) pts, r/o hyperparathyroidism, pheochromocytoma.
   c. *Operative*:
      i. Total thyroidectomy and central neck dissection for all pts w/ MTC.
      ii. Consider additional dissection (levels II–V) if tumor > 1 cm (or 0.5 cm in MEN IIb pts) or (+) LN metastasis in level VI.
   d. *Postop*:
      i. Does not uptake iodine; follow w/ calcitonin levels.
      ii. Adjuvant XRT not useful, but chemotx (usu. dacarbazine) may be considered in palliative setting.
6. *Anaplastic*:
   a. Least common, uniformly lethal. Mean age at dx older (65 yo) than other thyroid cancers. Assoc. w/ p53 mutation. Stage IV by definition. At dx, up to half have metastasized (usu. lung), most are locally unresectable. Death frequently (~ 1/2) from airway compromise. Median survival ~ 6 mo.

b. *Tx*:
   i. If CXR and CT scans suggest resectable dz, total thyroidectomy and selective LN dissection are appropriate for local control.
   ii. For unresectable tumor (majority), consider prophylactic tracheostomy.
   iii. Postop, pt should be referred for adjunctive care (i.e., combination hyperfractionated XRT and doxorubicin).

7. *Lymphoma*:
   a. More common after Hashimoto's thyroiditis.
   b. *Tx*: CHOP +/− thyroidectomy.
8. *Metastatic*:
   a. Renal cell CA followed by breast CA most common source of metastasis.
   b. MACIS (**M**etastasis, **A**ge, **C**ompleteless of Resection, **I**nvasion, **S**ize) score < 6 = 20-yr survival of 99%; > 8 = 20-yr survival < 25%.

E. **Thyroid nodules** [from Cooper DS, et al., *Thyroid.* 2006;16:109-42.]
   1. *W/u*: U/S and FNA (need 2 slides w/ 6 clusters w/ 10+ cells each) should be employed. Scintigraphic scans unnecessary.
   2. *Therapy*:
      a. *Operative*: differentiated thyroid carcinoma gen. an indication for complete thyroidectomy w/ compartmental nodal dissection.
      b. *Adjuvant*: check TSH and TG 3 wks postop. TSH > 30 required to benefit from I-131 ablation; all Hürthle cell carcinomas should be ablated. Pt should follow low-iodine diet for 2 wk prior to ablation. Adult dose is 100–200 mCi depending on stage (residual CA, [+] nodes, lung metastases). Synthroid is begun the day following ablation, then baseline total body scan 1 wk after ablation.
   3. *Surveillance*: protocol depends if low or high risk.
      a. *Low risk*: near total thyroidectomy and I-131 ablation; no clinical evidence of tumor; TG < 1 ng/mL on Synthroid; tumor < 4 cm, not of virulent subtype, no evidence of distant metastases; stage I and < 45 yo or stage II and > 45 yo; MACIS score < 6.
      b. *6-mo f/u*: *low risk*—stimulated TG (rTSH or off Synthroid), no I-131.
         i. If TG > 2 ng/mL, U/S of neck w/ bx if abnormality seen.
         ii. If bulky dz present, repeat surgery, followed by I-131 ablation.
         iii. If U/S negative, repeat I-131 ablation.
      c. *6-mo f/u*: *high risk*—Synthroid withdrawal w/ TG measurement.
         i. If TG > 2 ng/mL or significant rise from suppressed level → U/S neck w/ bx if abnormality seen.
         ii. If bulky dz present, repeat surgery, followed by I-131 ablation.
         iii. If U/S negative, repeat I-131 ablation.
      d. *12-mo f/u*:
         i. *If negative 6-mo evaluation*:
            - No scans, keep TSH suppressed and reevaluate at 12 mo.
         ii. *If positive 6-mo evaluation*:
            - Stimulated TG (rTSH or off Synthroid), no I-131 scan.
            - If TG > 2 ng/mL, U/S neck w/ bx if abnormality seen.
            - If bulky dz present, repeat surgery, followed by I-131 ablation.
            - If U/S negative, repeat I-131 ablation.
      e. *Ongoing f/u*: low risk w/ 2 negative f/u evals → annual suppressed TG; follow low but (+) TG. High risk w/ 2 negative f/u evals → annual suppressed TG; if TG > 2 ng/mL, obtain stimulated TG to see if there is further rise.
      f. *If suspect residual or recurrent dz*, pursue 1 tx w/ I-131, and if negative postablation, regard tumor now as "I-negative." Consider further eval w/ FDG PET under elevated TSH condition (rTSH or off Synthroid).

II. PARATHYROID

A. Embryology, anatomy, and physiology

1. *Embryology*: superior thyroids from 4th branchial pouch, and counterintuitively, the inferior parathyroids arise from the 3rd branchial pouch, and migrate caudally w/ the thymus, less constant in ultimate location.
2. *Anatomy*:
   a. Superior parathyroids usu. posterior to recurrent laryngeal nerve; inferior parathyroids are anterior to nerve.
   b. Blood supply generally from inferior thyroid artery of thyrocervical trunk.
      i. Unilateral adenomas feeding artery may be larger than contralateral, and useful for locating the gland.
   c. *Supernumerary glands*:
      i. 85% of pts have 4 glands. 10–15% of pts have supernumary glands. Most often in thyroid or thymus.
3. *Physiology*:
   a. *Parathyroid hormone*:
      i. Secreted by parathyroid chief cells in response to hypocalcemia levels.
      ii. In *bone*, works through cyclic AMP receptors to stimulate osteoclasts and inhibit osteoblasts.
      iii. In the *kidney*:
         - Increases distal nephron reabsorption of calcium.
         - Decreases proximal renal tubule resorption of bicarbonate, increasing chloride resorption.
           - *Chloride*: phosphorus ratio > 33 suggestive of hyperparathryoidism.
      iv. In the *gut*, PTH works indirectly through 1,25-dihydroxy vitamin D (PTH stimulates its hydroxylation from 25-hydroxy vitamin D in the kidney), promoting gut absorption of Ca^{++}, phosphorus.
   b. *Vitamin D*:
      i. D_3 (cholecalciferol): from UV-mediated activation of 7-dehydrocholesterol in skin and subsequently undergoes up to 2 hydroxylations:
         - *Liver* (first): to 25-hydroxycholecalciferol.
         - *Kidney* (second): to 1,25-dihydroxycholecalciferol.
      ii. D_2 (ergocalciferol): most common form in foods.
   c. *Calcitonin*: secreted by parafollicular cells; elevated in pts w/ medullary thyroid cancer. Stimulates calcium deposition in bone (net effect to decrease serum calcium levels), but is less clinically significant than PTH.

B. Hyperparathyroidism

1. *Primary*: elevated parathyroid hormone not caused by stimuli such as low serum calcium (i.e., parathyroid adenoma, hyperplasia, carcinoma).
2. *Secondary*: elevated parathyroid hormone in response to appropriate stimuli (i.e., low serum calcium).
3. *Tertiary*: persistence of elevated parathyroid hormone after initial stimuli have been removed. Often assoc. w/ renal transplantation.

C. Localization: Sestamibi and U/S useful for localization, pre- and intraop, respectively. Look for hidden *superior* parathyroid glands in tracheoesophageal groove along carotid sheath. Look for hidden *inferior* parathyroid glands in thymus.

D. Surgery (indicated if dx made as estimated long-term complications of asymptomatic dz ~ 20%)

1. *Adenoma* (80%): excise, bx at least 1–2 other glands.
2. *Hyperplasia* (15%—seen w/ MEN I, MEN IIa): remove 3.5 glands (or all, w/ reimplantation of 0.5 in forearm).
3. *Carcinoma* (5%): en bloc resection w/ thyroid lobe, regional lymphadenectomy.
4. *Intraop key that offending gland has been removed*: decrease in rapid PTH assay.

5. *Calciphylaxis may also be indication*:
   a. Results from dermal arteriolar calcification and patchy skin necrosis.
   b. Dx based on hx, exam, and calcium × phosphorus product ≥ 70.
   c. Skin lesions fail to heal skin grafts—most often amputation and 3.5 gland parathyroidectomy w/ 0.5 gland reimplant indicated.
6. When removing parathyroid for primarily parathyroid problem, if need to reimplant, do so in arm. If removing for other reason (i.e., vascular compromise from thyroidectomy), implant in SCM.

E. Hypoparathyroidism

1. Almost always from surgical removal of glands (i.e., thyroidectomy complication); sx from hypocalcemia, though hyperphosphatemia common as well.
2. *Tx*:
   a. Usu. hypoparathyroidism after thyroidectomy is transient (1–3 wk).
   b. *If pt has tetany*:
      i. Ensure adequate airway protection.
      ii. Calcium gluconate IV bolus (10–20 mL of 10% solution), then gtt 1 mL/kg/h (using 50 mL of 10% calcium gluconate in 500 mL of D_5W).
      iii. If refractory, check Mg^{++}. If low, give $MgSO_4$, 2–4 g/d IV.
   c. *Asymptomatic low-ionized calcium level*:
      i. Oral calcium, such as CitraCal (400 mg PO 2–4 times per day).
      ii. Add vitamin D (1,25-dihydroxycholecalciferol), 25,000–200,000 IU/d, if need to give above more frequently than 2 times per day.
      iii. Low-phosphorus diet (eliminate dairy, consider adding aluminum hydroxide gel).

III. PITUITARY

A. Embryology and vasculature

1. *Regions*:
   a. *Hypothalamus*: releases TRH, GHRH, GnRH, CRH into median eminence, through neurohypophysis to adenohypophysis.
   b. *Posterior pituitary* (neurohypophysis): releases:
      i. ADH in supraoptic nucei, regulated by osmolar receptors in hypothalamus (effects, mechanism).
      ii. Oxytocin in paraventricular nuclei in hypothalamus (effects, mechanism).
   c. *Anterior pituituary*: ACTH, GH, LH, FSH, TSH, prolactin.

B. Specific tumors

1. *Prolactinomas*
   a. *Dopamine*: inhibits prolactin secretion (bromocriptine effect).
      i. *Bromocriptine*: for prolactinomas, possibly for TSH, FSH/LH-secreting tumors
2. *Acromegaly* (growth hormone tumor)
3. *Nonfunctional tumors*: can cause *decrease* in adenohypophyseal hormones and mass effect such as bitemporal hemianopsia

C. Other syndromes

1. *Sheehan's syndrome*: postpartum infarction and necrosis of pituitary (etiology thought in part to be due from pituitary ischemia from obstetric hemorrhage a/o DIC). Sx (lactational failure, amenorrhea, adrenal insufficiency, hypothyroidism, etc.) may present soon after delivery or up to 20 yr postpartum. Certain aspects (i.e., gonadotropic) of pituitary function may be relatively spared. DI occurs in ~ 1% of cases.
2. *Nelson's syndrome*: see section IV. on adrenal below.

IV. ADRENAL (BENIGN AND NEOPLASIA)

A. Embryology and vasculature: adrenal cortex develops from mesoderm whereas medulla is of neuroendocrine origin. Arterial supply from inferior phrenic, aorta, and renal arteries. Venous drainage on right directly into IVC via multiple short veins, venous drainage on left into renal vein.

B. Adrenal insufficiency and perioperative management

1. To prevent, hydrocortisone 100 mg IV on induction, and q 8 h to total of 3 doses.

C. Syndromes

1. *Cushing's syndrome* (hypercortisolism):
   a. Most often from exogenous cortisol intake, followed by pituitary ACTH adenoma (Cushing's dz). Ectopic causes include medullary thyroid CA, thymomas, lung CA.
   b. *W/u*:
      i. *1st*:
         - Draw 24-h urine free cortisol.
         - Abstain from alcohol for 2 mo prior if possible.
         - Good to exclude hypercortisolism from depression, obesity.

      ii. *2nd*:
         - Get *low*-dose overnight dexamethasone suppression test; negative-feedback on pituitary.
         - 1 mg dexamethasone at 2300, check plasma cortisol at 0800.
         - Normal pts will suppress cortisol to < 3–5 mcg/100 cc; Cushing's pts will usu. not suppress.
         - False (+) possible w/ obesity, alcoholic, phenytoin, rifampin, estrogens, tamoxifen.
         - If still unsure, can confirm w/ CRH/dexamethasone suppression test.
            - Good for partially suppressible pituitary adenomas and nonsuppressible ectopic/adrenal lesions.
            - 0.5 mg dexamethasone q 6 h × 48 h, then 0800 bolus of CRH. Check cortisol at 15 min; 1.4 mcg/100 cc diagnostic for Cushing's syndrome.
         - If does suppress, then problem is from excess ACTH (pituitary) = Cushing's dz = most common noniatrogenic cause.
         - If does not suppress, then either have nonsuppressed pituitary or nonpituitary cause; go to next step.

      iii. *3rd*:
         - Get serum ACTH.
         - Normal = 10–100 pg/cc. If < 5, nearly pathognomonic for primary adrenal d/o.
         - If low, then primary adrenal problem (adenoma, hyperplasia, carcinoma).
         - If high, from pituitary (Cushing's dz—usu. 15–500) or ectopic source—often > 1000—go to next step (high-dose dexamethasone test).

      iv. *4th*:
         - If serum ACTH high, get *high*-dose overnight dexamethasone suppression test.
         - 2 mg dexamethasone PO q 6 h × 48 h, w/ 24-h urine for free cortisol and 17-OH steroids on second day. Also, can simply give 8 mg at 2400.
         - Cortisol will suppress if due to pituitary adenoma but not if from primary adrenal problem or ectopic ACTH source.
         - If suppresses, means pituitary source.
         - If doesn't suppress, means ectopic ACTH is problem. If still equivocal, go to CRH test.

      v. *5th*:
         - Get CRH test.
         - 1 mcg/kg ovine CRH given over 30 sec, then check plasma ACTH and cortisol q 15 min for 1 h.
         - If ACTH-independent, peak ACTH response will be < 10 pg/cc.
         - If ACTH-dependent, peak ACTH response > 30 pg/cc.
         - More useful perhaps is that w/ Cushing's dz, ACTH should increase > 35% whereas ectopic ACTH-producers rarely demonstrate any rise.
         - If ACTH increases, then pituitary adenoma.

- If ACTH doesn't change, then ectopic ACTH producer.

vi. *Note*: MIR and NP-59 scintigraphy can localize adrenal tumors, differentiating from hyperplasia.

c. *Etiology* (after exogenous administration)

i. Cushing's dz (pituitary adenoma) 68%, ectopic ACTH 12%, adrenal adenoma 10%, adrenal carcinoma 8%, adrenal cortical hyperplasia 1%, ectopic CRH < 1%, alcoholism < 1%. [Orth DN, *N Engl J Med.* 1995;332:791–803.]

ii. *Cushing's dz*: tx w/ transsphenoidal resection +/– XRT.

iii. *Adrenal adenoma*: adrenalectomy (if < 6 cm, can do posterior approach or laparoscopically) open anterior approach if > 6 cm or suspect carcinoma.

iv. *Adrenal carcinoma*: suggested by rapid progression of sx, wt gain, *virilization*, and elevated urinary 17-ketosteroids and plasma DHEA sulfate. Differentiation from CAH by presence of hypercortisolism.

- Only 50% produce hypercortisolism/Cushing's.
- MRI T-2 adrenal-to-liver ratio helpful:
  - *Adenomas* 0.7–1.4
  - *Carcinoma* (including metastatic dz) 1.4–3.0
  - *Pheochromocytoma* > 3.0

v. *Hyperplasia*: bilateral adrenalectomy (medical tx not first choice).

vi. *Pediatric*: most often adrenocortical neoplasia (adenoma vs carcinoma).

- Both carcinoma and congenital adrenal hyperplasia may cause virilization; latter typically assoc. w/ hypotension and hyperkalemia, however. See Chapter 20 on pediatric surgery.
- If < 15 yo, usu. malignant.
- *Tx*: adrenalectomy.

2. *Addison's disease* (hypocortisolism)

a. *Sx*:

i. *Chronic*: hyperpigmentation (most noticeable in non-sun-exposed areas), orthostatic hypotension.

ii. *Acute* (Addisonian crisis): hypotension, abdominal pain, N/V, fever, lethargy, hyperkalemia, hypoglycemia, altered MS, possible seizures, metabolic acidosis.

b. Critically ill pts who are excessively dependent on pressor agents for prolonged periods of time may be relatively cortisol-insufficient. Consider stress-dose hydrocortisone.

i. *UCSF protocol*: check baseline cortisol, then give 0.25 mg cosyntropin, then wait 45 min and draw another cortisol. Normal if either test > 20 or if increase > 7.

c. *Etiology*:

i. *Most often autoimmune* (may be assoc. w/ vitiligo, type I DM, Hashimoto's thyroiditis, etc., in autoimmune polyendocrine syndrome; Addison's + Hashimoto's referred to as Schmidt syndrome).

ii. *Hemorrhage* (e.g., Waterhouse-Friderichsen syndrome), infection (adrenal TB).

3. *Conn's syndrome* (primary hyperaldosteronism)

a. Classically high Na^+, low K^+, but 20% w/ normal K^+.

b. *Check renin level*: "Primary" = decreased renin. "Secondary" = elevated renin.

c. *Etiology*: aldosterone-producing adenoma >> bilateral adrenal hyperplasia >> adrenal carcinoma (secondary causes include renal artery stenosis, CHF, cirrhosis, pregnancy).

d. Suspect if diastolic HTN + K < 3.5 (< 3.0 if on diuretic).

e. Check 24-h urine K^+ and upright PRA and PAC.

f. *Screening (+) if 2 of 3*:

i. Spontaneous hypokalemia w/ inappropriate kaliuresis (> 30 mEq/d).

ii. Plasma renin activity (PRA) < 3.0 ng/cc/h.

iii. Plasma aldosterone concentration: plasma renin concentration ratio > 20.

g. *Confirmation*
   i. Supplement w/ KCl.
   ii. High Na^+ diet for 5 d, then . . .
   iii. Check 24-h urine aldosterone, Na^+, cortisol and upright PRA, serum K^+.
   iv. If elevated aldosterone, dx of primary hyperaldosteronism confirmed.
   v. Venous sampling, look for aldosterone: cortisol > 4:1.
h. *Source of primary aldosteronism*:
   i. First get adrenal CT or MRI.
      - Unilateral mass > 1 cm → dx = adenoma → unilateral adrenalectomy (give spironolactone, K^+ preop).
      - Otherwise, can get posture studies.
         - *If fall in aldosterone and 18-OH > 100 ng/dL → APA, consider to localize*:
            - Iodocholesterol (NP-59)
            - Adrenal venous sampling
            - Dexamethasone suppression
         - In general, bilateral adrenalectomy for adenomas is not performed, as resulting adrenal insufficiency is difficult to tx.
   ii. Idiopathic dz tx'd w/ spironolactone, triamterene, amiloride, or nifedipine.

4. *Incidentalomas*
   a. *Indications for resection*:
      i. Diameter > 4 cm.
      ii. Elevated 24-h urine free cortisol +/– (+) low-dose dexamethasone suppression test.
      iii. *Elevated aldosterone*: renin ratio.
      iv. Elevated urine *or* plasma metanephrines.
      v. Noncontrast CT w/ > 10 Hounsfield units *and* . . .
         - Delayed enhanced CT w/ < 50% contrast washout at 15 min *or* . . .
         - Chemical shift MRI w/ no signal drop on out-of-phase MRI.
      vi. Significant interval growth.

5. *Pheochromocytoma*
   a. *Pathology*:
      i. Derived from neural crest cells, which migrate from apex of neural tube to dorsal aorta, becoming symphathetic paraganglionic neurons, or to the adrenal gland, becoming chromaffin cells. Postnatally, extraadrenal chromaffin tissue usu. involutes. Produce epinephrine *and* norepinephrine. Epinephrine-producing cells are located near adrenal cortex exposed to high concentrations of cortisol that are required for induction of phenylethanolamine-N-methyltransferase (PNMT), required for methylation of norepinephrine to epinephrine. Extraadrenal pheochromocytomas usu. do not secrete epinephrine.
      ii. May be assoc. w/ MEN IIa, IIb (check calcium, calcitonin in addition to metanephrines); von Recklinghausen's dz (neurofibromatosis); Bourneville's dz (tuberous sclerosis); Sturge-Weber (meningofacial angiomatosis); von Hippel-Lindau (hemangioblastomas in retina, CNS, +/– renal cell CA).
      iii. Extraadrenal pheochromocytomas are referred to as paragangliomas. Typically arise in the retroperitoneum along aorta and iliac bifurcation along sympathetic chain; less commonly, they may be found in the bladder, near the trigone, and cause hypertensive crises w/ micturation. They are often multicentric, malignant in ~ 50% of the cases, may be assoc. w/ intraadrenal pheochromocytomas, are more common in children, and may be assoc. w/ the dz's listed above as well as Carney's triad (gastric epithelioid, pulmonary chondroma, paraganglioma). Cervical chemodectomas are considered distinct from these in that they are rarely functional and are usu. (–) for chromaffin staining
      iv. Like gastrinomas, thymomas, and phylloides tumors, malignancy is based on behavior, not histology.

v. *Related tumors*:
  - *Neuroblastoma*: immature derivative of sympathoadrenal tissue; see Chapter 20 on pediatric surgery.
  - *Ganglioneuroblastoma*: from immature ganglia cells.

b. *Dx*:
  i. *T_2-weighted MRI*: suspicious mass > liver ratio > 3 (< 1.4 = adenoma; 1.4–3 = carcinoma).
  ii. Clonidine will not suppress catecholamines < 500 pg/mL after 3 h w/ pheo.

c. *Localization*:
  i. T_2-weighted MRI have unique high-intensity signal.
  ii. ^{131}Iodine or ^{123}I-tagged metaiodobenzylguanidine (MIBG) may be used, but requires preparation w/ Lugol's solution.

d. *Tx*:
  i. Surgery indicated for all; laparoscopic approach increasingly accepted.
  ii. Control venous drainage first, minimize handling of gland.
  iii. Preop prep w/ alpha blocker (phenoxybenzamine) indicated for all, followed by addition of beta blocker if tachycardic. Ensure pt appropriately fluid-loaded before OR. Phentolamine useful intraop IV alpha blocker.

6. *Congenital adrenal hyperplasia (CAH)*: see Chapter 20 on pediatric surgery.
7. *Nelson's syndrome*
  a. Rapid enlargement of pituitary adenoma.
  b. 10% of postbilateral adrenalectomy.
  c. Visual disturbances, elevated ACTH, hyperpigmentation.
  d. Tx w/ surgery or irradiation although results frequently disappointing.

D. Pituitary-adrenal axis imaging

1. Pituitary best seen w/ gadolinium-enhanced MRI.
2. Adrenal best seen w/ thin-section CT or MRI.
  a. MRI benefit of suggesting carcinoma or pheochromocytoma.
3. If suspect ectopic, CT of chest may pick up bronchial carcinoids or small cell carcinoids.
  a. If no success, next image abdomen, pelvis, neck.
4. Inferior petrosal sinus sampling good to distinguish pituitary vs ectopic ACTH-producer.
  a. Sinus to plasma ACTH basal ratio of 2:1 or stimulated (CRH) 3:1 is sensitive/specific.

E. Antiadrenal medication

1. *Aminoglutethimide*: Aromatase inhibitor used in Cushing's syndrome (formerly also in breast CA) to reduce corticosteroid production. Blocks conversion of cholesterol to pregnenolone. Main side effects are hepatotoxicity and possible hypothyroidism.
2. *Mitotane*: an isomer of DDT, inhibits steroid production as well as peripheral metabolism and leads to destruction of adrenal tissue; used primarily for unresectable adrenocortical carcinoma.
3. *Metyrapone*: blocks cortisol synthesis by inhibition of 11-β hydroxylase. As this increases ACTH synthesis from pituitary, it has been historically used to help clarify source of increased ACTH (ectopic or pituitary), and occasionally for tx of Cushing's syndrome.

CHAPTER 14

UPPER GI AND GI PHYSIOLOGY

I. STOMACH

A. Anatomy and physiology

1. *Vasculature*:
   a. *Arterial*: celiac axis perfuses left and right gastric a.'s (latter comes from hepatic a.), as well as left (from splenic a.) and right (from gastroduodenal a.) gastroepiploic a.'s, which also contributes to short gastric a.'s. Most common anomaly is aberrant left hepatic a. originating from the left gastric a. (instead of the proper hepatic a.); thus proximal division of left gastric a. could potentially lead to left hepatic ischemia.
   b. *Venous*: right gastric and left gastric (coronary) veins drain into portal vein, and left gastroepiploic vein drains into splenic vein (which empties into portal vein). All other venous drainage nonportal.
2. *Vagus nerve anatomy and physiology*:
   a. *Anatomy*:
      i. *Anterior* (left) vagus gives early hepatic branch to supply liver, gallbladder, and duodenum. Main trunk of anterior vagus runs parallel to lesser curve of stomach approximately 1 cm into lesser omentum w/ branches going directly into stomach wall. At incisura, main trunk divides into smaller branches ("crow's foot"), which supply antrum and pylorus.
      ii. *Posterior* (right) vagus is larger and lies posterior and to right of esophagus in fatty tissue. Branches run to celiac axis and often to stomach fundus (this latter branch may arise in the thorax and is liable to be missed during vagotomy). Has variable position; may lie adjacent to esophagus or the anterior surface of aorta, or in between. Can palpate the lesser curve at the left gastric artery and apply caudal pressure to produce a "bowstring" effect of the nerve. Complete vagotomy hinges on division proximal to hepatic and celiac branches.
   b. *Physiology*: see section F. below on postvagotomy syndromes.
3. *Regions*:
   a. *Cardia*: Glandular elements predominantly secrete mucus.
   b. *Fundus and body*: contain *parietal cells (chief cells)*, which produce intrinsic factor (necessary for B_{12} absorption in small intestine), hydrochloric acid, and pepsinogen. Angle of His relates the fundus to the left esophagus. *Angularis incisura* relates the body to the antrum.
   c. *Antrum*: Contains *G cells* which make gastrin as well as *D cells*, which produce somatostatin.

B. Peptic ulcer disease (gastric)

1. Most common in elderly, men. 10% in United States harbor cancer. 85% colonized w/ *H. pylori*. Surgery reserved for cases refractory to medical therapy (3–6 mo), obstruction, hemorrhage, or perforation. *Divided into 5 types*: overall 10% represent malignancy. Risk ~ 5% if under 1 cm.
   a. *Type I*: lesser curvature, near incisura, *not* assoc. w/ high acid levels (many hypochlorhydric), assoc. w/ blood group A. Small, punched-out lesions, account for 60% of all gastric ulcers.
      i. *Tx*: distal gastrectomy (including ulcer) w/ Billroth I is primary. Billroth II is an acceptable alternative. Mortality ~ 3%, recurrence ~ 3%. Ulcer excision w/ highly selective or parietal cell vagotomy sometimes performed w/ mortality ~ 1%, but recurrence 5–25%.
   b. *Type II*: combination of duodenal and gastric (usu. near incisura) *are* assoc. w/ high acid levels, assoc. w/ blood group O. Account for ~ 25% of gastric ulcers.
      i. *Tx*: truncal vagotomy and antrectomy (including the ulcer), B-I preferred, but B-II acceptable reconstruction. Mortality 2%, recurrence 2%. Highly selective vagotomy w/ ulcer excision meets w/ recurrence 25%.
   c. *Type III*: prepyloric (may be multiple and usu. w/in 2–3 cm of pylorus) *are* assoc. w/ high acid levels. 15% of gastric ulcers.

i. *Tx*: truncal vagotomy and antrectomy (including the ulcer), B-I preferred, but B-II acceptable reconstruction. Mortality 2%, recurrence 2%. Highly selective vagotomy w/ ulcer excision meets w/ recurrence 44%.

d. *Type IV*: "Csendes ulcer," high on lesser curvature, w/in 1–2 cm of GE junction, *not* assoc. w/ high acid levels. Small, punched-out lesions, often assoc. w/ dysphagia and GERD.

i. *Tx*: variable. If < 2 cm from GE junction, can perform distal gastrectomy along lesser curve w/ ulcer and Roux-en-Y esophagogastrojejunostomy (Csendes procedure) may be appropriate. Ulcers > 2 cm from GE junction may be amenable to distal gastrectomy w/ vertical extension along lesser curvature to incorporate the ulcer (Pauchet, Shoemaker procedure) followed by B-I reconstruction. If large ulcer or much inflammation, a total or near-total (90%) gastrectomy w/ Roux-en-Y jejunal anastomosis is option. Less aggressive option: truncal vagotomy and antrectomy leaving ulcer in place (Kelling-Madlener procedure); multiple bx's should be taken if ulcer is not excised.

e. *Type V*: may occur anywhere in stomach, assoc. w/ NSAID usage.

f. *Emergent surgery*:

i. Hemorrhage, perforation, or obstruction, or an otherwise unstable pt may dictate a lesser procedure than described above.

- Intermittent bleeding from type I, II, or III ulcers → TV w/ distal gastric resection.
- Life-threatening hemorrhage from type I, II, or III ulcers → bx and oversew/excise ulcer + TV drainage procedure.
- Perforations (type I, II, III) in unstable pts, ulcer bx/excision w/ omentoplasty closure is indicated +/– vagotomy and drainage if pt tolerates the extra time.
  - *Note*: in the era of proton-pump inhibitors, pts w/ nonmalignant ulcers who have not been on PPI should be strongly considered to *not* have acid-reducing procedure; just repair the perforation, etc., then tx medically postop. Recurrence postop, after appropriate medical tx should receive an appropriate acid-decreasing procedure.
- Hemorrhage in type IV ulcers can be emergently addressed w/ ligation of left gastric artery, bx/oversewing ulcer through high anterior gastrostomy. Vagotomy and drainage may be added if tolerated.
- *Obstruction*: antrectomy and Billroth I (second choice, B-II). If severe scarring precludes these options, consider gastrojejunostomy.

C. Obesity surgery

1. *Definitions*:

a. *Overweight*: BMI > 25.

b. *Obese*: BMI > 30 (traditionally considered 20% over ideal body wt).

c. *Morbidly (severely) obese*: > 100 lb over ideal body wt *or* 2× or more than ideal body wt *or* BMI 40+ kg/m^2.

i. Possibly represents up to 5% of U.S. population.

d. *Super obese*: BMI > 50 (usu. 200 lb or more over ideal body wt).

2. *Physiology*:

a. Satiety mediated by CCK, ghrelin, leptin.

i. Ghrelin (from Proto-Indo-European root, *ghre*, "to grow"; also from growth hormone-releasing peptide) produced by gastric cells, stimulates appetite in the hypothalamus and is increased in low-calorie diets; gastric bypass operations, but not restrictive ones, decrease ghrelin levels. Obese persons generally have elevated plasma ghrelin levels.

ii. Leptin (from Greek, λεπτός, "small") produced by adipose tissue (coded for in chromosome 7), signaling satiety via receptors in hypothalamus. Interestingly, although leptin signals satiety, levels are usu. elevated in obese persons, suggesting possible receptor resistance. Leptin also appears to induce angiogenesis via increasing VEGF.

b. Surgery thus addresses caloric intake as well as potentially hormonal appetite drive.

3. *Indication for surgery*: BMI > 40 kg/m^2 or > 35% kg/m^2 obesity-associated comorbidities (HTN, DM, DJD, OSA, depression) in psychologically stable pt who has failed dietary therapy.

a. Proceed w/ particular caution if > 600 lb, nonambulatory, age > 60. Prader-Willi syndrome contraindication for surgery.

4. *Surgical therapy*: 2 procedures recommended by NIH: LAP-BAND and Roux-en-Y gastric bypass.
   a. *Restrictive*
      i. *Adjustable gastric banding* (LAP-BAND):
         - Adjustable band is placed laparoscopically ~ 1 cm below GE junction. Hospital stay ~ 1 d.
         - Add saline to band periodically w/ goal of 1–2 kg wt loss/wk.
         - Most pts experience loss of ~ 50% of excess wt for at least 3 yr.
         - > 1/2 of pts' HTN, DM resolve.
      ii. *Vertical banded gastroplasty*
   b. *Restrictive > malabsorptive*
      i. *Roux-en-Y gastric bypass*:
         - Most common bariatric procedure performed in United States. Can be laparoscopic or open.
         - Create 15- to 30-mL (average = 20-mL) pouch and jejunal limb 75–150 cm long (longer limb = more wt loss). Primary risk is gastrojejunostomy leak (< 2%). Can do laparoscopically or open.
         - Hospital stay ~ 3 d.
   c. *Malabsorptive > restrictive*
      i. Biliopancreatic diversion
         - Designed to inhibit absorption of fats and protein.
         - Can be laparoscopic or open.
      ii. Duodenal switch
         - Physiologically similar to biliopancreatic diversion.
5. *Complications*:
   a. Most significant complication w/ bypass procedures is anastomotic leak, which frequently first manifests as tachycardia (fever, peritonitis may be absent).
   b. Most common complication w/ banding procedures is migration of port, which can result in gastric obstruction, and even strangulation.
   c. Pts at high risk for pulmonary and thrombotic complications. Aggressive prophylactic measures appropriate.

D. **Gastric cancer:** see Chapter 12 on oncology.

E. **Postgastrectomy syndromes**

1. Up to 1/4 of pts develop attributable sx, the majority of which resolve w/ time a/o have unclear pathophysiologic basis. Reoperation is reserved for significant, refractory sx secondary to a well-defined, surgically amenable dx.
2. *Dumping syndrome*
   a. *Due to absence of pyloric "brake" from partial/total gastrectomy broadly classified into 2 forms*:
      i. *Early* (more common):
         - Fluid shifts from osmotic load (~ 30 min postprandial) cause N/V, possible diarrhea, diaphoresis, tachycardia, palpitations, etc. GI sx more common than cardiovascular.
         - Particularly common after gastrectomy + *Billroth II* reconstruction.
         - *Dx*:
           - Clinical picture frequently obvious.
           - Gastric-emptying studies (nuclear medicine) a/o provocation w/ 200 cc bolus of 50% glucose solution to reproduce sx may be considered.
         - *Tx*:
           - Frequent small meals high in protein, fat, fiber, and low in carbohydrate (esp. sugars) usu. sufficient. Separation of liquids and solids may be helpful as well.
           - Octreotide (somatostatin analogue) demonstrated to significantly decrease sx, esp. diarrhea.
           - Surgery required in < 1%.

        - Interposition of iso- or antiperistaltic 10- to 20-cm jejunal limb between stomach and small bowel most frequently used.
        - Alternately, Roux-en-Y reconstruction has been described.

    ii. *Late* (less common):
      - Rebound hypoglycemia and possible tachycardia, diaphoresis, confusion occur ~ 2 h postprandially due to excessive release of insulin in response to rapid carbohydrate load in small intestine.
      - Treat w/ diet modifications as for early dumping syndrome. Addition of pectin a/o acarbose to diet may yield additional benefit. Jejunal interposition surgery as for early dumping syndrome reserved for severe, refractory cases (rare).

3. *Afferent loop syndrome*
   a. Results from obstruction of afferent limb of *Billroth II*, and may mimic bile reflux gastritis, SBO/efferent limb obstruction, biliary dz, or pancreatitis. Mechanisms include kinking, internal herniation, anastomotic stricture, adhesions, or volvulus of afferent limb; antecolic limbs > 40 cm are predisposed to this complication.
   b. Incompletely obstructed pts present w/ postprandial crescendo pain relieved w/ bilious vomiting (w/out ingested food) $^1/_2$ to 1 h after meals. Megaloblastic anemia from bacterial stasis (bacteria bind w/ cyanocobalamin) may be seen. Elevation in LFTs a/o amylase may result from increase duodenal pressure. Complete obstruction may result in necrosis and perforation.
   c. *Dx*:
      i. Plain films +/– upper barium study may suggest the dx.
      ii. HIDA scan likewise can be of benefit.
   d. *Tx*: no effective medical solutions; surgical options include:
      i. Simply shortening the afferent limb or lysing adhesions (rarely performed).
      ii. Conversion to Billroth I anastomosis.
      iii. Conversion to Roux-en-Y.
         - Vagotomy should accompany Roux-en-Y to prevent marginal ulceration secondary to diversion of duodenal efflux.

4. *Retained antrum syndrome*
   a. Like the afferent loop syndrome above, this occurs exclusively in pts who have had *Billroth II* reconstruction after gastrectomy.
   b. Antral mucosa may extend up to 5 mm beyond pyloric musculature, and thus may be left in duodenal stump if gastrectomy does not extend far enough distally. W/ Billroth II reconstruction, this antral tissue is left exposed to alkaline secretions in the duodenal stump, w/ no buffering from acidic gastric juices. Resultingly, antral cells are stimulated to release large quantities of gastrin, leading to increased acid secretion by the parietal cells.
   c. Pts present w/ recurrent ulceration after *partial* gastrectomy and *Billroth II* reconstruction.
   d. *Dx*: although duodenal bx is the gold standard, a technetium scan may demonstrate abnormal uptake in duodenal stump.
   e. *Tx*: H_2 blockers or PPIs should be tried before considering surgical correction by either conversion to a Billroth I reconstruction or resection of retained antrum in duodenal stump.

5. *Efferent loop syndrome*
   a. Rare, usu. occurs after Billroth II reconstruction secondary to herniation of small bowel through mesocolic defect, although adhesions or other causes are occasionally responsible.
   b. Most often presents w/ intermittent abdominal (often LUQ) pain and distension, followed by bilious emesis, often w/ partially digested enteric contents.
   c. *Dx*: barium upper GI study demonstrates contrast in stomach, failing to pass through efferent limb.
   d. *Tx*: surgery is required to address causative problem—reduction of retroanastomotic hernia, closure of retroanastomotic space, lyse adhesions, revise anastomosis, etc.

6. *Bile (alkaline) reflux gastritis*
   a. Again, this occurs more commonly after Billroth II resection.

b. Presents w/ intense epigastric pain and bilious vomiting, frequently w/ wt loss and microcytic anemia as well.

c. *Dx*:

   i. Clinical hx suggestive.

   ii. HIDA scan useful to reveal bile flux into stomach/esophagus.

   iii. Endoscopy provides bx's as well as gastric aspirate for analysis (i.e., bile). Mucosa classically appears red and friable.

   iv. *Caveat*: difficult to correlate presence or magnitude of reflux w/ sx; many asymptomatic pts have evidence of bile reflux.

d. *Tx*:

   i. *Medical* tx not effective.

   ii. *Surgical* tx of choice is conversion to Roux-en-Y w/ limb at least 40 cm long.

   - If have Billroth II (usu. the case), can divide just proximial to gastrojejunostomy (leave that anastomosis intact), and bring down the proximal end to jejunum as Roux limb.

7. *Metabolic*

a. *Anemia*

   i. *Microcytic* (more common—affects ~ 1/3 gastrectomy pts)

   - Multifactorial (decreased intake, impaired absorption, poss. blood loss from inflamed mucosa).
   - *Tx*: oral iron supplementation.

   ii. *Megaloblastic* (less common)

   - Risk particularly high after > 50% gastric resection due to loss of intrinsic factor-facilitated B_{12} absorption in ileum. Check serum B_{12} level.
   - *Tx*: intramuscular B_{12} injections q 3 mo. Consider folate supplementation.

b. *Osteoporosis/osteomalacia*

   i. From impaired calcium malabsorption secondary to physiologic duodenal bypass a/o fat malabsorption leading to decreased absorption of vitamin D.

   ii. *Tx*: oral calcium (1000–2000 mg/d) and vitamin D (500–5000 U/d).

c. *Diarrhea*

   i. Steatorrhea from poor mixing of dietary fat w/ bile/pancreatic enzymes after effective duodenal bypass should be treated w/ pancreatic enzyme (and possibly fat-soluble vitamin) supplementation.

F. Postvagotomy syndromes

1. *Diarrhea*

a. 20–40% pts postvagotomy, but usu. abates after several months.

b. Mechanism poorly understood, possibly related to alterations in bile acid excretion/cycling.

c. *Tx*:

   i. *Medical*: cholestyramine (4 g PO 3 times per day w/ meals) binds bile salts and may help in persistent cases.

   ii. *Surgical*: interposition of 10-cm reversed jejunal segment ~ 80 cm from ligament of Treitz is most commonly performed procedure, but is required in < 1% of vagotomy pts.

2. *Gastroparesis*

a. Occurs to variable degree after total, but not highly selective/parietal cell, vagotomy.

b. Loss of antral pump results in *prolonged emptying of solids*.

c. Loss of receptive relaxation results in *more rapid emptying of liquids*.

d. Clinical sx range from subjective fullness to functional gastric outlet obstruction and bezoar formation.

e. *Dx*: w/u may begin w/ contrast upper GI study or scintigraphy to evaluate gastric emptying, but should include upper endoscopy at some point to evaluate anastomosis.

f. *Tx*: prokinetic agents such as metoclopramide (dopamine antagonist and acetylcholine-release potentiator) a/o erythromycin (activates motilin receptors) are given for established dx.

II. SMALL BOWEL

A. General

1. *Anatomy*
   a. *Average length 280 cm*: duodenum 20 cm, jejunum 105 cm, ileum 155 cm.
   b. *Jejunum vs ileum*:
      i. Jejunum larger diameter, thicker-walled, relatively long vasa recta in only 1–2 arcades.
      ii. "The jejunum tends to have a single marginal artery from which arise long, relatively straight branches of vasa recta. This pattern gradually blends into arcades [more distally], which travel close to the mesenteric ridge of the bowel and give rise to short branches in the ileum. The amount of fat along the mesenteric border tends to increase distally, at times encroaching the bowel in the distal aspects. The intestine tends to become thinner and paler distally, decreasing in diameter. . . . Peyer's patches are most numerous in the distal ileum, whereas plicae circulares are more prominent in the proximal jejunum." [Zuidema GD, Yeo CJ (eds.), *Shackelford's Surgery of the Alimentary Tract*, 5th ed. Philadelphia: WB Saunders; 2002: 206.]
2. *Physiology*:
   a. See Chapter 1 on fluids, electrolytes, metabolism, and nutrition for information about how and where specific nutrients are absorbed. In general, need at least 90–100 cm of small bowel to avoid short gut syndrome (parenteral nutrition dependence).

B. Duodenum

1. *Common benign pathology*
   a. *Duodenal peptic ulcers*:
      i. *Tx*:
         - *Acute bleeding*:
           - Mobilize via Kocher maneuver, apply manual pressure to posterior duodenal ulcer through anterior wall, then incise anterior surface of postpyloric duodenum ~ 2 cm. *Oversew in 3 locations*: superiorly and inferiorly in ulcer bed (targets gastroduodenal artery), and medially w/ U-stitch (targets transverse pancreatic artery). Close duodenum via pyloroplasty (read below), and add truncal vagotomy (gold standard) or HSV.
         - *Chronic bleeding refractory to medical tx*:
           - Truncal vagotomy and antrectomy (send specimen to ensure parietal cells seen in proximal margin and resect at least 1 cm distal to pylorus) is standard.
         - *Perforation* → (1) closure and omental patch +/– HSV *or* (2) closure and omental patch +/– TV.
         - *Obstruction* → (1) antrectomy and TV w/ B-I *or* (2) antrectomy and TV w/ B-II *or* (3) TV and Finney vs Jaboulay pyloroplasty *or* (4) TV and gastrojejunostomy.
         - *Intractability* → HSV (open vs laparoscopic).
   b. *SMA syndrome* (Wilkie's syndrome, cast syndrome): obstruction of third portion of duodenum caused by compression by SMA lying at an unusually shallow angle from the aorta (< 250), most often from rapid wt loss. Aortomesenteric distance also generally decreased (< 10 mm). CT scan is diagnostic means of choice. Medical tx consists of nutritional support (TPN, then frequent small feedings in "knee-chest" position, metoclopromide, etc.) Surgery (duodenojejunostomy) is reserved for refractory cases.
   c. *Duodenal diverticuli*: second most common location of intestinal diverticuli after the colon. More common in women, and persons older than 40 yo. Majority are periampullary, on the medial aspect of the C-loop. Usu. asymptomatic but may lead to hemorrhage, perforation, blind loop syndrome, cholangitis, a/o pancreatitis. Diverticulectomy via longitudinal incision and transverse closure (or whatever means compromises luminal diameter least) is most often appropriate tx.
2. *Malignant pathology*: adenocarcinoma is most common. Pts w/ familial adenomatous polyposis at high risk for periampullary polyps (and malignant transformation). Malignancy to the right of the SMA generally requires Whipple procedure.

C. Jejunum and ileum

1. *Benign pathology*
   a. *Crohn's dz*: see Chapter 15, section IB1. on inflammatory bowel dz.

b. *Sprue*: malabsorptive dz that may mimic intestinal lymphoma (conversely, consider intestinal lymphoma in "sprue" cases that do not completely respond to therapy). Frequently present w/ diarrhea/steatorrhea, wt loss, anorexia, abdominal distension, and anemia (iron- and B_{12}/folate-deficient). *Malapsorption of 2 of the 3 needed for dx*: fat, xylose, B_{12}. Bx usu. pursued.
   i. *Celiac sprue*: due to reaction to gluten (a protein found in wheat), w/ some genetic predisposition. 80% improve w/ gluten-free diet. The remainder may have another concomitant problem (i.e., lactase-deficiency) or lymphoma. Correctly dx'd cases refractory to diet therapy may (~ 50%) respond to glucocorticoids.
   ii. *Tropical sprue*: thought to be of yet-to-be-determined infectious etiology. Tx w/ 2–4 wk of abx (i.e., tetracycline) and B_{12}/folate +/– iron supplementation.

c. *Diverticular dz*:
   i. *False diverticula*: much less common than duodenal diverticula, decreasing in incidence in more distal bowel. Most frequently found along mesenteric border. Complications, such as bleeding, perforation, diverticulitis, and obstruction, are best tx'd w/ intestinal resection and reanastomosis.
   ii. *True diverticula* (contains all 3 components of bowel wall, including *muscularis*):
      - *Meckel's diverticula*:
         - Most common congenital anomaly of small bowel, resulting from failure of obliteration of vitelline (omphalomesenteric) duct.
         - *Classically follows the "rule of 2s:"* found in 2% of population; located on antimesenteric border of bowel usu. w/in 2 feet (45–60 cm) of ileocecal valve; may have 2 or more types of mucosa in the diverticulum (i.e., gastric > pancreatic >> colon, etc.).
         - Although usu. an incidental finding, the most common complication is hemorrhage (esp. in children) due to ulceration of normal ileum adjacent to gastric-mucosa (hence acid-producing) diverticulum. Much less commonly, pts present w/ obstruction or diverticulitis (more common in adults).
         - *Dx*: imaging test of choice is a Tc-99m-pertechnetate scan, which highlights ectopic gastric mucosa. Most useful in pediatric population (adults have less ectopic gastric mucosa). Sensitivity enhanced w/ pentagastrin a/o H_2 blocker. In adults (or children w/ negative scans), a small-bowel follow-through contrast study may be more helpful.
         - *Tx*: any symptomatic Meckel's diverticulum should be resected; incidentally found diverticula in children (and possibly adults [more controversial]) should probably be resected as well. If the adjacent ileum is bleeding, a segmental bowel resection and anastomosis is required; otherwise, depending on the width of the diverticulum, it may be feasible to resect just the diverticulum and primarily close the bowel (hand-sewn or stapled method).

d. *Short-gut syndrome*: sx may begin when < 120 cm of small bowel remain, and < 60 cm (often < 90 cm) requires TPN; intact ileocecal valve can lower threshold to ~ 45 cm. Numerous complications:
   i. *Diarrhea*: may be from hypergastrinemia (SB metabolizes gastrin) or bile acid malabsorption. Tx w/ fiber, H_2 blockers, PO opioids, a/o bile-acid binding medications as appropriate.
   ii. Malnutrition, fluid, and electrolyte deficiency.
   iii. *Urolithiasis* (calcium oxalate): excess binding of free oxalate in the colon results from presence of excess bile salts in colon (facilitate absorption); low dietary citrate augments propensity toward stone formation. Prevention of urolithiasis is undertaken w/ cholestyramine (binds bile salts), increased PO citrate, and avoidance of high-oxalate foods:
      - *High-oxalate foods*: beets, rhubarb, tofu, spinach, tomatoes, peanuts, nuts, poppy seeds, wheat germ, tea, cocoa/chocolate.
      - *Moderate-oxalate foods*: green beans, blueberries, blackberries, raspberries, strawberries, sweet potatoes, coffee, cocoa/chocolate.

2. *Malignant*: most common small bowel tumors—adenocarcinoma, carcinoid, GIST, lymphoma.
   a. *Adenocarcinoma*: predominantly occur in proximal small bowel (duodenum, proximal jejunum); tx w/ wide resection (10-cm margins) of bowel and mesentery.
   b. *Carcinoid*: see Chapter 12.
   c. *GIST*: see Chapter 12.
   d. *Lymphoma*: see Chapter 12.

III. THE ACUTE ABDOMEN

A. Typically sudden onset of abdominal pain that lasts > 6 h w/out improvement is surgical.

B. **General surgical causes**

1. Appendicitis, Meckel's diverticulitis, volvulus, SBO (in adults w/out h/o abdominal surgery, think about cancer, malrotation, internal hernias, Gallstone ileus, etc.), cholecystitis, pancreatitis, perforated peptic ulcer.

C. **Vascular causes**

1. AAA, mesenteric infarction, aortic dissection.

D. **Urologic causes**

1. Urolithiasis, pyelonephritis.

E. **Gynecologic causes**

1. Ectopic pregnancy, PID, mittelschmerz.

F. **Medical mimics**

1. DKA, Addisonian crisis, porphyria, sickle cell crisis, malaria, gastroenteritis.

CHAPTER 15

LOWER GI AND GI OBSTRUCTION, BLEEDING

I. COLON

A. Anatomy and physiology

1. Average 150 cm long, maximum diameter in cecum (average 7.5 cm; 10–12 cm portends perforation).
2. *Vascular*: right, transverse colon supplied by SMA: ileocolic, right colic, middle colic arteries. Left colon and sigmoid supplied by IMA: left colic, sigmoid, and superior rectal/hemorrhoidal arteries. Marginal artery of Drummond is a collateral vessel forming an arc between the SMA and IMA circulation along the mesenteric border of the colon; most vulnerable watershed area is the splenic flexure. Arc of Riolan (meandering mesenteric artery) is collateral between proximal SMA and proximal IMA of significance in the event of obstruction of either.
3. Primary function is to absorb water from stool.

B. Benign pathology

1. *Inflammatory bowel dz*: poorly understood, probably from genetic (i.e., genes NOD2/CARD15) as well as environmental influences (i.e., luminal bacterial exposure—*smoking* is strongest known factor) and mucosal immune system defect. In approximately 10–15% of cases, clinical and histologic features insufficient to distinguish Crohn's dz from ulcerative colitis. In such cases ordering serum p-ANCA (more often positive w/ UC) and ASCA (more often positive w/ Crohn's) assays may be warranted. [Information on medical management of both Crohn's dz and ulcerative colitis below in part from: Isaacs KL, et al., State of the art: IBD therapy and clinical trials in IBD. *Inflamm Bowel Dis*. 2005;11:S3–12.]
   a. *Crohn's dz*
      i. 50% involves small and large bowel, 30% exclusively small bowel, 20% exclusively large bowel.
      ii. Characterized by rectal sparing often, "skip lesions," transmural inflammation, linear ulcerations, "creeping" mesenteric fat, and granulomas. Smoking is risk factor. Incidence increasing.
      iii. *Medical management*:
         - *Aminosalicylates*: usu., active portion is bound to sulfa moiety until cleaved in the gut, activating it. Newer generations lack the sulfa component, making them better tolerated, able to be given in higher doses.
            - *Mesalamine/5-aminosalicylate/5-ASA* (*Pentasa*, slow-release) and *Asacol* (pH-dependent release) allow drug release in proximal gut, useful for small and large bowel dz. *Rowasa* is given as enema. *Sulfasalazine (Azulfidine)* may be given as regular and delayed-release oral tablets.
         - *Corticosteroids*: used to induce remission (not for maintenance), successful 70% of time after 1 mo. Tapered after improvement.
            - *Budesonide*: high topical potency, low systemic absorption w/ high first-pass effect. Its delivery is pH-dependent (due to coating), delivered to terminal ileum/cecum. Efficacy almost as good as prednisone.
         - *Immunosuppressant medications*
            - *6-mercaptopurine (6-MP)*: used as steroid-sparing drug to maintain remission, generally begun after corticosteroid-induced remission, w/ response lagging up to 4 mo. Potential myelosuppression warrants following CBC. Pancreatitis is another risk.
            - *Azathioprine (AZA, Imuran)*: precursor to 6-MP, can be used as alternate to 6-MP.
         - *Anti-TNF-α antibody*
            - *Infliximab*: chimeric mouse antibody to TNF-α, give for cases refractory to steroids or immunosuppressants (2/3 respond, 1/3 remit). Side effects to infusion in ~ 20%, and repeated doses may result in antichemeric antibodies; often given w/ immunosuppressants to prevent this.

iv. *Surgical management*:
- Most pts will ultimately require some surgical intervention.
- *Indications for surgery* (in decreasing order of frequency): obstruction, internal fistula, perianal dz, abscess, perforation, toxic megacolon.
- Resection and anastomosis has lower complication rate than strictureplasty, but risk of short gut syndrome should be borne in mind if large segments involved. Risk of Crohn's recurrence is not affected by choice of resection vs strictureplasty. Only resect grossly involved bowel.

b. *Ulcerative colitis*

i. Idiopathic inflammatory condition of colon clinically characterized by episodic diarrhea and rectal bleeding.

ii. Exclusively large bowel dz, although "backwash ileitis" may occur. Involves contiguous bowel, from anus retrograde. May lead to "lead pipe" colon. Microcrypts, pseudopolyps, mucosal ulceration.

iii. *Medical management* (approach as a pyramid):
- *ASA* best agent for induction as well as maintenance of mild dz. Total dose more important than route (PO vs rectal). Higher doses of mesalamine (> 1.2 g/d) may additionally afford some protection against colorectal cancer for UC pts.
- *Steroids* are indicated for moderate dz.
- *AZA* (precursor to 6-MP) is an immunomodulator, indicated to induce remission for moderate to severe dz, provide maintenance, and help avoid steroids.
- *Cyclosporine* may be added for severe cases, usu. as last line before surgery.
- Non-FDA-approved adjuncts include fish oil, nicotine, probiotics, and biologics.

iv. *Surgical management*:
- Less than 20% of pts after 20 yr of dz will have had surgery for UC.
- *Indications*: toxic megacolon, hemorrhage, perforation, failure of medical management, or malignancy. Dysplasia may be indication for surgery (esp. if assoc. w/ a lesion), but histologically can be difficult to differentiate from reactive atypia. Therefore, finding of dysplasia in acutely inflamed colon warrants repeat bx after inflammation subsides, according to some authors.
- *Procedure choice*:
  - *Three issues*: emergency or elective; should rectum be resected; should intestinal continuity be restored.
  - Total/subtotal colectomy and ileostomy usu. indicated for emergent indications (hemorrhage, perforation, etc.). < 15% will have continued sx after this, and a minority of these cases will need proctectomy.
  - Proctocolectomy w/ pouch-anal reconstruction is the usual procedure for elective cases.
    - Kock continent ileostomy rarely used for reconstruction anymore.
    - Ileostomy construction is safest procedure after proctocolectomy but requires appliance. *Indications* (contraindications for IPAA): Crohn's, prior extensive small bowel resection, perineal dz, anorectal dysfunction, malignancy in lower rectum, and poor systemic physiology.

2. *Diverticulitis*

a. *Colonic diverticuli*: M = F; 10% at 40 yo, 75% by 80 yo; 10% right colon; 80% asx, 95% involve sigmoid, 65% in sigmoid only; 10–20% will develop hemorrhage or diverticulitis.

b. *Diverticulitis*

i. Will occur in 20% of pts > 40 yo, caused by inspissated stool obstructing neck, increasing intraluminal pressure.

ii. 10–15% of cases will have free perforation, and generalized peritonitis; more common in immunosuppressed.

iii. *Sx*: pain, esp. LLQ; F, malaise; change in bowel habits; urinary sx (frequency, nocturia) from pericystic inflammation. 3–5% will have colovesical fistula, may have pneumaturia or recurrent polymicrobial UTIs. TTP, guarding; ileus or bowel obstruction; palpable mass, esp. on pelvic or rectal exam; guaiac-positive stool. Check CBC, UA.

iv. *Dx*: CT scan test of choice. Contrast enema less common. Flex sigmoidoscopy w/ minimal insufflation may be used to r/o perforated CRCA.

v. If surgery not chosen/indicated, colonoscopy mandatory after acute phase if bleeding or possible CRCA radiographically.

vi. *Tx*: cases can be broadly classified into uncomplicated and complicated.

- *Uncomplicated* (~ 75%): clinically, LLQ pain, fever, leukocytosis. Radiographically, CT w/ local inflammation w/out evidence of pericolonic abscess, bleeding, or free perforation.
  - Tx w/ bowel rest, IV vs oral abx (fluoroquinolone + metronidazole most commonly), and IV fluid resuscitation.
  - *Outpt*: if mild TTP, low-grade fever, can tx w/ oral abx 7–10 d; high-fiber diet w/ psyllium.
  - *Inpt*: NPO, IVF, +/– NGT.
    - Parenteral abx (for GNR and anaerobes) for 7–10 d, or until AF w/ normal WBC and NT exam.
    - Clear liquids, then low-residue diet 2–4 wk after acute attack; then high-fiber diet w/ psyllium. More effective for pain control than for decreasing complications.
  - Of those admitted, 50% will not be resolved w/ conservative therapy. 30% of inpts will develop free perforation. 9% will have urinary fistulas. 1% will have right-sided dz only.
  - If sx do not improve w/in 48 h, consider repeat CT scan w/ contrast. Abscess or extracolonic air/contrast suggest failure and need for operation.
- *Complicated* (~ 25%): clinically, peritonitis or obstruction. Radiographically, CT w/ perforation (or pneumoperitoneum on KUB), abscess, or fistula.
  - If no peritonitis, isolated abscess may be drained percutaneously, followed by semi-elective surgery.
    - Otherwise, surgical intervention indicated.
  - The Hinchey score stages of perforated dz:
    - *Stage characteristics*:
      - I—pericolic inflammation LLQ TTP.
      - II—pericolic retroperitoneal abscess LLQ TTP.
      - III—general purulent peritonitis diffuse TTP, rebound.
      - IV—general fecal peritonitis diffuse TTP, rebound.
- *Other*:
  - *Before any surgery done after resolution of acute inflammation,* a preop colonoscopy is performed if possible to exclude the possibility of carcinoma, as 10–20% of cases initially diagnosed as diverticulitis ultimately are found to harbor neoplasm.
  - Most surgeons recommend surgery for any repeat episodes of diverticulitis, or any episode in pts under 50 yo, but this remains controversial.
  - *Surgical strategies*:
    - *Single stage*: usu. elective cases w/ prepped bowel; resect, primary anastomosis.
    - *Two stage*: if anastomosis not safe due to bowel edema or gross contamination. First, resect colon, perform end colostomy and either mucous fistula or Hartmann pouch. (Alternatively: resection and anastomosis w/ prox diverting colostomy.) Second, reanastomosis after 2–6 mo.

II. ANORECTAL

A. Anatomy and physiology

1. *Rectum*: ~ 13 cm long, no taeniae (they merge together). Anterior 1/3 of proximal rectum covered by peritoneum. Peritoneal fold/reflection ~ 7 cm from anal verge.

2. *Anal canal*: 4 cm from anal verge to anorectal ring proximally. Lined w/ up to 14 columns of Morgagni, each of which contains cryptoglandular structures significant in anal fistula dz.
3. Proximal to dentate line, pink, lined by columnar epithelium. Distal to dentate line, lined by paler squamous epithelium.
4. *Internal sphincter palpable* ~ 1.5 cm distal to dentate line, essentially a thickening of smooth (involuntary) circular rectal muscle.
5. *External sphincter palpable* just distal to internal sphincter (intersphincteric groove between the 2), consists of voluntary, striated muscle from pelvic floor (contiguous w/ levator ani and puborectalis). Innervated by internal pudendal nerve and S4.
6. *Vascular supply to anorectal region*:
   a. *Proximal rectum*: *superior rectal (superior hemorrhoidal) artery*—last branch of IMA.
   b. *Distal rectum/anus*:
      i. *Middle rectal (hemorrhoidal) artery*—branch of internal iliac (hypogastric) artery.
      ii. *Inferior rectal (hemorrhoidal) artery*—branch of pudendal artery (which comes off of hypogastric artery).

B. Benign pathology

1. *Hemorrhoids*
   a. Cushions of soft tissue and blood vessels at right anterior, left lateral, and right posterior locations, which aid in fecal continence.
   b. *Internal* (proximal to dentate line, relatively insensate):
      i. *Sx*: bleeding a/o prolapse. Anal fecal/mucus leakage, pruritus also possible.
      ii. *Grades* (by degree of prolapse):
         - *1st degree*: no prolapse
         - *2nd degree*: spontaneously reduces
         - *3rd degree*: requires manual reduction
         - *4th degree*: cannot be reduced (strangulated)
      iii. *Dx*: DRE, anoscopy, and, particularly if pt > 40 yo, anemic, unimpressive hemorrhoids, or significant family h/o colorectal cancer, proximal endoscopy is indicated.
      iv. *Tx*:
         - Dietary fiber supplementation.
         - Most 2nd, 3rd degree → banding, although other options (sclerotherapy, heater probe, etc.) exist. Avoid banding if immunocompromised, due to risk of sepsis.
         - Surgical hemorrhoidectomy if refractory or 4th-degree internal hemorrhoids, and internal hemorrhoids w/ any of the following: symptomatic external hemorrhoids, fissure, fistula-in-ano, or large anal tags.
   c. *External* (distal to dentate line, covered w/ anoderm, sensate):
      i. *Sx*: relatively minimal (hygiene-related, usu.), unless thrombose (severe pain).
      ii. *Tx*:
         - Conservative management (i.e., dietary modification) usu. sufficient.
         - Consider excision if symptomatic and other indication for internal hemorrhoidectomy.
         - Excise/evacuate thrombosed external hemorrhoids w/in 72 h of thrombosis.
2. *Anal fissure*
   a. Painful linear ulceration of anal mucosa, usu. posterior midline, often assoc. w/ sentinel tag. Less often at anterior midline. *Sx*: pain w/ defecation +/– blood on stool/toilet paper.
   b. *Dx*:
      i. Physical exam should include gently spreading buttocks to visualize anus.
      ii. Invasive probing (anoscopy, etc.) usu. prohibitively painful in the clinic setting.
      iii. Location other than described above should prompt w/u for other etiology (i.e., Crohn's dz, STD, etc.).

c. *Tx*:

i. *Medical*

- Early dz (i.e., w/in 3 wk of onset) → dietary fiber and Sitz baths.
- Chronic lesions → above +/– topical NTG paste 3 times per day (0.2% preparation). Side effects such headaches may limit compliance. Try (2%) diltiazem if unable to tolerate NTG. Botox less frequently used: invasive, more expensive, poss. have higher recurrence rates.

ii. *Surgical*

- Failure of conservative tx → lateral internal sphincterotomy, which may be performed in an "open" or "closed" fashion; primary complication risk is fecal incontinence. Rate of recurrence should be no higher than 10%.
- Anorectal advancement flap if failure of LIS or significant stenosis of the anal canal.

3. *Perirectal abscess*

a. Cryptoglandular suppurative process that begins in the intersphincteric plane at the level of the dentate line, often spreading in one or more of several directions.

i. *Intersphincteric abscess*: abscess remains localized to original site. May manifest as deep anal pain, dyschezia in a pt w/out obvious visible source.

ii. *Perianal abscess*: caudad tracking of intersphincteric abscess toward external margin of anus; tender perianal mass. DDx should include thrombosed external hemorrhoid.

iii. *Intermuscular abscess*: cephalad tracking of intersphincteric abscess w/in confines of rectal wall. Sx often vague, may require CT, U/S, or EUA for dx.

iv. *Supralevator abscess*: cephalad tracking of intersphincteric abscess above levator. Sx often vague, may require CT, U/S, or EUA for dx.

v. *Ischiorectal abscess*: spread of abscess across external sphincter into ischiorectal fossa (alternately, pus may spread across internal sphincter into anal canal).

vi. *"Horseshoe abscess:"* circumferential spread of abscess in intersphincteric, supralevator, or ischiorectal spaces.

b. *Dx*: based on hx and physical exam. Occasionally, CT or other imaging useful for evaluating complex abscess anatomy.

c. *Tx*: wide incision and drainage.

i. *Intersphincteric*: drain via division of internal sphincter at level of abscess.

ii. *Perianal*: drain through incision in overlying skin.

iii. *Intermuscular*: drain through incision through rectal/anal mucosa.

iv. *Supralevator*: drain through incision through rectal mucosa.

v. *Ischiorectal*: drain widely through incision through overlying skin and soft tissue. Spreading w/ hemostat, finger, etc., appropriate to break up loculations.

vi. *Horseshoe*: drain through posterior midline incision extending from the coccygeal tip anteriorly to (but not through) the external sphincter. Counterincisions in the perineum for drainage may be appropriate.

4. *Perianal fistulas* (fistula-in-ano)

a. ~ 1/4 of perirectal abscesses develop this, less often from other dz (i.e., Crohn's dz).

i. *Intersphincteric* (most common): usu. follows path of perianal abscess (caudad to anal margin), although may track cephalad. Remains in intersphincteric space, medial to external sphincter.

ii. *Transsphincteric*: passes through external sphincter into ischiorectal fossa, ultimately opening into perineum.

iii. *Suprasphincteric*: uncommon and difficult to tx. Courses cephalad over puborectalis/levator before turning downward to perineum. To open tract, must divide all muscles necessary for continence. Additional high tracts parallel to rectum may be present.

iv. *Extrasphincteric*: rare, frequently due to noncryptoglandular dz (Crohn's, radiation, trauma, malignancy, etc.). Tract is lateral to both sphincter mechanisms, running from rectum to perineal skin. May be able to palpate indurated tract; may also have anal canal opening as well, depending on etiology.

b. *Dx*
   i. Exam under anesthesia w/ anoscopy, palpation (for induration), and probing internal opening along dentate line (for fistula from cryptoglandular dz) is required. If can't identify internal opening, inject external opening w/ H_2O_2 a/o methylene blue through angiocatheter or pediatric feeding tube.
      - *Goodsall rule*: if perineal opening anterior to line passing through ischial tuberosities, tract should pass to anal canal in a straight radial path (i.e., if skin opening is at 3 o'clock in the perineum, the anal canal opening should be roughly at 3 o'clock). If perineal opening posterior to the imaginary line, tract usu. courses around to open in the posterior midline anal canal. *Exception*: anterior fistula on the perineum > 3 cm (suggests prior horseshoe abscess) from anus frequently course to posterior midline, not in a straight radial path. Rule is more accurate for posterior than anterior abscesses. [Cirocco WC, Reilly JC, *Dis Colon Rectum*. Jun 1992;35(6):537–42.]

c. *Management*
   i. Must drain infectious (usu. cryptoglandular) source and fistula tract.
   ii. Intersphincteric fistulas → unroofed via division of interposed internal sphincter musculature (fistulotomy) over a probe. To preserve continence, setons should be used if > 1/2 of the internal sphincter is involved (or for anterior fistulas in females).
   iii. *Large, complicated fistulas (or recurrent) above sphincter mechanisms can be approached w/*:
      - Seton (i.e., thin Penrose drain that is sequentially tied tighter in outpt visits).
      - Fibrin glue.
      - Mucosal advancement flap: lift up rhomboid flap (wider at proximal base) including mucosa, submucosa, and internal sphincter, and advance to suture w/out tension over debrided base w/ fistulous opening ligated closed w/ absorbable suture.

5. *Rectal prolapse*
   a. Most frequently seen in multiparous older females, often accompanied by constipation a/o fecal incontinence.
   b. Important to differentiate full-thickness/complete prolapse (procidentia), which has *circumferential* folds, from mucosal prolapse, which has *radial* folds.
   c. W/u should address cardiopulmonary status, and also include barium enema or colonoscopy (look for lead points), anorectal manometry, cinedefecography, EMG, and colon transit studies.
   d. *Surgery*:
      i. *Transabdominal approach*: 0–5% recurrence.
         - *Rectopexy*
            - Use for complete prolapse; contraindicated in pts w/ constipation.
            - Mobilize and fix rectum to presacral fascia.
            - Ripstein procedure is rectopexy w/ Marlex mesh. Ivalon sponge may be used instead. Complication assoc. w/ these procedures is erosion of foreign body into bowel. Instead, using permanent suture is preferred.
         - *Resection and rectopexy* (Frykman-Goldberg procedure)
            - Use for complete prolapse w/ constipation.
            - Mobilize, resect redundant sigmoid colon, then suture rectal lateral ligaments to presacral fascia w/ permanent suture.
         - *Total abdominal colectomy* (w/ ileorectostomy or ileodescending colostomy)
            - Use for slow transit (colonic inertia) constipation w/ prolapse.
      ii. *Perineal approach*: 10–25% recurrence—reserved for pts too frail for transabdominal operations.
         - *Thiersch wire*
            - Places a nonabsorbable band (suture, tubing, etc.) SC around the anus as a cerclage. Procedure does not treat underlying disorder, and is assoc. w/ complications such as fecal impaction and pelvic sepsis from erosion of the prosthetic. Rarely performed.

- *Delorme procedure*
  - Use for mucosal prolapse *or* low complete prolapse *or* internal intussusception.
  - Resect 10–25 cm of circumferential sleeve of rectal mucosa. Plicate underlying muscular wall w/ absorbable sutures. Reanastomose mucosal edges. Can do under local/spinal/epidural + sedation.
- *Perineal rectosigmoidectomy* (Altemeier procedure)
  - Use for complete prolapse in the elderly or otherwise poor surgical risk.
  - Make full-thickness incision 1–3 cm above dentate line (w/ rectum prolapsed). Divide and ligate mesentery of involved bowel. Transect bowel and anastomose free edges. Plicate levator ani anteriorly.

6. *Rectovaginal fistula*
   a. Most common causes include trauma (esp. obstetric), neoplasm, irradiation, and inflammatory bowel dz. Pts typically complain of abnormal vaginal drainage (stool, air, mucous, blood, etc.).
   b. Broadly classified into high (require transabdominal repair) and low (amenable to perineal repair).
   c. *Tx*:
      i. *Medical*: some fistulas, particularly those from inflammatory bowel dz, may close spontaneously or w/ medical tx (i.e., infliximab for Crohn's dz).
      ii. *Surgical*:
         - *Low*:
           - Endorectal advancement flap.
           - Transperineal repair (fistula excision, muscle reapproximation, etc.).
         - *High*:
           - Transabdominal repair (fistula excision, layered repair, possible pedicled tissue interposition, possible bowel resection).
7. *Pouchitis*
   a. Pts who undergo colectomy w/ creation of a "pouch" may experience inflammation or "pouchitis," manifesting as diarrhea, bleeding, malaise, fever, etc.
   b. *Tx*: abx therapy (fluoroquinolone or metronidazole) generally effective. Refractory cases may benefit from topical mesalamine, or infliximab.
8. *Radiation proctitis*
   a. May occur wk to yr after rectal exposure to radiation (i.e., prostate CA XRT tx), manifesting w/ pain/tenesmus and bleeding.
   b. *Tx*: variety of topical therapies may be effective (steroids, sucralfate, 4% formalin).
9. *Pilonidal dz* (L. *pilus* = "hair" + L. *nīdus* = "nest")
   a. Pattern of acute or chronic inflammatory changes generally in the soft tissues of gluteal cleft in young adults, thought to be due in part to hair follicles.
   b. *Tx*:
      i. *Acute*: incision and drainage followed by packing of the abscess or sinus cavity is appropriate. Shaving the local region may help prevent recurrence.
      ii. *Chronic*: division of sinus tracts, curettage of sinus cavities, a/o excision of affected tissues. Marsupialization or flap coverage may be required.
10. *Hidradenitis suppurativa*: see Chapter 4 on infectious disease.
11. *Condyloma acuminatum* (Gk. *kōndylos* = "knuckle" + L. *acūminātum* = "pointed")
   a. "Genital warts" resulting from infection w/ HPV (6, 11, 16, 18, etc.), assoc. w/ anal intercourse and HIV. Rarely grows to giant "Buschke-Löwenstein" tumors, which may harbor SCCA; tx is wide local excision to include dermis. Poor surgical candidates → interferon/CO_2 laser/imiquimod.
   b. *Dx*: ddx—molluscum contagiosum (classically w/ umbilicated center), anal papillae, and secondary syphilis. Include anoscopy and proctoscopy to eval if in anal canal.
   c. *Tx*: recurrence is common.

i. Sharp excision w/ fine scissors provides suitable tissue for pathology and is minimally destructive.

ii. Topical podophyllin for perianal warts.

iii. Bichloracetic acid may be used for perianal or intraanal warts.

iv. Electrocautery excision a/o fulguration or CO_2 laser usage requires aspiration of vapors a/o masks.

III. APPENDIX

A. Anatomy and physiology

1. Blood supply from appendiceal artery from ileocolic artery from SMA.
2. Most commonly retrocecal position; find by tracing back taenia coli to confluence. Gravid uterus displaces cephalad.

B. Appendicitis

1. *Epidemiology/etiology*:
   a. M > F w/ bimodal age distribution, median age early 20s.
   b. From luminal obstruction most commonly from lymphoid hypertrophy (younger pts) > fecolith or stricture (older pts) > tumor.
2. *Presentation and dx*:
   a. *Clinical dx*: hx typically vague epigastric pain, gradually localizes, becomes more intense in RLQ, accompanied by N/V.
      i. Peritonitis inferred from pain w/ movement (i.e., walking) or pain w/ tapping heel.
      ii. Risk of rupture higher in very young and in elderly.
      iii. *Psoas sign*: pain w/ extension/hyperextension of right thigh.
      iv. *Obturator sign*: pain w/ passive external rotation of right hip w/ hip and knee flexed 90°.
      v. *Blumberg's sign*: eponym for rebound tenderness. *Note*: percussion may be just as useful, probably more humane (and specific for peritonitis).
      vi. *Rovsing's sign*: pain in RLQ w/ LLQ palpation.
   b. *Ddx*: urolithiasis, UTI (get *urinalysis* on all pts), gyn pathology (get *β-hCG* on all reproductive-age females, ectopic pregnancy, ovarian cyst, PID, etc.), diverticulitis, perforated peptic ulcer, IBD, etc.
   c. Radiographically, noncontrast helical CT (97% accurate) recommended for reproductive-age females, pts who will be observed, or those who may be d/c'd w/out reliable means for f/u (criteria: diameter > 6 mm, stranding in periappendiceal fat). U/S typically not useful except in children (criteria: diameter > 6 mm, no gas in lumen).
3. *Tx*:
   a. *Abx*:
      i. *Abx tx alone for early appendicitis* ("Ochsner treatment" [Ochsner AJ, *JAMA*. 1901;36: 1747–54]) not appropriate, although it is an important adjunct to timely operative intervention.
      ii. *Preferred*: ampicillin/sulbactam (Unasyn) 3 g IV q 6 h; piperacillin/tazobactam (Zosyn) 3.375 g IV q 6 h; ticarcillin/clavulanate (Timentin) 3.1 g IV q 6 h; ertapenem 1 g IV q d.
      iii. *Alternate*: cefoxitin 2 g IV q 8 h; cefotetan 2 g IV q 12 h; ciprofloxacin 400 mg IV q 12 h + metronidazole 500 mg IV q 6 h.
      iv. *Severe/life-threatening/ICU abx*: imipenem 500 mg q 6 h; meropenem 1 g IV 8 h.
   b. *Appendectomy*:
      i. First performed by Amyand in 1735. Term coined by Fitz in 1886.
      ii. ~ 20% negative celiotomy rate generally acceptable. Higher rates seen in females of reproductive age. Lower negative rates seen in males.
         - Finding of normal appendix should prompt intraop exploration for other sources such as Meckel's diverticulitis, Crohn's dz, sigmoid diverticulitis, perforated peptic ulcer, gynecologic source (i.e., PID, ovarian torsion), etc. Appendectomy should still be performed to diminish future diagnostic difficulty.
      iii. *Laparoscopic appendectomy*:
         - W/ experience, takes the same or less time than open w/ equal or lower complication rate and less hospital time.

- *Added benefit*: look for other pathology if appendix normal and search for mets if appy tumor found.
- Assoc. w/ significantly lower wound infection rates (but slightly higher rate of intraabdominal abscess) than open; however, it is more expensive than open.
- Advocated by many for reproductive-age females, for obese pts, and by some for pts over 50 yo.

iv. In pregnancy, premature labor generally responds to tocolytics.

v. *For complicated appendicitis*:

- *Pregnant pts*: appendix rises above iliac crest by 5 mo. Clinical suspicion of appendicitis warrants surgical exploration (laparoscopic or open) regardless of gestational age.
- *Perforated*: important to adequately resuscitate before performing appendectomy. Maintain postop abx for a wk, or at least until pt is afebrile w/ normal WBC.
- *Abscess* (L. *abscessus* = "a going away" or "separating off"): percutaneously drain, perform interval appendectomy if pt responds to drainage and abx (otherwise need to operate sooner, despite increased risk of complications such as fistula).
- *Phlegmon* (Gr. *phlegmonē* = "inflammation"): inflammatory mass not amenable to percutaneous drainage. Unless pt has frank peritonitis, nonoperative management (NPO, IV abx) is reasonable. If pt does not improve w/in 48–72 h, operation indicated. Otherwise, interval appendectomy in 6–8 wk appropriate.

c. *Postop care*:

i. If purulent peritoneal fluid, close fascia only, leave skin open, keep on IV abx until AF, normal WBC.

ii. If not ruptured or otherwise complicated, 1–2 doses of postop abx.

C. Appendiceal tumors

1. Malignancy found in ~ 1% of appendectomies. Carcinoid > malignant (metastatic > primary) > benign other. [Collins DC, *Am J Proctol*. 1963;14:365, and Schmutzer KJ, et al., *Dis Colon Rectum*. 1975;18:324.]
2. *Carcinoid*: majority in distal $^1/_3$ of appendix, forming a discrete rounded tumor, and usu. < 1 cm.
3. Malignant (usu. metastatic adenocarcinoma, most often w/ primary colorectal CA). High incidence of synchronous and metachronous colorectal CA.
4. Frozen section should be performed on tumor, suspicious lymph nodes.
5. Appendectomy often adequate. Right hemicolectomy indicated for carcinoids > 1.5–2 cm in diameter (or those involving the base at junction w/ cecum), adenocarcinoma, and adenomas w/ uncertain margins/invasion.

IV. GI HEMORRHAGE

A. General

1. > 80% self-limited. > 80% of GI bleed admissions are for upper GI sources (peptic ulcers, varices), ~ 15% for colon (diverticulitis, angiodysplasia), ~ 3% small bowel.
2. < 10% require surgery. For hemodynamically significant bleeds, mortality is 5–12%, related to hypotensive effects on comorbidities.
3. Hematemesis characteristic of upper GI bleed. Melena, hematochezia may represent upper or lower GI bleeding.
4. Good PMHx and medications essential. In pts w/ alcoholic liver dz, 1st episode equally likely to be variceal or nonvariceal, but after 1 episode of variceal hemorrhage, subsequent bleeds have at least 70% probability of being variceal.
5. *Initial management*:

a. 2 large-bore IVs, begin infusion of (usu.) lactated Ringer's. Foley, OGT/NGT. If significant hematemesis, intubate pt to protect airway.

b. *Identify source*:

i. Lavage stomach through OGT/NGT. If returns blood or "coffee grounds" (or if present w/ hematemesis), prepare pt for emergency endoscopy. If lavage (–) but index of suspicion is high, upper endoscopy reasonable given that a competent or spastic pylorus can prevent return of blood on lavage from duodenal bleed.

ii. If lavage (–) or otherwise upper source ruled out, manage for lower GI bleed (see section C. below).

B. Upper (proximal to ligament of Treitz)

1. *Peptic ulcer*
   a. Hemorrhage from stomach and duodenum equally common (together ~ 50% of upper GI sources).
   b. Approximately 1/2 of cases due to *H. pylori* (~ 1/3 due to NSAIDs). Highest risk ulcers for bleeding are in posterior duodenum.
   c. *Likelihood of endoscopic failure* (rebleeding):
      i. Visible vessel, 40–80%; nonbleeding clot, 20%; pigmented spot ulcer, 10%; clean ulcer, rare.
      ii. *Forrest classification:*
         - *FI*: active bleeding.
         - *FIIa*: visible vessel or pigmented protuberance in ulcer.
         - *FIIb*: adherent clot in ulcer.
         - *FIIc*: pigmented spot in ulcer.
         - *FIII*: clean ulcer.
      iii. Ulcer size > 2 cm independent risk factor for rebleed.
   d. *Medical management*
      i. Cease NSAIDs, *H. pylori*, PPI/H_2 blocker tx as indicated for outpt management; rescope in 6 wk.
      ii. *Endoscopy*: electrocoagulation, LASER, injection (epinephrine, sclerosant).
      iii. 20% of pts fail initial endoscopic management, w/ virtually all rebleeding beginning w/in 4 d.
         - Repeat endoscopy successful in ~ 1/2.
   e. *Surgical management*
      i. Required for ~ 10% of ulcer bleeding, specifically failures of endoscopic management or significant transfusion requirement (i.e., > 4–6 U PRBCs per 24 h). Endoscopic findings (i.e., visible vessel) on initial endoscopy not necessarily absolute indication for surgery, but depends on capability of available endoscopist. Aggressive surgical intervention for elderly pts w/ high-risk lesions should be considered.
      ii. *Duodenal ulcer*:
         - Enter duodenum through duodenotomy. Generally, suture ligation of posterior wall ulcer w/ permanent suture, but u-stitch or 4-quadrant ligation around ulcer perimeter may be necessary, or even cephalad and caudad stitching of gastroduodenal artery.
         - If the pt is stable enough, an antisecretory procedure should be added (*controversial*—if pt has not previously been on PPIs or tx'd for *H. pylori*, many assert that medical management should be entertained given the current efficacy of medical tx).
            - *Truncal vagotomy + antrectomy or pyloroplasty*: quick, 90% effective, but side effects include dumping syndrome and diarrhea.
            - *Parietal cell vagotomy*: more time-consuming, but fewer side effects.
      iii. *Gastric ulcer*:
         - Ulcer excision should be included in any procedure, partially because up to 10% of all gastric ulcers are malignant (not a significant concern w/ duodenal ulcers).
            - *Distal stomach* (most common—body/antrum/incisura):
               - Distal gastrectomy + B-I or B-II reconstruction (add TV pt relatively stable).
            - *Proximal stomach* (relatively rare):
               - Subtotal or near-total gastrectomy (high morbidity).
               - Local ulcer excision + distal gastrectomy (TV not necessary).

iv. *H. pylori ulcer*:
- Controversial. Many advocate simply oversewing the ulcer and medically treating the pt, although recurrence rates vary considerably.

2. *Portal hypertension/varices*
   a. *Pathology and presentation*:
      i. Up to 1/4 of cirrhotic pts have variceal bleeding at some point.
      ii. If no prior h/o variceal bleeding, a cirrhotic UGI hemorrhage is equally likely to be from peptic ulcers, gastritis, portal hypertensive gastropathy, or varices. After an initial variceal bleed, subsequent UGI hemorrhage ~ 75% likely to be from varices.
      iii. Variceal bleeding in a Child's C cirrhotic portends a 50% 30-d mortality, and 85% 1-yr mortality.
   b. *Medical tx* (80–90% effective):
      i. Pt should be moved to ICU, resuscitated, and prepared for upper endoscopy.
      ii. IV octreotide (somatostatin analogue) decreases splanchnic blood flow and is the medical adjunct of choice; vasopressin (+/– NTG) is often effective as well.
      iii. Endoscopic banding or sclerotherapy usu. effective.
         - *Exception*: sclerotherapy not good for gastric varices; surgery should be entertained if reasonable risk.
         - Sclerotherapy can be repeated 1–2 times in initial 48 h; if fails, Sengstaken-Blakemore tube should be inserted, and consideration for transjugular intrahepatic shunt (TIPS) or surgery. Mortality at this point likely exceeds 50%.
   c. *Surgical tx*: see Chapter 16 on hepatobiliary.
3. *Acute gastric mucosal lesion* ("stress gastritis" or "stress ulceration")
   a. *Pathology and presentation*:
      i. Generally seen in ICU setting, presenting w/ drop in hematocrit, hematemesis, a/o coffee-ground appearance to NGT aspirate.
      ii. *Endoscopy*: pale mucosa, erosions, and petechiae; most frequently in body of stomach (similar to NSAID gastropathy, but more clinically significant).
   b. *Medical tx*:
      i. Prophylax w/ H_2 inhibitors or PPIs to maintain gastric pH > 4.
      ii. If dx is contemplated, resuscitate, correct any coagulopathies, and transfuse as appropriate while preparing for endoscopy.
      iii. Endoscopic injection or coagulation may be useful for localized lesions, but dz usu. too diffuse.
      iv. Angiography (embolization vs vasopressin infusion) reserved for diffuse, refractory bleeding, but can be up to 80% (temporarily) effective if bleeding vessel can be found. Rebleeding common.
   c. *Surgical tx*:
      i. Rarely appropriate.
      ii. If only a few bleeding sites are found via gastrotomy (unusual), may be oversewed, followed by truncal vagotomy and drainage procedure.
      iii. More commonly, only appropriate surgical option is subtotal or near-total gastrectomy w/ Roux-en-Y gastrojejunostomy reconstruction. Mortality 60–90%.
4. *Mallory-Weiss tear*
   a. Tear in gastric mucosa near EG junction (most often lesser curvature), typically caused by intense retching/vomiting, most often in older (i.e., > 60 yo) males. ~ 10% of significant UGI hemorrhage. 90% self-limited, less if cirrhosis/coagulopathy.
   b. *Medical tx*:
      i. Endoscopy procures the dx, and usu. can stop the bleeding w/ injection or coagulation.
      ii. Up to 1/3 of pts rebleed after endoscopy w/in 24 h, but provision of PPI and correction of coagulopathy generally results in eventual cessation of bleeding.

c. *Surgical tx*:

i. Rarely needed. Oversewing of mucosal lesion through a cephalad gastrotomy effective.

5. *Dieulafoy lesion*

a. Also known as "constant-caliber vessel," an unusu. large submucosal or mucosal artery in the stomach, frequently along the mid-lesser curvature. Pathology is not generally due to an overlying ulcer. Bleeding is frequently intense, but often self-limited, w/ identification of the culprit lesion surprisingly difficult on endoscopy.

b. *Medical management*:

i. Endoscopy to dx cause of bleeding and identify vessel. Endoscopic tx prone to fail; endoscopist should mark the lesion w/ India ink to assist the surgeon (read below).

c. *Surgical management*:

i. Wedge resection of the involved gastric wall is appropriate management.

6. *Aortoenteric fistula*

a. Most common at proximal suture line after aortic aneurysm repair, but cases due to spontaneous inflammatory erosion reported. Typically involves duodenum or proximal jejunum, but colonic involvement possible. Classically herald bleeding followed hours to days later by catastrophic bleeding if urgent intervention is not undertaken.

b. *Medical management*:

i. Clinical suspicion should prompt upper endoscopy, which, if negative, should be followed by abdominal CT scan to look for an inflammatory process. If CT scan is negative (some argue *in lieu* of CT scan), angiography w/ lateral views should be the next step.

c. *Surgical management*:

i. Emergency celiotomy to achieve proximal aortic control followed by (typical scenario) removal of aortic graft and extraanatomic vascular bypass (i.e., axillary-bifemoral).

ii. See Chapter 11 for more details.

C. Lower (distal to ligament of Treitz)

1. Irrigate via NGT to r/o UGI source, followed by anoscopy/proctoscopy to r/o anorectal source (ulcer, hemorrhoid, neoplasm, etc.), which may be controlled. Upper GI hemorrhage may bleed briskly enough to present w/ hematochezia and signs of volume depletion. Hemodynamically unstable pts w/ hematochezia should undergo emergent upper endoscopy as well.
2. Significant bleed should be evaluated w/ colonoscopy or angiography (sensitive to 0.5 cc/min) as most precise and can be used therapeutically (coagulation or vasopressin/embolization, respectively) as well. Angiography should be reserved for massive bleeds; colonoscopy more appropriate for lesser, more intermittent bleeds. Angiography can also be used therapeutically (embolization or vasopressin infusion) as a bridge to surgery, or in lieu of surgery in high-risk pts. Tc-99m RBC scintigraphy can detect bleeding as slow as 0.1 cc/min, but rarely specific enough to determine which side of the colon is bleeding; its primary use is guiding subsequent angiography or colonoscopy.
3. If unstable after attempts at resuscitation (ongoing hemorrhage, transfusion of 6 or more units of PRBCs, etc.), go to OR. If unable to localize (do not rely on Tc-99m RBC scan alone), then perform subtotal colectomy; no role for "blind" hemicolectomy.
4. *Diverticuli* most common etiology (~ 50%), w/ often self-limited but intense arterial bleeding. Right colon diverticuli more prone to bleeding than left. 75–90% stop spontaneously, 10% recur w/in 1 yr, over 25% recur w/in 5 yr.

    a. *Tx*: endoscopic tx not advised. Persistent bleeding should be treated w/ segmental colectomy.
5. *Angiodysplasia* (arteriovenous malformations) next most common (5–20%) cause of lower GI bleeding in all pts and the most common cause in pts over 50 yo. They bleed less severely (venous) than diverticuli but are more likely to recur (75%). More common in right than left colon, and appear as small, flat, red submucosal lesions. Assoc. w/ aortic stenosis, ESRD, and von Willebrand's dz.

    a. *Tx*: endoscopic tx initially effective in > 75%, but rebleed rate 10–15%. Hemicolectomy (usu. right) reserved for refractory bleeding.
6. *Neoplasms* (polyps, malignancies) may be responsible for up to 20% of lower GI bleeds; under 20 yo, juvenile polyps are second most common cause.

    a. *Tx*: bleeding after endoscopic polyp bx can often be controlled by endoscopy. Polyps or malignancies should be addressed w/ an oncologically sound resection.

7. *Inflammatory/infectious* causes such as ulcerative colitis (bleeds much more frequently than Crohn's dz), postradiation enteritis (usu. 1–5 yr after radiation), and bacterial colitis commonly cause lower GI bleeding. Less common causes include AIDS, CMV, and Kaposi's sarcoma.
   a. *Tx*: depends on source. Rectal bleeding from radiation → tx w/ topical of formalin, steroids, or sucralfate.
8. *Vascular* etiologies usu. from bowel ischemia, but inflammatory vasculitides possible. R/o aortoenteric fistula if h/o AAA.
   a. *Tx*: aggressive restoration of cardiac output and bowel perfusion is mainstay for bowel ischemia, followed by revascularization procedure if indicated. See section B6. above on management of aortoenteric fistula.
9. *Hemorrhoids* frequently noted in pts w/ GI bleeds, but responsible for < 5% of significant bleeds.
   a. *Tx*: see Chapter 26 on key steps in key operations.

D. "Obscure etiology" GI hemorrhage

1. Small bowel is usual source of "obscure etiology" GI bleeding, and of 3% GI bleeding overall. ~ 1/2 due to angiodysplasia, except in pediatric population (*Meckel's diverticulum most common source of lower GI bleeding overall in children*). Other causes include leiomyoma, adenocarcinoma, lymphoma, Crohn's dz, metastatic neoplasm, hemobilia, etc.
2. W/u should follow algorithm for upper vs lower GI hemorrhage. If (–), a variety of modalities (CT scan, Meckel's scan [Tc-99m], capsule endoscopy, small bowel endoscopy, etc.) may be pursued depending on pt age, hx, physical, and clinical suspicion. Although angiodysplasia may be effectively treated w/ endoscopic injection/coagulation (if w/in reach of scope), most other etiologies require surgical intervention.

V. FISTULAS

A. Management by "SLATE" steps

1. ***S**tabilization* (immediately):
   a. Rehydrate, correct anemia, and occasionally may give albumin as well to increase to 3.0 mg/dL.
   b. Drain abscesses, other interventions to reduce septic sources.
   c. Control drainage (sump catheter), stomadhesive, etc., to protect skin.
   d. *Provide nutrition*: 1.3–1.5 × BEE and 1.2–2.0 g/kg nitrogen/d. May need to shift to lipid-based rather than carbohydrate-based enteral feed, or even parenteral nutrition. High-output fistulas should be met w/ 2 × RDA of water-soluble vitamins, esp. vitamin C.
   e. *Decrease secretion volume*: NGT not beneficial. H_2 blockers or PPI should be initiated. Sandostatin as 100–600 mcg/d divided 2–4 times per day will not result in a higher closure rate, but has been shown to decrease time to closure in those who do spontaneously close; also makes fluid/electrolyte replacement less arduous. Pt should be NPO, w/ TPN.
2. ***L**ocalize* (generally 7–10 d after dx):
   a. Water-soluble fistulogram via 5–8 pediatric feeding tube is single highest yield study. CT may be indicated if deep abscess suspected.
3. ***A**ssess*:
   a. *Define characteristics of fistula of prognostic importance w/ FRIENDS*:
      i. ***F**oreign body*: presence requires removal.
      ii. ***R**adiation*: less likely to heal spontaneously.
      iii. ***I**nflammation or **I**nfection*: *either reduces rate of closure.*
      iv. ***E**pithelialization*: reduces rate of closure.
      v. ***N**eoplasia and **N**utritional status*: cancer reduces rate of closure, and transferrin level > 200 at dx or after 3 wk therapy suggests reasonable spontaneous closure rate.
      vi. ***D**istal obstruction*: reduces rate of spontaneous closure.
      vii. ***S**ite and **S**ize* (length, width, and volume): most likely to heal (oropharyngeal, esophageal, duodenal stump, pancreaticobiliary, jejunal); least likely to heal (gastric, lateral duodenal ligament of Treitz, ileal). Tract length > 2 cm or bowel defect > 1 cm wide unlikely to close.
4. ***T**herapy* (definitive): typically resect and reanastomose affected segment.
5. ***E**nsure healing*: continue nutritional support and gradually resume enteric feeding.

VI. DIARRHEA, CONSTIPATION, AND BOWEL OBSTRUCTION

A. Diarrhea

1. *Infectious* (check fecal WBCs for enteroinvasive infections):
   a. Bacterial (enteroinvasive or enterotoxigenic *E. coli*, *Campylobacter*, *Salmonella*, *Shigella*, *C. difficile*)
   b. Protozoan (*Giardia*, *Cryptosporidium*, *Entamoeba histolytica*)
   c. Viral (Norwalk, etc.)
2. *Neoplastic*:
   a. Carcinoid
   b. Medullary thyroid CA
   c. *Zollinger-Ellison syndrome*: improves w/ PPI or H_2 blocker
   d. Somatostatinoma
   e. *VIPoma*: does not improve w/ PPI, H_2 blocker
3. *Vascular*: arterial or venous insufficiency
   a. Colonic ischemia classically w/ watery diarrhea followed by blood.
4. *Malabsorptive*:
   a. Pancreatic insufficiency
   b. Sprue (celiac or tropical)
   c. Intestinal lymphoma
   d. Short gut syndrome
5. *Medication*

B. Constipation: w/u (BE, defecography, serum tests, colonoscopy, physical exam) tailored to pt.

1. Medication (narcotic) or dietary (paucity of fiber and water)
2. Neurogenic
3. Endocrine (hypothyroid)
4. Anatomic (mass obstruction)

C. Obstruction

1. *General principles*: treat w/ bowel rest (NGT), resuscitation (IVF, Foley catheter).
   a. *Partial*: failure to improve after 3 d → OR.
   b. *Complete* (obstipated): all → OR.
2. *Etiology*: in United States postop adhesions are most common. In developing world, hernias are most common cause.
   a. *Mechanical*
      i. *Adhesions*: most often from pelvic operations, although any intraabdominal surgery can contribute.
      ii. *Hernia* (inguinal, ventral, *internal*—know the surgical hx!).
      iii. *Neoplasm*.
      iv. *Volvulus*: more common outside United States. Higher incidence w/ age, institutionalization, psychotropic meds.
         - *Sigmoid*:
            - ~ 70% of colonic volvulus.
            - *Plain films*: may show "coffee bean sign," or "bent inner tube" on AXR. Barium enema may show "bird's beak." CT scan rarely needed, but may reveal twisted mesentery.
            - *Tx*: decompression via rectal tube place w/ proctoscopy or colonoscopy usu. adequate for immediate tx, should be followed by sigmoid resection during the same hospital stay as frequently recurs (~ 1/2). Peritonitis or failure of rectal tube decompression mandates emergent operation.
         - *Cecal volvulus*:
            - Compared w/ sigmoid volvulus, pts usu. younger and higher percentage are females.

- AXR often similar to colonic volvulus, but often evidence of SBO as well. Although some references suggest the orientation and apex location of the colonic loop on AXR differentiates sigmoid from colonic volvulus, this is not reliable. Contrast enema can be useful to differentiate the 2 and look for colonic tumors.
- As not amenable to endoscopic decompression, the dx mandates surgery (tx = right hemicolectomy, as cecopexy frequently fails).

- *Cecal bascule* (French *basculer* v. = "to tip over," *bascule* n. = "rocker, see-saw"):
  - Extremely rare. Involves the distal cecum "flopping" over the more proximal segment, due to adhesive band or excessively large pouch of cecum. Surgical therapy may involve lysis of adhesion a/o cecopexy, depending on pathology.

b. *Ileus*: most often due to inflammation (postop, abscess, sepsis), electrolyte abnormality (hypomagnesemia, hypokalemia, etc.), or medication (narcotics). Reverse the primary process.

c. *Ogilvie's syndrome* (colonic pseudoobstruction):

i. Incompletely understood physiologic (not anatomic) colonic dilatation w/ variable degrees of clinical obstructive picture. Usu. assoc. w/ rx (i.e., narcotics), orthopaedic trauma (esp. pelvic or hip), or retroperitoneal inflammation.

ii. *Dx*: clinical obstruction (although diarrhea may be present) w/ radiographic evidence of colonic dilatation (may be pancolonic or predominantly right-sided) and no evidence of mechanical blockage. Small bowel not involved as w/ ileus unless pt has incompetent ileocecal valve.

iii. *Tx*: cessation of implicated factors (i.e., narcotics, calcium channel blockers, anticholinergics) if able. Cecal diameter > 10 cm ↑↑ risk of perforation (law of LaPlace—see Chapter 11) and mandates urgent intervention. Consider naloxone (0.4 mg IV) if narcotic-related.

- *Medical*:
  - Rectal tube a/o colonoscopy to decompress colon.
  - Neostigmine, 1–2.5 mg IV over 3 min may be successful and can be repeated in 30 min. Caveat is possibility of bradycardia: should be given in monitored (i.e., ICU) setting w/ atropine available (1 mg IV prn).
- *Surgical*:
  - Exploration is indicated for failure of above measures or if evidence of bowel ischemia or perforation (i.e., peritonitis) or cecal diameter > 10 cm postcolonoscopy.
  - *Cecostomy*: performed if no evidence of colon necrosis (has been described under local anesthesia).
  - Loop colostomy.
  - Segmental resection w/ end ileostomy, mucous fistula: performed if necrosis encountered.

VII. OSTOMIES

A. May be created as end or loop for either colon or ileum. See Chapter 26 for operative details. Note that although traditionally it is recommended to place through rectus musculature to prevent parastomal herniation, the data are conflicting on the efficacy of this.

B. Complications

1. *Parastomal hernia*: treat the first time w/ local repair (i.e., mesh repair of parastoma fascia). Treat recurrence by re-siting the stoma.
2. *Stomal prolapse*: most often seen w/ transverse loop colostomies, usu. involving the distal end. An effective and relatively noninvasive means of treating is to staple the prolapsed segment (similar to an Altemeier procedure for rectal prolapse). [Maeda K, et al., *Tech Coloproctol.* 2004;8:45–6; Tepetes K, et al., *Tech Coloproctol.* 2005;9:156–8.]
3. "*High output*:" just like fistulas, ileostomies can lead to considerable fluid loss. Treat initially w/ psyllium fiber, Imodium, possibly tincture of opium. Aggressively replace fluid losses to avoid renal failure. [For those interested in more details, Cataldo PA, MacKeigan JM, *Intestinal Stomas*, 2nd ed. 2004; New York: Marcel Dekker Inc., is a well-balanced, thorough reference.]

CHAPTER 16

HEPATOBILIARY AND PANCREAS

I. LIVER (NONBILIARY)

A. Embryology and vasculature: begins as ventral foregut bud. Portal vs 70% blood flow, 50% O_2. Hepatic a. usu. comes off celiac axis. Left hepatic a. may come off left gastric a., and right hepatic a. may come off SMA.

B. Anatomy

1. *Couinaud system* describes 8 segments w/ independent arterial, venous, and biliary flow.
   a. Cantlie's line (from IVC to gallbladder fossa) divides liver into right, left lobes—corresponds internally w/ course of middle hepatic vein.
      i. Falciform ligament divides left lateral segments (II, III) from left medial segment (IV).
   b. Segments named in relation to hepatic vein drainage.
      i. Caudate lobe immediately anterior to IVC, w/ caudal aspect posterior to portal vein and cephalad aspect posterior to middle and left hepatic veins.
   c. Portal vein structures encased in fibrous sheath continuous w/ Glisson's capsule.
2. *Lobes and sections* (segments that compose them):
   a. *Right lobe*: V, VI, VII, VIII
      i. *Right anterior segment*: V, VIII
      ii. *Right posterior segment*: VI, VII
   b. *Left lobe*: II, III, IV
      i. *Left lateral segment*: II, III
      ii. *Left medial segment*: IV

C. Physiology

1. *Bilirubin*: direct increased when liver unable to normally excrete conjugated bilirubin and it leaks into systemic blood supply. Indirect increased when unable to conjugate/clear the pigment it receives. Icterus apparent w/ $T_{bili} > 2$ mg/dL.
2. *Alk phos*: bone, placenta, liver produces. Elevation suggests biliary obstruction if no bone dz or pregnancy.
3. *Determining resectability of liver*:
   a. Best indicator of synthetic function of liver is INR.
   b. *Indicators that generally preclude resection*:
      i. Bilirubin twice normal generally precludes surgery.
      ii. Child-Pugh B or C (total score > 7)—mortality w/ A = 3.7% vs B, C = 16.7%.
      iii. Indocyanine green clearance at 15 min.
         - < 10% retention, any resection should be feasible; 10–20%, bisegmentectomy possible; 20–29%, do not recommend > unisegmentectomy.
      iv. Wedged hepatic pressure (hepatic venous gradient) > 10 mm Hg suggests nonresectable physiology.
      v. *Lidocaine metabolite (monoethylglycinexylidide [MEGX]) test*:
         - Metabolite decreases as functional liver mass decreases.
         - C_{13}-aminopyrine test is a breath test based on same principle.
      vi. Signs of portal hypertension (i.e., bleeding esophageal varices) are a relative contraindication to resection. [Franco, et al., Resection of hepatocellular carcinomas: Results in 72 European patients with cirrhosis, *Gastroenterology*. 1990; 98:733–8; Bismuth, et al., Liver resection versus transplantation for hepatocellular carcinoma in cirrhotic patients, *Ann Surg*. 1993;218:145–51; Bruix J, et al., Surgical resection of hepatocellular carcinoma: prognostic value of preoperative portal pressure, *Gastroenterology*. 1996;111:1018–22.]

D. Benign disease

1. *Cirrhosis*
   a. Scar tissue in liver parenchyma, leads to resistance to blood flow, w/ formation of portosystemic shunts (esophageal varices, hemorrhoids, umbilicus).
   b. *PEx*: jaundice, dark urine, peripheral edema, caput medusa, spider angiomata, gynecomastia, testicular atrophy, palmar erythema.
   c. Albumin, coag factors (fibrinogen, prothrombin, V, VII, IX, X) decreased.
   d. PT elevated w/ fat absorption (hence, vitamin K absorption) decreased, impaired due to biliary obstruction as well as synthetic abnormalities of coag factors.
   e. Cardiac output increased, SVR decreased, may lead to cardiac failure.
   f. See Table 16.1.

TABLE 16.1. Child-Pugh Classification

	1 Point	2 Points	3 Points
Encephalopathy	None	Moderate (I, II)	Severe (III, IV)
Ascites	None	Slight	Moderate
Bilirubin (mg/dL)	< 2.0	2.0–3.0	> 3.0
Albumin (g/dL)	> 3.5	2.8–3.5	< 2.8
INR	< 1.7	1.7–2.3	> 2.3

To calculate Child-Pugh class, add points from each row: A = 5–6, B = 7–9, C = 10–15.

2. *Liver failure and portal hypertension*
   a. *Relevant anatomy and physiology*
      i. *Anatomy*:
         - Portal vein results from SMV and splenic veins (splenic v. receives blood from IMV) confluence behind pancreatic neck. Left gastric (coronary) vein empties gastric lesser curvature and distal esophagus into portal vein near origin.
         - *Collaterals can develop in*: coronary/short gastric v.'s → azygous v. (esophagogastric varices); recanalized umbilical v. (from left portal v.) → epigastric v.'s (caput medusae); retroperitoneal v.'s; hemorrhoids.
      ii. *Physiology*:
         - Cirrhosis (hepatocellular necrosis resulting in fibrosis and nodular regeneration) results in hepatocellular failure and portal hypertension.
         - Portal pressure > 5–8 mm Hg stimulates formation of portosystemic collaterals.
         - Hepatic artery can increase in blood flow to compensate for decreased portal blood flow (buffer response), but the reverse is not true.
         - Advanced liver dz results in increased levels of endogenous vasodilators (prostacyclin, NO, etc.) w/ peripheral dilation and hyperdynamic state, activating sympathetics and renin-aldosterone axis.
   b. *Classification and etiology*
      i. *Prehepatic*:
         - Portal vein thrombosis (most common; in absence of hepatic dz, collateral flow to liver may develop, called cavernomatous transformation of portal vein).
         - Splenic vein thrombosis (left-sided or sinistral portal hypertension; usu. secondary to pancreatitis or pancreatic neoplasm). Isolated gastric varices result. Splenectomy alone curative.
      ii. *Intrahepatic*:
         - *Presinusoidal*: schistosomiasis most common; many nonalcoholic cirrhosis cases begin here also; primary biliary cirrhosis.

- *Sinusoidal*: alcoholic (deposits collagen in space of Disse); postnecrotic viral.
- *Postsinusoidal*: alcoholic (regenerating nodules compress hepatic veins); Budd-Chiari syndrome (hepatic vs thrombosis); right heart failure; constrictive pericarditis; vena caval web.

c. *Medical management*

i. *Ascites*:

- *W/u*:
  - Paracentesis for cell count, cx, total protein, and albumin.
    - Serum-ascites albumin gradient (SAAG): $Alb_{serum} - Alb_{ascites}$
      - *SAAG > 1.1*: ascites assoc. w/ sinusoidal hypertension (cirrhosis, CHF, Budd-Chiari, hepatitis, etc.)
      - *SAAG < 1.1*: ascites assoc. w/ altered peritoneal permeability (infection, extrahepatic malignancy, other inflammatory d/o)
- *Nonoperative management*
  - *Salt-restriction* (impaired ability to clear free water; sodium-avid physiology). < 2 g/d.
  - *Aldosterone-antagonist* (spironolactone) crucial. 100–400 mg/d. Titrate up q wk prn.
    - Furosemide may be added for extra diuresis.
  - *Large-volume paracentesis* (LVP)—ensure INR < 2 and plt > 40,000 before procedure; give albumin (6 g/L) if > 5 L removed.
  - *TIPS* (not usu. offered if $T_{bili} > 5$, INR > 2, significant CHF, encephalopathy, or portal vs thrombosis).
    - Decreased recurrence compared to LVP.
    - Increased rate of encephalopathy.
    - Does not improve overall survival.
    - Best viewed as a bridge to transplantation.
  - *Spontaneous bacterial peritonitis*: prophylaxis (after an episode of SBP or GI hemorrhage) and tx (dx = > 250 PMNs/mm^3 and single, nonanaerobic, bacterial species) is w/ FQ (ofloxacin, ciprofloxacin, etc.).
- *Operative management* (*Note*: refractory ascites has 25% 1-yr survival.)
  - Liver transplant is tx of choice.
  - *Shunts* (particularly partial shunts, read below): selective shunts are contraindicated.

ii. *Varices*:

- *Prevention of bleeding*
  - Beta blockers (nonselective, such as propanolol or nadolol).
    - Don't prevent varices, but are indicated to prevent bleeding in already extant varices.
  - Titrate to reduce resting pulse by 25% or to 55 bpm.
    - Addition of nitrates may confer additional protection.
  - Endoscopic ligation.
    - Reserved for pts w/ large varices who cannot tolerate beta blockers.
    - Combined w/ beta blockers, effective for prevention of *recurrent* bleeding.
- *Tx of acute bleeding*
  - *Medications*:
    - *Octreotide* (has replaced vasopressin as DOC): 100 mcg IV bolus, then 250 IV mcg/h.
    - Beta blockade.
  - *Endoscopy*: may tx w/ banding or sclerotherapy.
  - *TIPS*: see entry i. above.
  - *Sengstaken-Blakemore tube*: may be used to tamponade bleeding varices up to 48 h (useful as temporizing measure until transfer or surgery).

iii. *Hepatorenal syndrome*: results from loss of vasodilatory compensation for heightened renin-aldosterone axis.

- *Type I*: rapidly progressive (doubling Cr to > 2.5 in < 2 wk). Refractory to medical management, poor prognosis.
- *Type II*: not rapidly progressive.
- Avid sodium retention in both forms. Low urine Na^+ and FENa (< 1%) are characteristic. Serum BUN/Cr and Cr clearance may overestimate actual GFR in cirrhotics. Intravascular volume expansion, low-dose dopamine, fenoldopam have been advocated. IV fluid management should not rely upon large amounts of salt solution, but instead albumin, glucose solutions, and FFP. Body compensates for elevated vasoconstrictive aldosterone by increasing vasodilatory prostaglandins—thus, NSAIDs should be avoided, esp. in pts w/ hyponatremia. Continuous hemodialysis may be indicated for fulminant hepatic failure.

iv. *Hepatic encephalopathy*:

- Shunting of portal blood into systemic circulation results in impaired metabolism of suspect agents such as ammonia, mercaptans, short chain fatty acids, "false" neurotransmitters such as octopamine and serotonin, and γ-aminobutyric acid.
- *Sx*: may include confusion, stupor, hyperreflexia, asterixis, or even coma.
- Precipitating factors may include GI hemorrhage, constipation, azotemia, sepsis, hypoxia, CNS depressants, and shunt procedures (TIPS, surgical portosystemic shunts).
- *Tx steps include*: control of precipitating factors; limiting protein intake to 20–30 g/d, transitioning to 60–80 g/d later; lactulose 15–45 cc PO 2–4 times per day titrated to 2–3 soft stools/d (may also be given as enema 300 cc lactulose + 700 cc water 2–3 times per day). Oral abx such as neomycin (1 g PO 2 times per day) or metronidazole (250 mg PO q 6 h) may be useful as well. Zinc deficiency should be corrected.

v. *Coagulopathy*: coagulation factors synthesized by liver (II, VII, IX, X, protein C, protein S) decreased, resulting in prolonged PT. As synthetic function of liver compromised, vitamin K administration less effective than replacement of factors w/ FFP or PCC (see Chapter 2 on hematology).

d. *Surgical management*: for failure of medical/endoscopic management. 10% of variceal bleeds fail initial medical tx, and 30% of initial successes rebleed. Mortality > 25% regardless of type of surgery.

i. *Types of surgery*:

- *Hepatic transplant*: tx of choice for varices/portal HTN in cirrhotic pts w/ high Child-Pugh score, but limited by supply, and feasibility in acutely bleeding pt.
- *Esophageal stapling*: emergent procedure, which is fast and simple, but has high-rebleed rate and same overall mortality as shunt procedures.
- *Shunts*:
  - *Total/nonselective*: completely divert portal flow, thus risk of variceal rebleed essentially nil. However, 3/4 of pts develop fulminant hepatic failure a/o encephalopathy.
    - End-to-side portacaval shunt (Eck fistula)—largely abandoned.
    - Side-to-side portacaval shunt—rarely performed.
  - *Partial*: limits amount of diversion via a *reinforced* portacaval or mesocaval anastomosis.
    - Generally the best option for control of ascites, and effective for varices as well.
    - *Mesocaval*: longer than portocaval, thus possibly more thrombogenic.
    - *Portocaval*: preferred operation is H-graft using 3 cm of 8-mm ribbed Gore-Tex.
    - Physiologic goal is decrease of portal pressure by 10 mm Hg, decrease of PV/IVC gradient by 10 mm; generally can appreciate thrill in IVC at anastomosis.
    - Assoc. w/ significantly lower the rebleed rate than TIPS.
  - *Selective*: divert only gastroesophageal varices, not the portal vein; contraindicated if ascites as can actually increase sinusoidal pressure.
    - *Warren distal splenorenal shunt*: ligate, divide splenic vein, and anastomose to distal left renal vein.

- Also divide gastroepiploic vv., coronary v., and branches w/ pancreatic vv.
- Gastroesophageal varices then drain via short gastrics → left renal v. → IVC.
- Advantageous in that maintains hepatic perfusion (minimal encephalopathy or exacerbation of liver insufficiency), but technically difficult, and, as mentioned above, may promote ascites.

- For pts w/ portal vein occlusion and ascites, consider interposition splenorenal shunt, proximal splenorenal (Linton) shunt (allows drainage of SMV → splenic → left renal), or gastric devascularization.

3. *Hepatic cysts*
   a. *Noninfectious*
      i. Usu. solitary. 50% of cases assoc. w/ polycystic renal dz (see Chapter 5).
      ii. Solitary lesions w/ cuboidal epithelium = cystadenomas = premalignant → resect.
      iii. Multiloculated cysts, if not echinococcal, are generally neoplastic.
      iv. Virtually no role for aspiration as simple cysts reaccumulate rapidly, neoplastic cysts mandate removal, and parasitic cysts are at risk of rupture.
      v. Most simple cysts can be managed w/ laparoscopic unroofing (~ 1/3) of cyst, w/ placement of omentum in the cavity. Multiple cysts can also be unroofed w/ fenestrations created to drain underlying cysts.
   b. *Infectious*—echinococcosis (hydatid dz)
      i. Most common cause of acquired hepatic cysts, endemic in Greece, portions of Europe, South America, Australia, and southern and western Africa.
      ii. Usu. caused by *E. granulosus* (cystic dz), more rarely by *E. multilocularis* (alveolar dz, generally limited to Alaska and Canada and less amenable to surgery). Eggs in dog feces ingested by cows, sheep, etc., or humans, then filtered in liver, or more rarely, lungs.
      iii. Most pts present w/ abdominal pain, although symptoms of complications such as infection, anaphylaxis, biliary obstruction, etc. ~ 3/4 of cysts are solitary and in right lobe.
      iv. *Dx*:
         - Eosinophilia and mildly elevated LFTs may be present.
         - Indirect hemagglutination test and Casoni skin test w/ ~ 85% sensitivity.
           - Latter actually can sensitize the pt to become falsely positive or anaphylactic in future assays.
         - Complement fixation ~ 70% sensitive.
         - Plain radiographs may demonstrate calcification of cyst walls in 1/2 of pts. CT scan, U/S, liver scan all ~ 100% sensitive. ERCP rarely demonstrates daughter cysts or "sand."
      v. *Tx*:
         - *Surgical resection is tx of choice.*
           - Liver resection/radical surgery and pericystectomy w/ similar mortality rates, but the former has lower recurrence rates. Laparoscopic pericystectomy often feasible for peripheral, readily accessible lesions.
           - Adjunctive pre- and postop benzimidazole is recommended.
           - Ablation via aspiration and injection of scolecite (hypertonic saline, chlorhexidine, 80% alcohol, 0.5% cetrimide; formalin no longer widely used). If bile is aspirated, sclerosants not used. Process repeated, then cyst unroofed. Anaphylaxis possible if ruptures or spills. Procedure rapidly waning in popularity. 80–90% effective.
           - Drainage or obliteration alternative tx.
           - Mebendazole recommended in early cases or cases not amenable to surgery.
4. *Hepatic infections*
   a. *Abscesses*
      i. *Pyogenic*
         - More common in United States, often multiple sites w/in liver.
         - Often from cholecystitis, appendicitis, obstructing pancreaticobiliary neoplasm, PID, trauma, and rarely colon cancer. Immunodeficiency increases risk.

- Causative organisms *E. coli, Streptococcus* > *Bacteroides* > *Klebsiella, Enterococcus.*
- Treat by drainage and abx.

ii. *Amebic*

- More common in developing world, usu. isolated lesion in right lobe of liver.
- More common in men and in younger pts (< 40 yo).
- 7–14 d of metronidazole is usual tx.
  - If no marked improvement or resolution w/in 48 h, may have wrong dx or may be superinfected → aspirate or drain.
  - Other indications for percutaneous drainage: rupture into thorax/abdomen; tx failure after 3–5 d of abx; bacterial superinfection; abscess in left liver lobe (risk of rupture into pericardium).

b. *Cholangitis*

i. *Charcot's triad*—RUQ pain, jaundice, fever.

ii. *Raynauld's pentad*—above plus shock, obtundation.

iii. Mandates resuscitation w/ IVF, IV abx, and emergent decompression via ERCP.

c. *Parasitic*

i. *Clonorchis sinensis, Opisthorchis viverrini*: flukes, which spend part of life cycle in biliary tree, endemic in portions of Asia (esp. China, Thailand, Korea, Vietnam, depending on species), acquired from eating raw freshwater fish. Although usu. asymptomatic, heavy infections can result in biliary obstruction and cholangitis. Tx of acute dz is w/ praziquantel or albendazole. Chronic infection is risk factor for cholangiocarcinoma.

ii. *Fasciola hepatica, F. gigantica*: liver flukes w/ worldwide distribution, acquired by eating contaminated freshwater plants such as watercress. Although their life cycle varies from the *C. sinensis* and *O. viverrini*, they also can cause biliary obstruction and cholangitis. Unlike most trematodes, *Fasciola* is resistant to praziquantel: triclabendazole is the drug of choice.

iii. *Ascaris*: roundworm rarely lodges in ampulla of Vater, causing pancreatitis and biliary obstruction.

d. *Viral*: see hepatitis section in Chapter 23.

5. *Solid lesions*

a. Check AFP, CEA, CA-19-9 for possibility of malignancy. U/S should be first radiographic test.

b. *Hemangioma*

i. Most common solid hepatic tumor; F > M, 6:1.

ii. Majority are subcapsular. If greater than 4 cm, may be palpable or cause pain. Rupture is rare. Large lesions may act as AV fistula causing CHF. Kasabach-Merritt syndrome (thrombocytopenia from platelet sequestration) has been reported.

iii. *Dx*:

- *U/S*: well-defined, hyperechoic, hypervascular.
- *CT*: peripheral enhancement w/ IV contrast.
- *MRI*: T1 = isodense; T2 = hyperdense w/ peripheral enhancement w/ gadolinium.
- *Tc-99m RBC scan*: good test—sensitive, specific. Core needle bx contraindicated, but some assert FNA is acceptable risk.

iv. *Tx*: symptomatic lesions may be surgically removed; radiotherapy or embolization is reserved for poor surgical candidates. Pts w/ large lesions and h/o usage of estrogens should be counseled against continuing estrogen.

c. *Focal nodular hyperplasia*

i. 2× more common in females (avg. age at dx 40 yo). Like adenomas (below), genesis or enlargement may be linked to oral contraceptives. Unlike adenomas, no malignant potential.

ii. Most pts are asx, though some complain of RUQ mass a/o discomfort.

iii. *Dx*:

- *U/S*: not helpful.
- *CT*: w/ contrast often reveals characteristic central stellate scar.
- *Angiography*: hypervascular pattern.

- *MRI*: T1/T2 = isodense; T1 central low-signal scar that enhances w/ gadolinium.
- *Tc-99m sulfur colloid scan*: variable.

iv. *Tx*: OCPs should be discontinued, and symptomatic lesions should be excised.

d. *Hepatic adenoma*

i. Virtually limited to women and linked to OCP usage. Majority are solitary lesions, and about 1/2 are asx.; may progress to hepatocellular carcinoma.

ii. Pts generally present w/ RUQ pain or intraabdominal hemorrhage; bleeding occurs more frequently during menstruation.

iii. *Dx*:

- *U/S*: not helpful; usu. increased blood flow.
- *CT*: hypodense; contrast may yield heterogeneous appearance.
- *Angiography*: ranges from hypovascular to hypervascular.
- *MRI*: frequently hypodense.
- *Tc-99m sulfur colloid scan*: generally nonenhancing.
- CT and U/S are nonspecific, and angiographic appearance ranges from avascular to hypervascular. FNA may be warranted, but not core needle bx.

iv. *Tx*: as lesions may regress off of oral contraceptives, asx or mildly symptomatic lesions smaller than 6 cm may be observed off of OCPs. Lesions larger than 6 cm are more likely to bleed or be malignant and should be removed.

e. *Hepatic resection*: see Chapter 26 for principles and techniques of hepatic resection.

II. BILIARY

A. Biliary stricture

1. *Benign causes*: chronic pancreatitis, primary sclerosing cholangitis, acute cholangitis, trauma; most common iatrogenic from laparoscopic colectomy.

a. Unrecognized injury may lead to cholangitis, secondary biliary cirrhosis, portal hypertension.

i. Iatrogenic cases often present w/in 1 wk postop w/ pain, fever, and jaundice (T_{bili} > 2.5 mg/dL) from biloma/peritonitis.

- CT- or U/S-demonstrated bilomas should be perc drained. ERCP or sinogram can demonstrate anatomy. PTC may be useful to place stent.
- Cystic duct leaks can be treated w/ perc drainage, +/– ERCP ampulla stent to decrease resistance.
- Lateral bile duct injury can be stented w/ T tube.

b. Strasberg classification of biliary injury [Strasberg SM, et al., *J Am College Surgeons*. 1995; 180:101–25.]

i. *Type A*: bile leak from injured minor ducts (cystic duct, duct of Lushka, etc.).

ii. *Type B*: occlusion of non-CBD part of biliary tree, usu. an aberrant right sectoral hepatic duct.

iii. *Type C*: transection, but not ligation, of right hepatic sectoral duct.

iv. *Type D*: lateral injury to an extrahepatic bile duct.

v. *Type E*: major injury to CHD (subdivide w/ Bismuth classification → E1–5).

c. Bismuth classification of stricture (proximal) injuries are more difficult [Bismuth H, *The Biliary Tract. Clinical Surgery International*, vol. 5. Edinburgh: Churchill Livingstone; 1982: 209–18.]

i. *Type 1*: injury > 2 cm distal to bifurcation hepatic duct.

ii. *Type 2*: injury < 2 cm distal to bifurcation of hepatic duct.

iii. *Type 3*: involves hilum, but right and left hepatic ducts still communicate.

iv. *Type 4*: destruction of hilum, discontinuity between right and left ducts.

v. *Type 5*: separate inserting sectoral duct +/– CBD injury.

vi. In acute injury, unless have experience w/ anastomosing nondilated ducts, place drains and transfer; definitive repair (often definitively performed 6–8 wk later). *Usual surgical interventions as follows*:

- *Type A*: drain + suture repair of cystic duct, drain. Drain + ERCP stent an alternative.
- *Type B*: if symptomatic, repair w/ hepaticojejunostomy (if anastomosis not possible, consider hepatic resection).
- *Type C*: drain + one of the following: hepaticojejunostomy, resection, or ligation.
- *Type D*: drain + ERCP stent is usu. sufficient. Alternatively, drain + suture (absorbable) repair over T tube (through separate incision in duct if possible). If tissue loss, or > 50 of duct, or thermal injury, then Roux-en-Y hepaticojejunostomy better option.
- *Type E*: short strictures may be stented by PTC or ERCP. If stents not an option or if they fail or if have duct discontinuity, operation required.

B. Primary sclerosing cholangitis (PSC)

1. Progressive cholestatic dz characterized by stenosis and beading of intra- and extrahepatic biliary tree. Unlike PBC (see section C. below), more commonly affects men. ~ 1/2 to 3/4 pts also have inflammatory bowel dz, but only ~ 5% of pts w/ IBD have PSC (some speculate abd colonic mucosal barrier may be linked to etiology). Often presents w/ abdominal pain, fever, hepatomegaly, pruritus, etc. Assoc. w/ HLA-DR8 and HLA-DR3. May lead to cholangiocarcinoma, particularly in pts w/ high EtOH ingestion.
2. *Dx*:
   a. Hyperbilirubinemia, perinuclear antineutrophil cytoplasmic antibodies (p-ANCA, ~ 75% seropositive) suggestive.
   b. *Radiology*:
      i. *U/S*: intra- and extrahepatic ductal dilatation, possible increased echogenicity (but normal in 1/2 of cases).
      ii. *MRI*: T2 imaging w/ wedge-shaped high signal intensity areas characteristic.
      iii. *Cholangiography*: multiple strictures and dilatations ("beading").
3. *Tx*:
   a. *Medical*: prednisone, methotrexate, cyclosporine, pentoxifylline, abx all reported.
      i. Ursodeoxycholic acid useful for sx related to hyperbilirubinemia as well. Extrahepatic strictures may be tx'd w/ balloon dilatation. Supplement fat-soluble vitamins.
   b. *Surgery*: drainage procedures (porto- or choledochoenterostomy) doomed to failure. Particularly in children, liver transplantation may provide good long-term relief.

C. Primary biliary cirrhosis (PBC)

1. Probable autoimmune condition affecting small-to-medium bile ducts w/ progressive cholestasis and ultimately liver failure. More common in *women* (unlike PSC above) and assoc. w/ HLA-DR8, elevated levels of IgM, hepatic granulomas, increased ESR, frequent concurrent autoimmune conditions (autoimmune thyroiditis, scleroderma, etc.). 90+% w/ antimitochondrial (98% specific). Antinuclear Ab in 20–50%. Often initially presents w/ fatigue. 10% w/ severe pruritus that does not correlate well w/ degree of hyperbilirubinemia, thought to be related to increased production of endogenous opioids.
2. *Dx*:
   a. Hyperbilirubinemia, *antimitochondrial Ab*, etc., suggestive.
   b. *Radiographic findings*: U/S of liver demonstrates increased echogenicity. PTC/ERCP.
   c. Bx w/ nonsuppurative cholangitis w/ basement membrane damage, lymphocytic infiltration.
3. *Tx*:
   a. Ursodeoxycholic acid initial tx. Methotrexate, cyclosporine, corticosteroids, colchicines sometimes used. Pruritus tx'd w/ cholestyramine/colestipol. Rifampin, dronabinol, and plasmapheresis reported to be helpful as well. Refractory cases w/ cirrhosis are definitively tx'd w/ liver transplantation.

D. Congenital conditions

1. *Choledochal cysts*
   a. More common in Asia (partic. Japan) and women. Vast majority have long (> 1 cm) common channel (CBD and pancreatic duct).
   b. "Classic" presentation of RUQ pain, jaundice, and abdominal mass only occurs in ~ 10%.

c. *Dx*:
   i. U/S or CT can procure dx, but cholangiography needed to establish type of cyst and facilitate operative planning.
d. *Classification and tx* (*note*: all cysts are resected—given 25–30% lifetime cancer risk otherwise; also, simply draining into enteric limb assoc. w/ cholangitis)
   i. *Type I* (50%)—fusiform dilatation of entire CBD.
      - *Tx*: cholecystectomy, resect extrahepatic biliary tract, Roux-en-Y hepaticojejunostomy.
   ii. *Type II* (< 10%)—saccular diverticulum of CBD.
      - *Tx*: same as for type I.
   iii. *Type III* (< 10%)—intraduodenal choledochocele involving sphincter.
      - *Tx*: excise, sphincteroplasty vs sphincteroplasty/sphincterotomy alone.
   iv. *Type IV* (35%)—intra- and extrahepatic cysts.
      - Resect extrahepatic biliary tract, Roux-en-Y hepaticojejunostomy.
      - If cysts in 1 lobe only, consider lobectomy. If both lobes, transplant.
   v. *Type V* (< 10%)—intrahepatic cysts (Caroli dz).
      - Cholecystectomy w/ common bile duct exploration.
      - If cysts in 1 lobe only, consider lobectomy. If both lobes, transplant.

2. *Biliary atresia*: see Chapter 20.

E. Cholelithiasis and complications

1. *Cholelithiasis*: present in ~ 15% of U.S. population, usu. asymptomatic. Sx develop at rate of 1–2% per yr, reaching a plateau of about ~ 20%. Asymptomatic cholecystitis is not generally an indication for cholecystectomy except in some pt populations (i.e., heart bypass pts; they develop stones more frequently and have significant cholecystitis complications due to immunosuppression).
   a. *Cholecystitis*: 95% of cases related to gallstone impaction. RUQ pain and U/S demonstrating gallbladder wall thickening (> 3.5 mm) a/o pericholecystic fluid are diagnostic. Tx w/ abx and laparoscopic cholecystectomy (or open if unable to safely proceed laparoscopically). Intraop cholangiogram generally recommended if abnormal LFTs (particularly bilirubin and alkaline phosphatase) or dilated CBD (> 6 mm, although the normal diameter increases w/ age).
   b. *Acalculous cholecysitis*: accounts for 5% of cases of cholecystitis, generally occurs in older males who are critically ill; etiology possibly related to reperfusion injury or other inflammatory d/o. Dx is suggested by GB wall edema and pericholecystic fluid, but HIDA is test of choice. Gold standard is also laparoscopic cholecystectomy, although percutaneous cholecystostomy tube should be strongly considered for the unstable pt.
2. *Choledocholithiasis*
   a. *Primary*:
      i. Form in the biliary tree, not from the gallbladder.
      ii. Usu. brown pigment stones, which appear soft, "earthy," and are assoc. w/ chronic biliary stasis and infection.
      iii. Stasis may be from sphincter of Oddi dysfunction, papillary stenosis, or biliary stricture.
      iv. *Definitive tx depends on cause*:
         - *Hepaticojejunostomy*: use Roux-en-Y, w/ nonrefluxing end-to-side anastomosis and limb length of at least 45 cm.
         - *Sphincteroplasty*: see Chapter 26 on key steps for key operations.
   b. *Secondary*:
      i. Form in gallbladder, then pass into biliary tree. Usu. either cholesterol stones or black pigment stones.
      ii. Treat w/ cholecystectomy (and clearance of CBD w/ IOC/exploration or ERCP).
3. *Mirizzi syndrome*: compression of common hepatic duct by stone lodged in Hartmann's pouch or cystic duct.
   a. *Classified as follows*:

i. *Type I*—no fistula present.
   - *Type IA*—presence of the cystic duct.
   - *Type IB*—obliteration of the cystic duct.

ii. *Types II–IV*—fistula present.
   - *Type II*—defect smaller than 33% of the CBD diameter.
   - *Type III*—defect 33–66% of the CBD diameter.
   - *Type IV*—defect larger than 66% of the CBD diameter.

4. *Biliary pancreatitis*: see section III. below on pancreas.
5. *Cholangitis*: medical emergency from bacterial infection of obstructed (cancer, stone, parasite, etc.) biliary system. Charcot's triad = fever, RUQ pain, jaundice. Raynold's pentad = fever, RUQ pain, jaundice, hypotension, altered mental status.
6. *Gallstone ileus*: results when cholecystoenteric fistula develops (usu. duodenum, occ. colon), allowing gallstone(s) to enter intestinal lumen. Point of obstruction is usu. ileocecal valve. Treat by milking stone back to normal bowel, then creating an enterotomy through which to deliver the stone. Most fistulas will close spontaneously, and the dissection required to perform chlolecystectomy and fistula is excision, which is generally not recommended during the initial surgery, particularly in unhealthy pts.
7. *Bouveret's syndrome*: gastric outlet caused by proximal migration of gallstone from fistula.
8. *Bile leak*: often presents w/ abdominal pain, possibly fevers a/o jaundice. Check LFTs and RUQ U/S or CT. If biloma present, can percutaneously drain. ERCP should demonstrate leak, and if involves cystic duct, stenting should decompress sufficiently to allow healing. Injuries to CBD or right/left typically require exploration.

a. *Evaluation of jaundice*

i. *After H&P, check bilirubin*:
   - Indirect (*unconjugated*) hyperbilirubinemia—*nonsurgical*.
     - Increased production (hemolysis, burns, transfusion rxn's).
     - Impaired hepatocyte uptake or conjugation (Gilbert's, Crigler-Najjar, viral hepatitis, neonatal jaundice, drug inhibition).
   - Direct (*conjugated*) hyperbilirubinemia—*usu. surgical*.
     - Impaired transport and excretion (Dubin-Johnson, Rotor's, cirrhosis, amyloidosis, cancer, hepatitis, pregnancy, TPN cholestasis).
     - Biliary obstruction (choledocholithiasis, Mirizzi's, benign stricture, periampullary CA, cholangiocarcinoma, primary sclerosing cholangitis, parasitic, Caroli's dz).
     - *Note*: high levels of indirect bilirubin eventually result in elevated direct bilirubin levels as well as after the bilirubin is conjugated.
   - *Direct hyperbilirubinemia w/u*:
     - If suspect intrahepatic dz, check hepatitis panel, liver bx, other tests.
     - If suspect common duct stones, check U/S.
       - If see dilated ducts, pursue ERCP for stone extraction.
       - If see normal ducts, some recommend MRCP.
     - If suspect malignant obstruction, check CT scan.
       - If see mass or dilated ducts and suspect proximal obstruction → ERCP.
       - If see mass or dilated ducts and suspect distal obstruction → PTC.

b. *ERCP*

i. *Indications*:
   - *Preop*:
     - Worsening biliary pancreatitis
     - Cholangitis
     - Stent placement for stricture (benign or malignant)
     - Symptomatic cholelithiasis in pts unfit for surgery

- *Postop*:
  - Bile leak
  - Retained CBD stone

ii. *Note*: open surgical papillotomy can be performed as well through duodenotomy. Key point is to perform papillotomy at 10 o'clock position to avoid bleeding.

III. PANCREAS

A. Benign disease

1. *Acute pancreatitis*

a. *Etiology*: gallstones, alcohol, trauma (including ERCP), hypercalcemia, hypertriglyceridemia, paramyxovirus (mumps), medications (diuretics [thiazides, furosemide], steroids, azathioprine, sulfonamides, NSAIDs), autoimmune (polyarteritis nodosa, SLE), scorpion envenomation [Bartholomew C, Tityus trinitatus of Trinidad. *BMJ*. 1970;1:666–8.] Rare causes include pancreas divisum, cystic fibrosis, pancreatic malignancy, helminth (i.e., *Ascaris*) obstruction, etc.

b. *Presentation and w/u*:

- *Clinical*: epigastric pain radiating to the back is classic. Hemorrhagic pancreatitis may (rarely) demonstrate Cullen's sign (periumbilical ecchymosis) or Grey Turner's sign (flank ecchymoses) or Fox's sign (inguinal ecchymosis).
- *Biochemical*:
  - *Amylase*: generally rises w/in 2–12 h of sx onset, normalizing w/in 1 wk.
    - *Hyperamylasemia ddx*: pancreatic injury or inflammation, small bowel injury, appendicitis, parotiditis, orchitis, hereditary macroamylasemia (molecule too large to be renally excreted), renal failure.
  - *Lipase*: generally rises w/in 4–8 h of sx onset, normalizing in 1–2 wk.
    - Slightly more sensitive and specific for pancreatitis; no need to order lipase *and* amylase.
- *Radiographic*: imaging not usu. needed for the dx. Timing of contrast CT is controversial, in part because most cases are not severe, and even if necrosis does occur, it is not fully radiographically manifest for 4–5 d. Some order CT initially to distinguish from other conditions such as perforated ulcer or identify/quantify necrosis. More commonly, however, it is ordered if pt deteriorates, is thought to be septic, or fails to improve after a wk.

c. *Scoring systems*:

- Most cases are mild and resolve w/in several days.
- Ranson's criteria (3+ predictive of severe attack w/ > 10% mortality; pt should be in ICU). See Table 16.2.
- APACHE II score (8+ at 48 h predictive of severe attack w/ > 10%; pt should be in ICU).
  - Factors include obesity, organ failure markers, hypotension, tachycardia, hypoxia, etc.
  - An online calculator is available at *http://sfar.org/scores2/apache22.html*.
- CRP > 150 mg/mL also suggests severe dz.

TABLE 16.2. Ranson's Score for Pancreatitis

Nonbiliary Pancreatitis		Biliary Pancreatitis	
Initial	48 h	Initial	48 h
> 55 yo	Hct decrease > 10%	> 70 yo	Hct decrease > 10%
WBC > 16k / mm^3	BUN increase > 5 mg/dL	WBC > 18k / mm^3	BUN increase > 2 mg/dL
Glucose > 200 mg/dL	Ca^{++} < 8 mg/dL	Glucose > 220 mg/dL	Ca^{++} < 8 mg/dL
LDH > 350 IU/L	Fluid sequestration > 6 L	LDH > 40 IU/L	Fluid sequestration > 4 L
AST > 250 U / 100 mL	Base deficit > 4 mmol/L	AST > 250 U / 100 mL	Base deficit > 5 mmol/L
	PaO_2 > 55 mm Hg		

d. *Tx*: all cases are managed w/ the first 2 steps mentioned below. Moderate to severe cases, however, are biphasic. The first (inflammatory) phase is managed conservatively w/ these same first 2 stages, and surgery, which may actually worsen the inflammatory response, is avoided if possible. The second stage involves managing the sequelae, which are generally determined in the first 4–5 d; surgery and other invasive interventions are more frequently used in this phase.

   i. *NPO w/ NGT decompression* (some authors argue the latter is not necessary).

      - Nutritional support for prolonged cases has traditionally been via TPN; however, several studies now support enteric (at least trophic) feeds via nasojejunal tube both for alimentation and to prevent bacterial translocation.

   ii. *IVF resuscitation + Foley catheter.*

   iii. *Abx*: infected pancreatic necrosis merits tx w/ carbapenems, while prophylactic use (i.e., for sterile pancreatic necrosis) is controversial, w/ literature supporting both sides. One reasonable compromise is carbapenem usage if > 30% necrosis.

   iv. *ERCP*: reserved for biliary pancreatitis that deteriorates or fails to improve after 48 h.

   v. *Surgery*:

      - Delay surgery for after first 2 wk if at all possible; increased mortality w/ early operative intervention.
      - *Infected* pancreatic necrosis is the main indication for surgery, although some pts who fail to respond to optimal medical therapy may benefit from debridement. Many surgeons rely upon CT-guided FNA to determine if necrotic material is infected, while others base the decision to operate on clinical and radiographic evidence.
      - Pancreatic necrosectomy followed by temporary closure and planned redebridement in 24–48 h vs necrosectomy and placement of irrigation (i.e., Davol) drains are the 2 usual approaches.

   vi. *For cases of biliary pancreatitis*, cholecystectomy should be performed before discharge ($^1/_3$ of pts will have recurrence w/in 8 wk otherwise). In mild cases, surgery is generally undertaken once the pt is pain-free, w/ no abdominal tenderness; most also wait for normalization of amylase a/o lipase. If ERCP is not performed preop, intraop cholangiogram should be performed.

e. *Sequelae/complications*:

   i. *Acute fluid collection*: fluid around pancreas typically < 4 wk following onset of inflammation that lacks capsular wall. If not infected, manage w/ observation, as most spontaneously resolve.

   ii. *Pancreatic pseudocyst*: fluid (pancreatic "juice") collection(s) in/around pancreas > 4 wk following onset of inflammation. Most resolve w/ time, but collections persisting > 6 wk or > 6 cm in diameter are more likely to require intervention to avoid complications such as infection, gastric compression, or hemosuccus pancreaticus. Drainage (cystgastrostomy, cystjejunostomy, or, rarely, cystduodenostomy) is performed once pseudocyst has substantial capsule.

   iii. *Pancreatic abscess*: infected peripancreatic fluid (either acute fluid collection or pseudocyst). Most are successfully managed w/ abx and percutaneous drainage.

   iv. *Pancreatic necrosis*: see section d. above on general tx.

   v. *Pancreatic ascites*: direct communication of pancreatic duct from trauma or rupture of pancreatic pseudocyst. Management is usu. conservative, w/ percutaneous drainage, converting the condition to a *pancreatic fistula*.

   vi. *Pancreatic fistula* (see entry ii. on pancreatic pseudocyst and entry v. on pancreatic ascites above): initial tx is w/ TPN a/o nasojejunal feeds +/– IV octreotide, replacement of electrolytes (i.e., sodium, bicarbonate). Fistulas that persist beyond 6 wk despite appropriate medical tx are definitively managed w/ distal pancreatectomy (leak in tail), or Roux-en-Y limb (leak in head, body), although endoscopic stenting may be a viable option for some. If pancreatic duct is dilated (i.e., 8 mm), lateral pancreaticojejunostomy is often appropriate.

   vii. *Pancreatic pleural effusion*: manage as pancreatic ascites/fistula.

   viii. *Hemosuccus pancreaticus*: hemorrhage resulting from pseudocyst erosion into peripancreatic vessel. Tx w/ endovascular embolization of involved vessel, possibly followed by surgical exploration and packing.

2. *Chronic pancreatitis*
   a. Most commonly from recurrent alcoholic pancreatitis, resulting in pain and potentially exocrine a/o endocrine insufficiency.
   b. *Surgical tx can be divided into 2 broad approaches*: ductal drainage (theorizing that problem is ductal hypertension) or resection (theorizing that nerve proliferation or sensitization is responsible for pain *or* if duct is too small to drain).
      i. *Resection procedures* (have generally fallen out of favor)
         - *Whipple*: sometimes performed for benign, inflammatory mass in head w/ nondilated duct. Entails pancreaticoduodenectomy followed by jejunostomy/gastrostomy + gastrojejunostomy + choledochojejunostomy. Although the procedure has significant potential for morbidity, good outcome for pain relief up to 90%.
         - *Traverso-Longmire*: essentially a pylorus-preserving pancreaticoduodenectomy to avoid postgastrectomy complications of a Whipple.
         - *Subtotal pancreatectomy*: generally less than 80% (if remove 95%, leaving thin rim along duodenum and CBD, termed Child's resection). Generally performed for distal dz (pseudocyst, failed pancreaticojejunostomy, nondilated duct, etc., and assoc. w/ majority of pts developing IDDM afterward.
      ii. *Drainage procedures*
         - *Partington-Rochelle* (modification of Puestow, *vide infra*): side-to-side pancreaticojejunostomy w/out resection of pancreatic tail or spleen. Generally requires duct diameter of at least 8 mm (mucosa to duct anastomosis), although success has been reported w/ 5 mm (mucosa to capsule anastomosis).
         - *Mercadier*: drainage of pancreatic body into Roux-en-Y jejunal loop via side-to-side anastomosis.
         - *Rumpf's extended drainage*: a modification of Partington-Rochelle w/ a transduodenal pancreatoplasty, indicated if prepapillary obstruction from stricture—largely abandoned now w/ availability of ERCP/interventional endoscopy.
      iii. *Combination procedures* (procedures of choice for vast majority, good results up to 95% reported).
         - *Puestow*: although generally referred to as a drainage procedure, the original Puestow (1956) denoted longitudinal opening of pancreatic duct lateral to mesenteric vessels AFTER resection of pancreatic tail and splenectomy. Followed by invagination of open duct and pancreas into Roux-en-Y limb of jejunum. 60–80% effective.
         - *Beger*: a duodenum-preserving resection of pancreatic head, w/ an end-to-end pancreaticojejunostomy of the body as well as a side-to-side anastomosis of the rim of pancreatic head. Mostly used in cases w/ inflammatory mass in pancreatic head, obstruction of CBD, or duodenal stenosis.
         - *Extended Beger*: if multiple strictures in left pancreas in addition to mass in head, can do head resection as described above, plus side-to-side anastomosis of pancreatic duct and interposed jejunal loop.
         - *Frey*: less technically challenging than the Beger, this cores out pancreatic head overlying ducts, maintaining 5 mm of tissue posteriorly and medially, and also opens main duct in body and tail. Lateral pancreaticojejunostomy is then performed. Duct is anastomosed to mucosa unless diameter < 8 mm, in which case capsule is anastomosed to mucosa (some have reported success w/ ducts as small as 3.5 mm). Ideally indicated for pseudocysts, CBD obstruction, pancreatic ascites, fistulas, and recurrent pain after lateral pancreaticojejunostomy, but contraindicated if cancer can't be excluded.

B. Developmental anomalies

1. *Pancreas divisum*:
   a. *Etiology/presentation*: failure of fusion of dorsal and ventral ducts (ventral duct [duct of Wirsung] assoc. w/ CBD and migrates inferiorly to dorsal duct [duct of Santorini] to drain via major papilla). Result is the normally smaller duct of Santorini draining the pancreatic body through minor papilla instead of the duct of Wirsung through the ampulla of Vater; it should be noted that variations of this anomaly are common (up to 5–10%). Usu. asymptomatic, but may result in pain/pancreatitis.

b. *Dx*: made via ERCP/MRCP, but all efforts must be made to r/o other possible causes of pancreatitis.

c. *Tx*:

i. *Endoscopic*: balloon dilatation or papillotomy may be used in minimally symptomatic pts. Stents have been successfully employed as well, but long-term studies are lacking. Botulinum toxin injection into the minor papilla has also been reported.

ii. *Operative*: surgery is indicated for pts w/ pancreatitis (or in pts w/ pain in whom stenting is technically not possible). Most often, dorsal duct (minor papilla) sphincterotomy is performed. Lateral pancreaticojejunostomy is indicated for dilation of duct of Wirsung. Distal pancreatectomy is reserved for extensive pathologic changes (atrophy, fibrosis, etc.) in the tail.

2. *Annular pancreas*: see "double bubble" on x-ray, as w/ duodenal atresia or malrotation. Perform duodenojejunostomy w/out resecting pancreas.

C. W/u of pancreatic lesions

1. *Solid*—consider as malignant until proven otherwise:

a. *CT w/ 3-mm cuts should be obtained*: adenocarcinomas are often slightly hypodense, but this is not diagnostic.

i. *CT criteria for unresectability include*: evidence of distant/extrapancreatic spread; obliteration of fatty plane between mass and superior mesenteric vein; encasement of SMA.

ii. *Pts w/ unresectable dz need bx for palliative tx (chemo, XRT); this is best obtained by EUS. Pathologic dx is not required preop, however.* In pts w/ strong possibility of having an inflammatory mass instead of cancer, endoscopic FNA may be considered, but carries a 10% risk of being false-negative due to sampling error.

b. Endoscopic U/S a/o ERCP useful to identify lesions < 2 cm. Endoscopically placed stents may also be used to provide symptomatic relief, tx cholangitis, or help correct hepatic dysfunction preop, but should be plastic, not metal, if surgery is planned.

c. In pts w/ tumors > 2 cm that appear resectable on CT, laparoscopy sometimes used to confirm resectability before proceeding w/ open operation (assuming one would not need to perform open biliary a/o gastric bypass regardless of findings).

2. *Cystic*: pseudocyst >> neoplasms > congenital.

a. *Hx*: pancreatitis (esp. alcoholic, chronic) or trauma suggests pseudocyst.

b. *CT characteristics*: septations suggest neoplasm.

c. *ERCP/MRCP*: pancreatic duct communication suggests pseudocyst or intraductal papillary mucinous neoplasm.

d. *Aspirate*: high amylase suggests pseudocyst whereas mucin or high CEA a/o CA 19-9 suggest neoplasm.

e. *Bx*: epithelial cells in cyst wall exclude pseudocyst.

CHAPTER 17

HERNIAS

I. INGUINAL HERNIAS

A. In men, indirect hernias 2× more common than direct. Direct hernias even less common in females; females have femoral hernias more commonly than men (but still relatively uncommon).

1. Indirect and femoral hernias both 2× more common on the right. (Right testis descends more slowly on right, and sigmoid colon may tamponade left femoral canal.)
2. Infant females may have fallopian tube/ovary in inguinal ring. 1% of pediatric female inguinal hernias assoc. w/ testicular feminization; obtain buccal smear for chromatin testing in female infants w/ inguinal hernia. If no chromatin found, leave gonad in canal to generate estrogen until puberty, then take out to prevent malignant degeneration.
3. Young males (up to 3 yo) should undergo contralateral groin exploration esp. if presenting hernia is on left.

B. **Anatomy**

1. *Conjoined tendon*: fusion of fibers from internal oblique and transversus abdominis aponeuroses. Inserts on pubic tubercle, pectineal ligament, and superior pubic ramus.
2. *Genital nerve*: motor to cremaster muscle *and* sensory to lateral scrotum/labia (not leg). Arises from L1 to L2. Lies on iliopubic tract, accompanying cremaster vessels, generally divided w/ impunity. Runs along spermatic cord, often in inferoposterior aspect of cord along w/ external spermatic vessels. In males can be divided w/ impunity; females may experience undesirable hypesthesia of labia majora, however.
3. *Hesselbach's triangle*: although not exactly the same boundaries as initially described in 1814, circumscribes area through which *most* direct hernias protrude. Superolateral = inferior epigastric vessels; medial = lateral border of rectus sheath; inferior/base = inguinal ligament.
4. *Iliopectineal arch*: medial thickening of iliopsoas muscle deep to inguinal ligament; external oblique aponeurosis and fibers of inguinal ligament insert into it and also serve as lateral attachment of iliopubic tract.
5. *Ilioinguinal nerve*: mixes w/ fibers of iliohypogastric nerve to provide sensation to groin, penile base/scrotum, medial upper thigh. Arise from T12 and L1. Found superficial and superior to spermatic cord in 60%, but may be behind or in cremasteric muscle.
6. *Iliopubic tract*: transverse aponeurotica at upper border of femoral sheath; aponeurotic band extending from iliopectineal arch to superior pubic ramus. Passes medially, contributing to inferior border of internal ring, then crosses femoral vessels to form anterior margin of femoral sheath. Attaches to pectineal ligament and is often confused w/ inguinal ligament. More simply, a ridge-like thickening of aponeurotic tissue along superior rim of inferior pubic ramus immediately deep/posterior to inguinal ligament, essentially where transversalis fascia attaches to the ramus.
7. *Inguinal ligament* (Poupart's ligament): thickened inferior aspect of external oblique aponeurosis. Extends from AS iliac spine to pubic ramus; middle $^{1}/_{3}$ has a free (shelving) edge, lateral $^{2}/_{3}$ attached to iliopsoas fascia.
8. *Lacunar ligament* (Gimbernat's ligament): inferiormost portion of inguinal ligament, which recurves to attach to pectineal ligament.
9. *Pectineal ligament* (Cooper's ligament): formed from tendinous fibers of internal oblique, transversus, and pectineus muscle. More simply, a somewhat broad ridge of thickened ligamentous tissue found immediately posterior to iliopubic tract (which itself is immediately posterior to the inguinal ligament), in the medial portion of the groin. Division of the transversalis fascia is mandatory to view this structure.
10. *Reflected inguinal ligament* (Colles' ligament): thick band formed mostly by fibers of lacunar ligament and fibers of internal oblique, transversus abdominis, and pectineus muscle; formed by aponeurotic fibers from inferior aspect of external ring. Fixed to periosteum of superior pubic ramus.
11. *Semiarculate line of Douglas*: in lower $^{1}/_{4}$ of abdominal wall, aponeuroses of internal oblique and transversus abdominus pass anterior to muscle, which is bounded posteriorly by transversalis muscle only.
12. *Shelving edge of inguinal ligament.*

C. Hernia nomenclature and types

1. *Incarcerated hernia*—irreducible.
2. *Taxis*—manipulation of the hernia resulting in reduction.
3. *Strangulated hernia*—vascularity of viscus is compromised.
4. *Richter's hernia*—contents of the sac consist of only a portion of the intestinal wall of the intestine; esp. precarious in that strangulation can occur w/out obstruction.
5. *Sliding hernia*—internal retroperitoneal organ (cecum, sigmoid colon for indirect, bladder for direct) forms part of the wall of the hernia sac.
6. *Indirect hernia*—dilated persistent processus vaginalis, emerges lateral to inferior epigastric vessels, and lies along anteromedial aspect of cord. Properitoneal fat may be found w/in, inappropriately called "cord lipoma." If remains completely open and contains testicle, is termed communicating hydrocele. *Note*: 80% of newborns and 50% of 1-yr-olds have patent processes vaginalis; only 20% of adults remain patent.
7. *Direct hernia*—protrusion through inguinal floor, via Hesselbach's triangle (*almost* always medial to inferior epigastric vessels, which are the last branch of external iliacs).
8. *Femoral hernia*—herniation between femoral vein/sheath laterally and lacunar ligament medially; limited anteriorly by inguinal ligament and posteriorly by Cooper's ligament. Often contains node(s) of Cloquet/Rosenmüller.
9. *Pantaloon hernia*—defect w/ herniation both medial and lateral to epigastric vessels.
10. *Littre's hernia*—any inguinal hernia that contains a Meckel's diverticulum.

D. Repairs (for full details of each procedure, see Chapter 26)

1. *Marcy*: repair myopectineal orifice–tightening of internal ring. Performed for indirect hernia w/ minimal pathology of deep ring. Involves placing 1–2 sutures in transverse aponeurotic arch and iliopubic tract just medial to spermatic cord. For females w/ indirect hernia, first divide round ligament and eliminate sac, then fully close ring. In other words, high ligation of sac and suture tightening of internal ring. Purportedly first performed in 1871.
2. *Bassini*: as originally described (1889), internal oblique, transversus abdominis, and transversalis fascia (Bassini's triple layer) are approximated to inguinal ligament and iliopubic tract inferiorly w/ a double layer of interrupted sutures (Cooper's ligament may be included in most medial bites). Early in operation, emphasis is given to longitudinal, then transverse division of cremasteric muscle (to facilitate visualization of floor) as well as incision of transversalis fascia parallel to inguinal ligament (taking care not to injure underlying epigastric vessels). North American modification results in mere high ligation of sac and approximation of conjoined tendon and internal abdominal oblique to shelving edge of inguinal ligament. Alternately described as relaxing cut above conjoint tendon, then bring inferior edge down to sew directly onto shelving edge of inguinal ligament.
3. *Shouldice*: (1953) similar to original Bassini repair but instead of using interrupted sutures to approximate structures, the structures are imbricated (Latin for "shingle") w/ running suture w/ the superior edge lapping over the inferior edge. In the deeper row, Bassini's "triple layer" is approximated to iliopubic tract from medial to lateral. This is followed by running lateral to medial w/ the same suture, but suturing internal oblique and transversus abdominis to shelving edge of inguinal ligament. Third and fourth rows are finally created w/ a second suture approximating superior structures to inferior aspect of divided external oblique fascia. Relaxing incision may be used. In other words, incise transversalis fascia parallel to fibers, lift up superior edge, then bring inferior edge up to sew it to conjoint tendon. Next, bring superior edge down to suture it to shelving edge of inguinal ligament.
4. *McVay (1942)–Lotheissen (1897) Cooper ligament repair*: repairs deep ring, Hesselbach's triangle, and femoral canal. Transverse aponeurotic arch is sutured to Cooper's ligament medially and to femoral sheath laterally—requires excision of medial portion of iliopubic tract. The nonmesh procedure of choice for femoral hernias, although small femoral hernias in females may be adequately treated w/ simple infrainguinal direct suture closure or "corked" w/ plug/Marlex. Ideal tx is likely properitoneal prosthetic repair. *Relaxing incision* along border of rectus sheath and external oblique is necessary for Cooper ligament repair.
5. *Lichtenstein's tension-free repair*: sew mesh to Cooper's ligament, then tack down to conjoined tendon above and shelving edge of inguinal ligament below, reinforcing transversalis fascia floor (for direct hernias), and can tighten "legs" of mesh to reconstruct internal ring (for indirect hernias).
6. *Stoppa GPRVS*: essentially replaces transversalis fascia w/ large piece of mesh in the preperitoneal space after reduction of hernia.

7. *Laparoscopic*:
   a. Results in fewer recurrences compared to open suture, but not mesh repairs.
   b. Takes longer, possibly fewer infections, possibly earlier return to work.
   c. *Two approaches*:
      i. *Transabdominal preperitoneal* (TAPP): dissect, identify structures listed below, then cover myopectineal orifice w/ mesh, which is fastened medially to rectus, superiorly to transversus abdominis arch, inferiorly to Cooper's ligament, laterally to the iliopubic tract. Peritoneum is reapproximated afterward.
      ii. *Totally extraperitoneal* (TEP): necessary to visualize abdominal wall, bladder, Cooper's ligament, and iliopubic tract, inferior epigastric artery/vein, gonadal vessels and vas deferens. Access begun w/ incision through skin and rectus muscle, then balloon dissection performed superficial to posterior rectus fascia. Further dissection occurs in the space of Retzius (between vesicoumbilical fascia posteriorly and the posterior rectus sheath and pubic bone, anteriorly).
   d. *Causes for recurrence*: inadequate dissection, inadequate prosthetic size, mesh migration.
8. *Open preperitoneal* (Nyhus): esp. good for strangulated hernias as can provide direct access to peritoneal contents for bowel resection w/out additional incision. Also useful for femoral and recurrent hernias. In essence, divide abdominal wall layers down to peritoneum, reduce hernias. For indirect hernias, close space between transversalis fascia and iliopubic tract w/ sutures or mesh. For direct hernias, approximate transversalis fascia/transverse aponeurotic arch to iliopubic tract. For femoral hernias, Cooper's ligament to iliopubic tract.

E. Complications

1. *General*
   a. *Neuralgia*: pain, paresthesias, a/o numbness result from partial nerve division or entrapment in mesh or scar tissue, but most largely subside w/in 2 mo. Completely transecting nerve can avoid this for nerves at risk, yielding only a variable degree of numbness.
   b. *Injury to vas deferens*: may present as painful spermatic granuloma; tx by granuloma excision and repair of vas.
   c. *Recurrence*: most repairs report 1–10% recurrence rate.
   d. *Ischemic orchitis/testicular atrophy*: most often from venous, not arterial, insufficiency. Initially presents as swollen, firm cord, epididymis, and testis, most often 2–5 d postop; symptoms may last several mo. Decrease risk by not dissecting medial to pubis and not dissecting distal hernia sac (except in sliding hernias).
2. *Laparoscopic*
   a. *Triangle of doom*: defined by vas deferens medially, spermatic vessels laterally, and external iliac vessels inferiorly. Contains external iliac artery/vein, deep circumflex iliac vein, genital branch of genitofemoral nerve, as (covered by fascia) femoral nerve. Stapling in this area can cause significant bleeding a/o neuralgia.
   b. *Triangle of pain*: defined by spermatic vessels medially, iliopubic tract laterally, and inferior edge of skin incision. Contains lateral femoral cutaneous nerve and anterior femoral cutaneous nerve. Stapling in this area can cause neuralgia.
   c. *Circle of death* ("corona mortis"): vascular ring formed by anastomosis of aberrant branch of obturator artery w/ a branch of internal iliac artery. Injury can lead to considerable bleeding.

II. <u>NON-INGUINAL HERNIAS</u> (*Note*: paraesophageal hernia discussed in Chapter 8)

A. Epigastric hernia: risk factors include obesity and pregnancy. Differentiate from diastasis recti, as the latter does not present risk of significant complication.

B. Ventral hernia

1. Mesh repair standard of care:
   a. *Polypropylene mesh (Marlex)*: excellent incorporation, relatively resistant to infection, high fistula rate if placed directly on bowel.
   b. *PTFE (GoreTex)*: material of choice for placing on bowel (i.e., dual-sided mesh) if necessary, but virtually impossible to clear infection.
   c. *Mersilene*: not recommended for ventral hernia repair.
   d. *Vicryl/Dacron*: useful for contaminated wound for temporary closure—will granulate, take skin graft.

2. Ramirez (1990) first described component release (ext oblique and posterior rectus fascia) for abdominal closure; can get up to 20 cm at level of umbilicus. [Ramirez OM, et al., *Plast Reconstr Surg.* 1990;86(3):519–26.]

C. **Spigelian hernia**: lies between aponeurotic edge of transversus abdominus and lateral border of rectus sheath. Majority are w/in 6 cm of level of iliac crest. Often difficult to appreciate on abdominal exam; CT generally procures dx. Repair through incision directly over hernia or through preperitoneal or laparoscopic means.

D. **Petit's hernia**: like Grynfeltt's hernia, is a lumbar hernia. Petit's is inferior and represents an upright triangle bounded by latissimus dorsi, iliac crest, and external oblique muscle; it is covered only by superficial fascia. Repair requires prosthesis or myoaponeurotic flap.

E. **Grynfeltt's hernia**: like Petit's hernia, a lumbar hernia. Grynfeltt's is superior and represents an inverted triangle defined by 12th rib, internal oblique muscle, and sacrospinalis muscle; it is covered by latissimus dorsi. Repair requires prosthesis or myoaponeurotic flap.

F. **Parastomal hernia**: for first-time hernias, moving site of stoma and mesh repair of hernia is preferred. For recurrent hernias, mesh repair is recommended. [Rubin MS, et al., *Arch Surg.* 1994;129(4):413–8.]

G. **Obturator hernia**: most common variant of pelvic hernias, and is generally seen in elderly, cachectic females, often strangulated upon presentation. Compression of obturator nerve may result (50%) in hip, knee, and medial thigh pain, esp. w/ internal rotation of thigh (Howship-Romberg sign). Mass may be palpable in upper medial thigh, or on pelvic/rectal exam. Exploration through lower midline incision useful to assess bowel and repair hernia. Can often be repaired w/out mesh.

H. **Umbilical hernia**: black > white children. F > M adults. Risk factors include multiple pregnancies and ascites; latter condition may result in rupture requiring emergent portal decompression. Strangulation of colon, omentum not uncommon. Infants w/ defects 2 cm or smaller may be observed while defects larger than 2 cm or any defect in a child older than 3 yo should be repaired. The Mayo "vest-over-pants" imbrication remains the standard for small hernias; prosthetic repair for larger defects is appropriate.

CHAPTER 18

SPLEEN

I. **ANATOMY**

A. Tethered by gastrosplenic, gastrocolic, splenorenal, and phrenosplenic ligaments, must take down superior, lateral, and inferior ligaments to mobilize. Splenic artery branches off celiac axis, and divides into 6 segmental end branches. Accessory spleens in ~ 25%, from failure of anlagen to fuse—most often in hilum, splenic ligaments, omentum, mesentery, and rarely along left ureter or left gonad. Histologically arranged into inner white pulp (w/ lymphatic follicles and immunologic function), marginal zone (filters material from white zone), and outer red pulp (w/ sinuses; serves phagocytic function).

II. **TRAUMA:** see Chapter 9.

III. **NONTRAUMA INDICATIONS FOR SPLENECTOMY** (splenectomy, splenorrhaphy details in Chapter 9.)

A. **ITP:** splenectomy reserved for the 75% of adults who fail steroid +/– IVIgG, +/– Rho(d) immunoglobulin tx; > 85% get good response to surgery. Thrombocytopenia and intracranial bleed are indications for emergent splenectomy. Nuclear medicine scans such as SPECT imaging useful to identify accessory spleens in refractory cases.

B. **TTP:** if pt fails plasmapheresis and FFP +/– steroids +/– aspirin (~ 30–50%).

C. **Gaucher's dz:** deficent β-glucosidase leads to glycosylceramide accumulation in RES. Can cause hypersplenism or mechanical sx from splenomegaly. *Partial* splenectomy recommended (over total splenectomy) to lessen risk of malignancy and accelerated bone dz.

D. **Felty syndrome:** constellation of rheumatoid arthritis, autoimmune neutropenia (often w/ recurrent infections), and splenomegaly. Splenectomy can improve neutropenia.

E. **Pyruvate kinase deficiency, thalassemias, and elliptocytosis:** splenectomy can help w/ hemolytic anemia if significant.

F. **Spherocytosis:** from RBC lack of spectrin; splenectomy only useful tx. Eval for cholelithiasis (55%), do concomitant cholecystectomy as appropriate.

G. **Splenic vein thrombosis (often from pancreatitis):** can lead to "left-sided ("sinister") portal hypertension" manifesting w/ isolated gastric varices. Splenectomy, not shunt, is indicated.

H. **Part of total gastrectomy or other surgery.**

I. **Sarcoidosis:** granulomatous dz of spleen may lead to anemia, which is improved w/ splenectomy.

J. **Hairy cell leukemia:** tx first w/ interferon a/o cladribine, reserving splenectomy for failures (primarily palliative at that point—very rare).

K. **Giant hemangiomas:** rarely may lead to platelet entrapment and Kasabach-Merritt syndrome as in the liver.

L. **Infections:** formerly, splenic abscesses warranted splenectomy, but majority can be handled w/ percutaneous drainage and abx.

IV. **CONSEQUENCES OF SPLENECTOMY**

A. **Howell-Jolly bodies:** nuclear remnants in RBC.

B. **Heinz bodies:** denatured hgb remnants (think Heinz ketchup = red = hgb).

C. **Pappenheimer bodies:** iron granules.

D. **Leukocytosis.**

E. **Thrombocytosis:** conventionally, aspirin given if > 1,000,000, although little data to support.

F. Loss of tuftsin (helps PMNs phagocytose) and properdin (helps initiate alternate complement pathway) and major site of IgM synthesis. Leads to OPSS (below).

G. **Risk of "overwhelming postsplenectomy sepsis."**

1. Avoid splenectomy if pt less than 4 yo if possible.
2. Mortality > 50% in children, decreases w/ age.
3. Typically occurs in first 2 yr postop, but can occur > 5 yr later.

4. *Streptococcus pneumoniae* (50–90%), *H. influenzae*, *N. meningitidis* should all be vaccinated against; last not as commonly indicated though. *E. coli*, β-hemolytic strep, and *Pseudomonas* are other potential pathogens. (Encapsulated bacteria require opsonization for optimal elimination.) Increased risk for severe malaria, babesiosis.
5. Risk greater if splenectomy for heme/onc dz than trauma or if pt less than 4 yo.
6. Prodrome of F, C, ST, D, V → hypotension, DIC, death.
7. No data to support prophylactic abx in adults.
   a. *Children < 5 yo*: amoxicillin 20 mg/kg PO q d or penicillin VK 125 mg PO 2 times per day (*alt*: TMP-SMX, clarithromycin).
   b. *Children > 5 yo*: penicillin VK 250 mg PO 2 times per day × 1 yr postsplectomy (*alt*: TMP-SMX, clarithromycin).
   c. *All children*: self-tx w/ ampicillin-clavulanate for febrile illness while awaiting eval by physician.

H. Most common complication is LLL atelectasis, followed by subphrenic abscess. Placement of drain in splenic fossa unnecessary (unless pancreatic injury/leak), and contributes to risk of subphrenic abscess.

CHAPTER 19

BREAST

(See Chapter 12 for breast cancer.)

I. ANATOMY AND VASCULATURE OF BREAST AND AXILLA

A. Vascular and lymphatic

1. *Vascular*: 60% blood supply from subclavians via internal mammary perforators. 30% blood supply from axillary artery via lateral thoracic artery → external mammary artery. 10% from aorta via posterior intercostals. Batson's plexus refers to anastomotic network connecting intercostal veins w/ vertebral veins, thought to be important for vertebral metastases.
2. *Lymphatic drainage*: majority to level I—lateral to pectoralis minor. Level II refers to nodes deep to pectoralis minor (aka "Rotter's nodes"). Level III medial to pectoralis minor.

B. Nerve

1. Long thoracic n. (innervates serratus anterior) 1–3 cm anterior to thoracodorsal n. (innervates latissimus).
2. Transverse intercostobrachial n. crosses axilla transversely to provide sensory function to medial arm.
3. Lateral pectoral nerve runs under and medial to pectoralis minor to innervate pectorals.

C. Anatomic anomalies

1. 2–6% women w/ polymastia (typically in axilla) or polythelia (typically inferior to primary nipple).
2. < 10% women w/ benign nipple inversion.

II. BENIGN DISEASE

A. Mastodynia

1. 66% of women. Do H&P; if abn, manage accordingly. If WNL, do mammogram; tx lesions accordingly.
2. If no lesion, 5–10% will respond to medical tx; primrose oil (gamma-linoleic acid) or Danazol (FDA-approved).

B. Nipple discharge

1. May be physiologic, from meds, or pituitary tumors. Pathology usu. papilloma.
2. More worrisome if spontaneous (doesn't require squeezing/induction), bloody, unilateral from 1 duct, assoc. w/ mass, or if age > 60 yo.

C. Breast abscess

1. Abx and aspiration likely to be successful unless > 20 cc volume, > 5 cm diameter, or > 1 wk delay dx, in which case I&D probably required. [Ervilmaz R, et al., *Breast*. Oct 2005; 14(5):375–9; Schwarz RJ, et al., *Am J Surg*. 2001; 182(2):11–9.]

D. Fibroadenomas

1. Most common lump if < 30 yo. R/o cystosarcoma phylloides. Observe, or if sx (or > 2–3 cm), excise.
2. No increased cancer risk.

E. Fibrocystic dz

1. 50% U.S. females meet clinical definition; 70% meet histologic criteria.
2. 58% premenopausal females have microcysts, 21% have macrocysts. Of female w/ cysts, 54% will refill, and 10% refill after aspiration.
3. Intraop, classically have appearance of "blue domed cysts."
4. Appropriate to cytology and excise if atypical pathology or if persistently symptomatic.

F. Breast lumps

1. If cystic, aspirate, f/u w/ mammogram; if nonbloody (which does NOT require cytology) or if disappears, just observe (some would add if strong fam hx, bx too).

2. If mass recurs × 2, or aspirate is bloody, or if persists, or if get positive cytology, or if initial size was > 5 cm, bx.
3. If is solid, but clinically benign *and* mammogram/sonogram (–) *and* CNBx/FNA benign, then observe (triple test—neg predict value 100%).
4. If solid but indeterminate or mammo suspicious and CNBx or FNA malignant or benign, bx.

G. Mondor's dz

1. Superficial thrombophlebitis of the breast.
2. *Tx*: NSAIDs, warm compresses.

H. Benign lesions and breast CA risk

1. *No increased risk*:
    a. Apocrine metaplasia.
    b. Duct ectasia.
    c. Mild epithelial hyperplasia of unusual type.
2. *1–4× increased risk*:
    a. Moderate (3–5+ cell layers above BM—normally only 2)—florid (> 70% luminal filling) hyperplasia.
    b. Sclerosing adenosis.
    c. Papilloma.
    d. Radial scar/complex sclerosing lesion.
    e. H/o fibroadenoma (some say no risk w/ fibroadenomas, though).
3. *4–5× increased risk*:
    a. Hyperplasia w/ atypia (indication for tamoxifen).
4. *8–10× increased risk*:
    a. Lobular or ductal carcinoma *in situ*.

III. DIAGNOSTIC MODALITIES

A. Mammogram: indications include screening, palpable mass (> 25 yo), mastodynia (> 35 yo), bloody nipple d/c, skin/nipple retraction.

1. < 35 yo only get for dx. 35–40 baseline mammogram. 40–50 q 1–2 yr. 50–74 annual (highest yield). > 75 controversial.
2. *BI-RADS*:
    a. 0—incomplete, do complete w/u.
    b. 1—no findings, regular f/u.
    c. 2—benign findings, regular f/u.
    d. 3—probably benign findings, 6-mo f/u (1–2% bx +).
    e. 4—indeterminate finding, bx (core or open, 20–30% +).
    f. 5—highly suspicious finding, excise (85% CA).

B. U/S: useful to eval cystic vs solid, for palpable masses a/o mammo abn or screening in young females w/ dense breasts; also consider for high-risk pts.

C. FNA: 10-cc syringe w/ 22-g needle. False neg 1–35%, False pos 1–18%.

D. Core needle bx: for histo of masses. False neg 5%. Rare false pos. Can do mastectomy based on results. Stereotactic core needle bx another option.

E. Mammotome: get 8× volume as w/ core needle bx; can do w/ U/S or stereotactically.

F. Open bx: for atypical ductal hyperplasia or BI-RADS 5 lesions.

CHAPTER 20

PEDIATRIC

I. VITALS, FLUIDS, AND OTHER PEDIATRIC BASICS

A. **See Table 20.1.**

TABLE 20.1. Normal Vital Signs

Age	Wt (kg)	Heart Rate	Systolic BP	Resp. Rate
0–1 mo	2–4	120–180	60–70	30–60
2–12 mo	4–10	80–160	70–100	20–50
12–24 mo	10–13	80–140	75–110	20–40
2–6 yo	13–25	80–120	80–110	20–30
6–12 yo	20–40	70–110	85–120	20–30
> 13 yo	> 40–60	55–105	90–120	12–20

Modified with permission from Cline DM, et al. *Emergency Medicine, Fifth Edition*. New York, NY: The McGraw-Hill Companies, Inc., 2000, page 754.

B. **Fluid management**

1. *Per h*: 4 mL/kg for 1st 10 kg (40 mL) *PLUS* 2 mL/kg for 2nd 10 kg (20 mL) *PLUS* 1 mL/kg thereafter.
2. *Per 24 h*: 100 mL/kg for 1st 10 kg (1000 mL) *PLUS* 50 mL/kg for 2nd 10 kg (500 mL) *PLUS* 20 mL/kg thereafter.

C. **Nutrition** (*Note*: infants should gain ~ 30 g/d)

1. *Calories*:
   a. *< 1 yo*: 100–120 kcal/kg/d
   b. *1–3 yo*: 100 kcal/kg/d
   c. *4–6 yo*: 90 kcal/kg/d
   d. *7–10 yo*: 70 kcal/kg/d
2. *Protein*:
   a. *< 1 yo*: ~ 3 g/kg/d
   b. *9 yo*: ~ 2 g/kg/d
   c. *18 yo*: ~ 1 g/kg/d
3. *Carbohydrate*: neonate: min. 5 mg/kg/min, increase up to 10 mg/kg/min
4. *Fat*: begin 0.5 g/kg/d, increase up to 3 g/kg/d

D. **See Table 20.2.**

II. HEAD AND NECK

A. **Thyroglossal duct cyst**: results from failure of obliteration of the tract created by the descent of the thyroid from the foramen cecum. Presents as midline neck mass. Tx is Sistrunk procedure, which removes the cyst/tract along w/ the midportion of the hyoid bone, up to the level of the base of the tongue. Important to ensure pt has normal thyroid tissue elsewhere in the neck (i.e., w/ radionuclide scan) before removing what may represent an incompletely descended thyroid.

B. **Branchial cleft cyst**

1. Head and neck structures develop from branchial (*pharyngeal*) *arches*, derived from neural crest cells. Failure of regression of the clefts gives rise to fistulas (more commonly seen in children), sinuses, or cysts (more commonly seen in adults).
   a. *First branchial arch*: develops structures for mastication, innervated by CN V.

TABLE 20.2. Resuscitation

Broselow-Luten	Wt (kg)	Fluids	Equipment
Grey	3–5	3 Kg: Bolus: 60 crystalloid; 30 colloid Maint: $D_5W+{}^1/_4$ NS+20 mEq KCl at 12 mL/h 4 Kg: Bolus: 80 crystalloid; 40 colloid Maint: $D_5W+{}^1/_4$ NS+20 mEq KCl at 16 mL/h 5 Kg: Bolus: 100 crystalloid; 50 colloid Maint: $D_5W+{}^1/_4$ NS+20 mEq KCl at 20 mL/h	Use Pink/Red zone equipment, except Foley (5 Fr) and BP cuff neonatal/inf.
Pink	6–7	Bolus: 130 crystalloid; 65 colloid Maint: $D_5W + {}^1/_4$ NS + 20 mEq KCl at 28 mL/h	Laryngoscope: 1 straight ETT: 3.5 uncuffed, insert to 10–10.5 cm Chest tube: 10–12 Fr Foley: 8 Fr NGT: 5–8 Fr Vasc: 22–24 Ga Intraoss: 18–15 Ga BP cuff: inf/child
Red	8–9	Bolus: 170 crystalloid; 85 colloid Maint: $D_5W + {}^1/_4$ NS + 20 mEq KCl at 35 mL/h	Same as Pink (above).
Purple	10–11	Bolus: 210 crystalloid; 105 colloid Maint: $D_5W + {}^1/_4$ NS + 20 mEq KCl at 40 mL/h	Laryngoscope: 1 straight ETT: 4.0 uncuffed, insert to 11–12 cm Chest tube: 16–20 Fr Foley: 8–10 Fr NGT: 8–10 Fr Vasc: 20–24 Ga Intraoss: 15 Ga BP cuff: child
Yellow	12–14	Bolus: 260 crystalloid; 130 colloid Maint: $D_5W + {}^1/_4$ NS + 20 mEq KCl at 45 mL/h	Laryngoscope: 2 straight ETT: 4.5 uncuffed, insert to 13.5 cm Chest tube: 20–24 Fr Foley: 10 Fr NGT: 10 Fr Vasc: 18–22 Ga Intraoss: 15 Ga BP cuff: child
White	15–18	Bolus: 325 crystalloid; 165 colloid Maint: $D_5W + {}^1/_4$ NS + 20 mEq KCl at 55 mL/h	Laryngoscope: 2 straight ETT: 5.0 uncuffed, insert to 14–15 cm Chest tube: 20–24 Fr Foley: 10–12 Fr NGT: 10 Fr Vasc: 18–22 Ga Intraoss: 15 Ga BP cuff: child
Blue	19–23	Bolus: 420 crystalloid; 210 colloid Maint: $D_5W + {}^1/_4$ NS + 20 mEq KCl at 65 mL/h	Laryngoscope: 2 straight or curved ETT: 5.5 uncuffed, insert to 16.5 cm Chest tube: 24–32 Fr Foley: 10–12 Fr NGT: 12–14 Fr Vasc: 18–20 Ga Intraoss: 15 Ga BP cuff: child

(Continues)

TABLE 20.2. Resuscitation *(continued)*

Broselow-Luten	Wt (kg)	Fluids	Equipment
Orange	24–29	Bolus: 530 crystalloid; 270 colloid Maint: $D_5W + {}^1/_4$ NS + 20 mEq KCl at 70 mL/h	Laryngoscope: 2 straight or curved ETT: 6.0 cuffed, insert to 17–18 cm Chest tube: 28–32 Fr Foley: 12 Fr NGT: 14–18 Fr Vasc: 18–20 Ga Intraoss: 15 Ga BP cuff: child
Green	30–36	Bolus: 660 crystalloid; 330 colloid Maint: $D_5W + {}^1/_4$ NS + 20 mEq KCl at 75 mL/h	Laryngoscope: 3 straight or curved ETT: 6.5 cuffed, insert to 18.5–19.5 cm Chest tube: 32–38 Fr Foley: 12 Fr NGT: 18 Fr Vasc: 16–20 Ga Intraoss: 15 Ga BP cuff: sm. ad.

Above information adapted from *Broselow™ Pediatric Emergency Tape*, ©Copyright Vital Signs, Inc., 2002 Ed. A, Armstrong Medical Industries, Inc., Lincolnshire, Illinois.

i. *1st BA cleft anomalies*: present anterior to external auditory canal, passing through parotid gland and facial nerve branches.

b. *Second branchial arch*: develops structures for facial expression, innervated by CN VII.

i. *2nd BA cleft anomalies*: most common place for cleft anomalies; present anterior.

C. Tracheoesophageal fistula: see Chapter 8.

III. **HEART**: see Chapter 7.

IV. **PULMONARY**

A. Diaphragmatic hernia: 80% left, 20% right. Exceedingly rarely bilateral. Results from failure of pleuroperitoneal canal to close. ~ 60% survival, largely limited by pulmonary hypoplasia and pulmonary hypertension.

1. Usu. presents w/ respiratory insufficiency and cyanosis, which may not be immediately apparent postpartum; up to 20% may deteriorate more than 24 h after birth. Dx may be made w/ prenatal U/S or postnatal CXR w/ gastric air bubble or intestinal air in the chest. Mediastinal shift or polyhydramnios (from gastric obstruction) may also be seen.
2. *Bochdalek hernia* = left posterolateral diaphragm.
3. *Morgagni hernia* = anterior central herniation.
4. Congenital diaphragmatic hernia often assoc. w/ pentalogy of Cantrell (omphalocele, anterior diaphragmatic hernia, sternal cleft, ectopia cordis, intracardiac defect [ventricular septal defect or diverticulum of left ventricle]).
5. *Tx*: fetal surgery not supported by data. Postnatal intubation and NGT placement are routine. Acute decompensation may reflect PTX, which will be contralateral to diaphragmatic defect. Ventilation w/ permissive hypercapnea may be sufficient if ECLS is not pursued.
   a. Surgery should be delayed for 24 to 72 h after dx to physiologically stabilize the pt.
   b. Repair diaphragm w/ interrupted nonabsorbable sutures is via subcostal or thoracotomy approach. Large defects may require prosthetic (Gore-tex, Permacol) patch or muscle flap closure; patch repairs assoc. w/ higher recurrence rate. Excise hernia sac if present.

B. Pulmonary sequestration

1. Both forms receive systemic arterial blood supply and do not connect to tracheobronchial tree.
2. *Intralobar* sequestrations most often drain into pulmonary veins and are most often on the left (~ ${}^2/_3$), in medial or posterior segments of lower lobes. Blood supply most frequently from infradiaphragmatic aorta in inferior pulmonary ligament. Resection via segmentectomy or lobectomy is usu. indicated because of risk of infection and bleeding.
3. *Extralobar* sequestrations drain into systemic (azygous) veins, are on left (~ ${}^3/_4$), and are more common in males. 40% are assoc. w/ other anomalies (pectus excavatum/carinatum, diaphragmatic

hernia, congenital heart defects, enteric duplication cysts, etc.). Resection not usu. indicated except in cases of diagnostic uncertainty.

C. Congenital cystic adenomatous malformations (CCAMs)

1. Lesion w/ proliferation of bronchial structures w/ relative paucity of alveolar tissue, and, unlike sequestrations, typically has bronchial and arterial/venous flow from pulmonary vasculature.
2. *Three types*:
   a. *Type I* (macrocystic): single or multiple cysts > 2 cm diameter, may result in shift of remaining parenchyma. ~ 50% of cases, no assoc. anomalies.
   b. *Type II*: multiple small (< 1 cm) cysts, often assoc. w/ other congenital anomalies (renal, cardiac, skeletal, etc.). Prognosis depends on assoc. anomalies.
   c. *Type III*: bulky, appears solid, but has microscopic cysts, often results in mediastinal shift, and is assoc. w/ nonimmune hydrops and poor prognosis. Nonimmune hydrops → 100% fatal.
3. Poor prognosis if involves more than 1 lobe or if type II or III. Small risk of malignant transformation. Resect all.

D. Congenital lobar emphysema

1. Due to insufficient cartilaginous support of bronchus, resulting in bronchial collapse, air trapping, and overdistention. LUL affected in ~ 50% of cases, w/ RML and RLL each about 25%.
2. May be asymptomatic, w/ incidental dx of radiolucency. Observation may be pursued, but resection indicated if sx (dyspnea, recurrent pneumonia). In neonates w/ large CLE, may mimic tension PTX—should be differentiated, as thoracotomy and resection, not chest tube (w/ potential of penetrating the lung), would be indicated.

E. Bronchogenic cysts

1. Usu. solitary, w/ $^2/_3$ in lungs (generally communicate w/ bronchus), and $^1/_3$ in mediastinum (gen. do not communicate w/ bronchus).
2. May be asymptomatic or present w/ pneumonia, cough, dyspnea, hemoptysis, etc. Tx is resection for sx as well as the (small) risk of malignant transformation.

V. <u>GASTROINTESTINAL</u>: type of lesion

A. Stomach

1. *Pyloric stenosis*:
   a. Classically presents in first-born males (M:F = 4:1) about 1 mo of age w/ "projectile" vomiting. Caused by both hyperplasia and hypertrophy of pyloric musculature.
   b. Often results in hypokalemic, hypochloremic metabolic alkalosis.
   c. Clinically, an "olive" may be palpated in RUQ; dx confirmed w/ U/S (dx = 16 mm × 4 mm).
   d. For majority of resuscitations, give bolus of NS (20 mL/kg) followed by D_5 $^1/_2$ NS w/ 20 KCl at 6 mL/kg/h. Take to OR once pt is euvolemic w/ serum bicarb less than 30 and normal K^+.
   e. Tx is open vs laparoscopic Ramstedt pyloromyotomy (incision longitudinally across pylorus down to mucosa, then close transversely). (See Chapter 26 on key steps for key operations.)

B. Intestinal atresia

1. Usu. due to interruption of blood flow, commonly secondary to gastroschisis herniation; multiple in 10% of cases. Jejunoileal > duodenal (see section 7. on duodenal atresia below) > colonic > pyloric.
2. Prenatally, polyhydramnios present; maternal U/S → dilated stomach a/o duodenum.
3. Postnatally, see emesis (usu. bilious, depends on level) w/in 48 h, +/– abdominal distension (depends on level).
4. KUB → if demonstrates "double bubble," then dx is duodenal atresia. If demonstrates multiple loops of dilated bowel, need to order contrast study. Contrast enema reveals microcolon.
5. *Type I* = intact bowel and mesentery w/ septum. *Type II* = ends connected via fibrous cord and intact mesentery. *Type IIIa* = ends in discontinuity w/ wedged gap of mesentery. *Type IIIb* = terminal ileum wrapped in spiral fashion around ileocolic vessel → "apple peel" or "Christmas tree" lesion (results from loss of majority of SMA w/ gut supplied by ileocolic and right colic arteries via anastomoses from IMA). *Type IV* = "string of sausages."
6. *Tx of jejunoileal atresia*:
   a. Obtain BE preop, as up to 15% of pts have multiple atretic segments. *Note*: 10% of pts w/ jejunoileal atresia have cystic fibrosis—diagnostic testing for this entity is appropriate.

b. Anastomosis of atretic ends is performed. Size discrepancy between proximal and distal segments may be addressed by a resection (if limited to short length) or enteroplasty.

7. *Duodenal atresia*:

a. Failure of recanalization by 8th wk gestation. Most always at or just distal to ampulla of Vater. Most often forms a diaphragm/web of mucosa/submucosa that is stretched into "windsock" configuration, although can result in 2 ends. Assoc. anomalies common (annular pancreas, biliary atresia, malrotation); 30% assoc. w/ trisomy 21 (r/o cardiac anomalies). *Ddx* = malrotation w/ volvulus (surgical emergency), annular pancreas.

b. *Dx*: AXR classically reveals a "double-bubble" sign (air in stomach and duodenal bulb). If air is noted elsewhere in small bowel, an upper GI study should be obtained to r/o midgut volvulus.

c. *Tx*: Duodenal web is *not removed* via duodenotomy, because of risk of injury to major ampulla. Duodenoduodenostomy or duodenojejunostomy is performed via open or laparoscopy approach.

C. Pancreas

1. Pancreas divisum (see Chapter 16)
2. Annular pancreas (see Chapter 16)

D. Colon

1. *Hirschsprung's disease*

a. Common etiology of neonatal intestinal obstruction. Due to absence of ganglion cells in distal segment of bowel, w/ resultant failure of relaxation in that segment.

b. Presents w/ constipation, distention, possibly diarrhea. *Always think of this w/ failure to pass meconium w/in 48 h of birth.*

c. Contrast enema often procured to demonstrate transition zone, but false negatives not infrequent in infants.

d. Do transrectal bx for *absence* of ganglia cells AND acetylcholinesterase. Bx must be at least 1 cm proximal to dentate line.

e. Initially manage w/ rectal irrigation or temporary colostomy.

f. Definitive management is pull-through procedure in first 3 wk of life (primary surgery) or, if following colostomy, around 6 mo of age.

g. Hirschsprung's pts are at lifelong risk of high morbidity/mortality enterocolitis.

E. Anorectal

1. *Imperforate anus*

a. Slightly more common in males, mechanism unknown. Sometimes assoc. w/ VACTERL (esp. tetrology of Fallot, VSD), Down syndrome, duodenal atresia, a/o Hirschsprung's dz.

b. Original classification based on relation of rectal end to the levators. Newer dichotomy is based on tx (need for colostomy).

i. *Need for protective colostomy*: rectourethral, rectovesical, or vaginal fistula; cloaca; anorectal agenesis (no fistula); rectal or vestibular atresia. Note, these infants usu. have a "flat" bottom.

ii. *No need for protective colostomy*: cutaneous fistula; anal stenosis; anal membrane.

c. *Dx*:

i. Clinical. Look for perineal fistula; if present, observe up to 48 h for meconium; if (+), then pt has a "low" lesion. Invertograms have been supplanted by prone, cross-table film.

ii. Eval for VACTERL w/ NGT, echocardiogram, abdominal/renal U/S, plain films of vertebrae, +/– lumbar MRI.

d. *Tx*:

i. Maintain NPO w/ parenteral nutrition until operation.

ii. If need protective colostomy (see entry bi. above), perform colostomy (and urinary diversion if indicated [rare]).

- Postop, irrigate mucous fistula to remove meconium and perform distal colostogram to define anatomy. PSARP is generally performed between 2 and 12 mo of age.

iii. If rectocutaneous fistula (i.e., no need for protective colostomy), perform primary posterior sagittal anoplasty (PSARP) w/in first few wks of life.

F. Intussusception

1. Usu. in age group 4 mo to 3 yo (peak = 8 mo). In children of this age range, usu. at ileocecal junction w/ no identifiable lead point, but significant mesenteric/gut lymphadenopathy. Tends to follow viral URI/gastroenteritis.
2. Typically presents w/ crampy, intense abdominal pain w/ emesis in an otherwise healthy child, causing child to flex hips/knees during episodes of pain, and punctuated by periods of relative calm.
3. "Currant jelly" stool that reflects ischemic bowel producing mucus admixed w/ clotted blood is frequently reported. A palpable mass in the abdomen may be noted, a/o relative lack of fullness in RLQ—"Dance's sign."
4. *Radiology*: all → 3-way KUB: if air/stool throughout colon, unlikely dx—suspicious if lack of air in RLQ. Often followed by air contrast enema. If low index of suspicion → *U/S*: "target" sign of intussuscepted bowel on transverse view and "pseudokidney" on longitudinal view. If low index of suspicion → *CT*: "target" or "bullseye" w/ mass in RLQ and SBO proximally. If high index of suspicion → contrast, saline, or *air enema* (can do under fluoro) can be diagnostic as well as therapeutic (80% effective), but should be bypassed if pt is unstable or has peritonitis (go to OR). Manage 1st recurrence w/ repeat enema, but if recurs twice, should go to OR. If intussusception is known to not involve colon (involves small bowel only), A-C enema not likely to be therapeutic, and therefore not indicated.
5. *Operation*:
   a. *Indications*: peritonitis, failure of enema to reduce, high index of suspicion of nonviable gut, complete SBO, lack of colonic involvement, and multiple recurrences.
   b. *Procedure*: laparoscopy may be used for incomplete reduction, but generally a transverse incision in right abdomen is made to access the bowel, which is milked from distal to proximal for reduction (push, don't pull). Adhesions, if any, are lysed, and the appendix is removed. Bowel is resected if reduction can't be achieved, if lead point is identified, or if intestine is nonviable.
6. *Prognosis*: recurrence is ~ 5% after either enema reduction or operative intervention.
7. *Caveat*: in older children, the risk of the lead point being a malignancy increases.

G. Malrotation

1. GI tract develops outside coelomic cavity from gestational wk 4–10, then begins counterclockwise rotation of 2 segments around the SMA. The duodenojejunal segment first rotates 270° and then is fixed at the ligament of Treitz. The cecocolic segment then rotates. At completion, intestines are fixed to the retroperitoneum via a broad mesentery, the duodenal C-loop, and right/left colon. If the fixation is incomplete, intestines can rotate around a narrow stalk and strangulate the superior mesenteric vessels.
   a. Will always occur to some degree w/ omphalocele, gastroschisis, and congenital diaphragmatic hernia.
   b. Assoc. to lesser degree w/ intestinal atresia and Hirschsprung's dz.
2. *Three specific anomalies*:
   a. *Nonrotation*: most common variant. Neither segment rotates appropriately, but are closely apposed, sharing a mesentery w/ a narrow base that is prone to volvulus. Duodenum courses "vertically" (cephalad–caudad) along right side of abdomen.
   b. *Duodenojejunal anomalies*: frequently manifest as duodenal obstruction from Ladd's bands extending down to colon, across duodenum. Comparatively broad mesenteric base.
   c. *Cecocolic anomalies*: Cecum and proximal colon are medially situated. Prone to volvulus as w/ nonrotation due to narrow mesenteric base.
3. *Dx*:
   a. *Clinical*: most severe presentation is w/ bilious emesis from volvulus. Hematemesis, melena, a/o sepsis may ensue as bowel becomes compromised and the child becomes increasingly ill.
   b. *Roentgenographic*:
      i. *Plain films*: may demonstrate gas pattern consistent w/ obstruction, or relatively gasless abdomen due to intraluminal transudate.
      ii. *UGI*: demonstrates obstruction (if present) and malrotation (incomplete duodenojejunal rotation). Normally, LOT to left, but will be on right w/ malrotation.
      iii. *BE*: less useful than UGI, as cecal position relatively variable in children, and may be normal in some children w/ malrotation.
      iv. *U/S*: can demonstrate absence of usual position of SMV to the right of SMA.

4. *Tx*:
   a. *Incidental malrotation*
      i. *Ladd procedure* [Ladd WE, *NEJM*. 1932;206:277–83.]
         - *Eviscerate*: via supraumbilical midline incision.
         - *Lyse Ladd's bands*: divide these peritoneal bands as they compress 2nd/3rd portion of duodenum.
         - *Widen mesenteric base*: move small bowel to lie along right gutter and colon to the left (ileocecal valve will be oriented opposite direction as usual).
         - *Verify duodenal patency*: perform additional dissection as necessary to properly orient and decompress duodenum. Also, r/o atresia/stenosis or tx if present.
         - *Appendectomy*: to avoid future diagnostic quandaries.
   b. *Malrotation w/ volvulus*
      i. Resuscitate w/ IVF, NGT/OGT then to OR emergently.
      ii. Operative steps same as above, except that immediately after evisceration (before lysing Ladd's bands), detorse bowel by counterclockwise rotation. Examine bowel for areas of viability/ischemia/necrosis. Condition of bowel may warrant second look 24 h later, or immediate resection +/– primary anastomosis.
5. *Prognosis*:
   a. Recurrent volvulus in 5–10% of pts after Ladd procedure, and ~ 5% risk of adhesive obstructive dz.

H. **Meconium ileus variants:** *note*, the below diagnoses are variably assoc. w/ cystic fibrosis, which is diagnosed w/ pilocarpine iontophoresis sweat test. Positive = chloride concentration > 60 mEq/L, but less reliable in infants. Testing for mutated *CFTR* gene required for definitive dx.
   1. *Meconium plug*: most affected pts are normal, but is assoc. w/ CF as well as Hirshsprung's, maternal diabetes, hypothyroidism, preterm delivery. Usu. presents as distal intestinal obstruction; water-soluble contrast enema diagnostic and therapeutic.
   2. *Meconium ileus (simple)*: virtually pathognomonic for CF in white children in North America. Terminal ileum dilated w/ inspissated meconium. Typically, KUB shows dilated small bowel w/ meconium mass and small bowel gas often interpreted as "soap bubble" or "ground glass" appearance. Water-soluble contrast enema effective tx in 75%. Failure of enema is indication for operation, as is 3rd occurrence (2 recurrences). In OR, evacuate meconium via enterotomy in dilated ileum. Irrigate proximally and distally w/ saline or 4% *N*-acetylcysteine through a red rubber catheter. Meconium can be milked into colon or out through enterotomy. Enterotomy may be closed, partly diverted w/ Bishop-Koop or Santulli ostomy, or end small bowel enterocutaneous ostomy. Rarely, a T tube may be placed for postop irrigation.
   3. *Meconium ileus (complicated)*: refers to meconium ileus w/ perforation, resulting in peritonitis. May present w/ obstruction or calcified cyst if occurred prenatally, or superinfection, ascites, or dense adhesions.

I. **Foreign body ingestion/aspiration**
   1. *Ingestion*:
      a. *3 most common places to lodge in the esophagus*: cricopharyngeus (most common), mid-esophagus (region of left mainstem bronchus), diaphragmatic hiatus.
         i. Evaluate w/ CXR and retrieve w/ rigid or flexible esophagoscope.
      b. 95% of ingested foreign bodies safely pass once distal to the esophagus, usu. w/in 48 h. Those who have blunt objects w/out projections beyond the esophagus may be sent home w/ appropriate precautions including instructions to return if no passage w/in 5 d. Surgery is reserved for no passage after 5 d, or significant N/V/pain/bleeding. Emetics and cathartics are contraindicated.
      c. Long, blunt, slender objects (tools, pencils, etc.) pass less frequently, and should more frequently be followed in the hospital w/ serial x-rays.
      d. Ingestion of sharp objects (glass, needles, etc.) mandates hospitalization for serial abdominal exams and daily KUBs. As long as object continues distal travel w/out peritonitis or significant bleeding, observation is reasonable and usu. successful.
      e. Battery ingestion poses a significant risk of alkali burn or mercury poisoning and requires emergent removal. Remove them endoscopically if in the stomach. If distal (i.e., duodenum), q 6 h films must document rapid transit if the pt is to avoid celiotomy.

2. *Aspiration*
   a. Right mainstem bronchus most common due to relatively shallow angle w/ trachea compared w/ left.
   b. CXR often demonstrates hyperinflation; less often the foreign body will be demonstrated.
   c. Rigid bronchoscopy for definitive dx and removal.

J. **Necrotizing enterocolitis (NEC)**
1. Most common neonatal GI emergency. Primary risk factor is prematurity.
2. 80% of cases occur during first postnatal mo, but rarely in the first several days. Typically involves distal ileum and right colon, but may affect entire GI tract. 80–90% are successfully treated w/ supportive care alone (nonsurgically).
3. Frequently presents w/ nonspecific sx such as bradycardia, dyspnea, irritability, labile temperatures, poor feeding, a/o hematochezia/melena. This may progress to sepsis and DIC.
4. Classic roentgenographic finding is pneumatosis intestinalis, although portal gas, free air, and ascites may also be seen.
5. *Tx*:
   a. Begin w/ NGT, fluid/blood products resuscitation, broad-spectrum IV abx for 3 wk.
   b. *Operation*:
      i. *Absolute indication*: perforation.
      ii. *Relative indication*: worsening clinical picture (i.e., progressive sepsis, worsening neutropenia/thrombocytopenia/acidosis/sepsis), palpable abdominal mass, abdominal wall cellulitis, radiographic fixed loop of intestines.
   c. Resect nonviable bowel and create enterostomies as needed. In severely ill, unstable pts, bedside placement of peritoneal drains under local anesthesia may be sufficient.
   d. Mortality 10–50% of operative candidates. Primary long-term sequelae include short gut syndrome and strictures.

VI. **GASTROINTESTINAL DIFFERENTIAL DIAGNOSIS**: type of symptoms

A. **Vomiting**
1. *Malrotation*
   a. Etiology of bilious emesis in newborn until proven otherwise.
   b. May see "double bubble."
   c. Ladd's procedure:
      i. Divide Ladd's bands.
      ii. Counterclockwise rotation of gut.
      iii. Place small bowel on right, large bowel on left.
      iv. Appendectomy.
2. *Duodenal atresia*
   a. Assoc. w/ Down syndrome.
   b. May see "double bubble" on AXR (r/o malrotation!).
3. *Annular pancreas*
4. *Pyloric stenosis*
5. *Intussusception*
   a. Most common cause of intestinal obstruction to age 2 yo.
   b. 95% of pediatric cases w/ no identifiable mass to act as lead point.
   c. Ileal "intussusceptum" into colonic "intussuscipiens" most common.
   d. Most resolve w/ air or barium enema.
   e. If require laparotomy, push mass out from distal bowel rather than pull out proximal bowel.

B. **Abdominal distension**
1. Intestinal obstruction
2. Pneumoperitoneum
3. Pseudocyst (assoc. w/ CF, meconium ileus)
4. Mesenteric cysts or intestinal duplication

5. Hydrocolpos/hematocolpos
6. Instestinal inflation (TEF, or secondary to CPAP)
7. Hydrops (Rh dz w/ anasarca and hepatosplenomegaly)

C. Scaphoid abd ddx

1. CDH
2. Esophageal atresia
3. Duodenal atresia

D. Diarrhea

1. Intussusception

E. Constipation

1. Meconium ileus
2. Hirschsprung's dz
3. Intestinal neuronal dysplasia

F. Blood in stool

1. Intussusception
2. NEC
3. Volvulus

G. Respiratory distress

1. Esophageal atresia +/– TEF
2. Congenital diaphragmatic hernia
3. CCAM
4. CLE
5. PTX
6. Congenital heart dz

VII. ABDOMINAL WALL

A. Umbilical hernia

1. Caused by incomplete contraction of umbilical ring.
2. More often in African Americans, premature babies, twins, mucopolysaccharide storage disorders (esp. Hurler's syndrome).
3. Majority spontaneously close by 2 yo. Surgical repair indicated after age 5 or if > 2-cm diameter after age 2.

B. Omphalocele

1. Proposed etiology is failure of lateral/cranial/caudal mesoderm ingrowth and fusion during gestational wk 4–7.
2. Assoc. w/ pentalogy of Cantrell (diaphragmatic hernia, ectopia cordis, sternal cleft, etc.), bladder extrophy, cloacal extrophy, imperforate anus, and meningomyelocele. 10–30% chromosomal anomalies (i.e., 12, 13, 18, 21). 35–81% w/ major congenital anomaly(ies), most frequently cardiac ($^1/_5$, such as TOF, ASD, VSD). In addition to VACTERL, also assoc. w/ Beckwith-Wiedemann (visceromegaly, neonatal hypoglycemia, macroglossia).
   a. *VACTERL w/u should include* echocardiogram; renal U/S; plain films of chest, pelvis, and spine; karyotype/chromosomal analysis; thorough physical exam.
3. If not already diagnosed in utero, presents postnatally as > 4 cm umbilical defect (< 4 cm = "cord hernia") w/ eviscerated organs covered w/ amnion (minority rupture in utero or during delivery).
4. *Tx*:
   a. Place OGT. Do not mask ventilate (intubate).
   b. Excise sac, correct malrotation (usu. present), explore abdominal contents.
   c. Primarily close abdomen if defect small enough and sufficient peritoneal domain exists.
   d. Alternatives for closure include patch, skin flaps, or silo (serially tighten, then close in delayed fashion).

e. If pt not stable for anesthesia, consider applying Silvadene to sac to create eschar and allow for epithelialization; repair ventral hernia when able (usu. at 1 yo).

5. *Prognosis*: usu. limited by assoc. anomalies (~ 80% long-term survival).

C. Gastroschisis

1. Thought to be related to defect from early right umbilical vein involution w/ resultant weakness to the right of umbilicus (95+% of cases are on the right). Not assoc. w/ other anomalies, other than intestinal atresia (10–15%), probably secondary to incarceration in utero, and undescended testes.
2. Presents postnatally, defect almost always just to right of umbilicus w/ eviscerated organs *not* covered by amnion. Organs covered by generally thick rind from exposure to amniotic fluid (this will resolve w/ time in the abdomen). Variable degrees of malrotation present.
3. *Tx*:
   a. Place NGT to prevent distention.
   b. Wrap eviscerated contents in bowel bags or saline-moistened gauze.
   c. Generally need to enlarge defect to facilitate reduction.
   d. Repair atresias if possible, but inflammation may preclude this, requiring revisit 6–8 wk after reduction. Correct malrotation as indicated.
   e. Tension-free closure of abdomen may require use of patch, flaps, etc.
   f. Anticipate prolonged ileus (up to 6 mo postop) w/ early institution of TPN. NEC also more common than in omphalocele pts as gastroschisis pts more frequently born premature.
4. Prognosis excellent w/ appropriate early management.

D. Eagle-Barrett (prune belly) syndrome: 1 in 50,000 live births, more common in males.

1. Triad consists of absent/deficient abdominal wall musculature, cryptorchidism, urinary tract malformations (usu. ureteral dilatation). Some pts lack 1 or more of the classical components. Pt at risk for complicated UTI due to frequent vesicoureteral reflux. Increased risk for postop respiratory complications due to compromised respiratory mechanics. Malrotation common. Orchidopexy should be performed by 2 yo; abdominoplasty may be performed concurrently.

VIII. GENITOURINARY AND ADRENAL

A. Sexual development

1. See Tables 20.3 and 20.4.

TABLE 20.3. Tanner Score (Male)

Male	Testis	Pubic Hair	Penis	Other
Stage 1 Prepubertal	< 4 cc or 2.5 cm long	No coarse, pigmented hair	No growth	
Stage 2	4 cc, 2.5–3.2 cm long (9.5–13.5 yo)	Minimal coarse, pigmented hair at base of penis (9.9–14 yo)	Earliest increased length and width (10.5–14.5 yo)	
Stage 3	12 cc, 3.6 cm long (11.5–16.5 yo)	Coarse, dark curly hair over pubis (11.2–15 yo)	Increased length and width (10.1–14.6 yo)	Possible gynecomastia (13.2 yo avg) Voice breaks (13.5 yo avg) Muscle mass increases
Stage 4	4.1–4.5 cm	Adult quality, but not to junction of thigh w/ perineum (12–15.8 yo)	Continued growth in length and width (11.2–15.3 yo)	Axillary hair (14 yo avg), voice changes, acne vulgaris (14.3 yo avg)
Stage 5	> 4.5 cm	Adult quality Spread to medial thigh but not linea alba	Mature size by 16.5 yo	No further height gain after 17 yo

TABLE 20.4. Tanner Score (Female)

Female	Breast	Pubic Hair	Other
Stage 1 Prepubertal	Papilla elevation only	Villus hair only (not coarse)	
Stage 2	Breast buds palpable, areolae enlarge (8.9–12.9 yo)	Minimal coarse, pigmented hair, mainly on labia (9.0–13.4 yo)	With increasingly earlier puberty, these changes may appear 1–2 yr earlier
Stage 3	Elevation of breast contour, areolae enlarge (9.9–13.9 yo)	Dark, coarse, curly hair over mons (9.6–14.1 yo)	Axillary hair (13.1 yo avg), acne vulgaris (13.2 yo avg)
Stage 4	Areola forms secondary mound on breast (10.5–15.3 yo)	Adult quality, no spread to thigh/perineal junction (10.4–14.8 yo)	
Stage 5	Adult breast contour, areola recedes to contour of breast	Adult quality, spread to medial thigh, but not linea alba	No further height gain after 16 yo

B. Congenital adrenal hyperplasia (CAH)

1. Most common cause of female fetal virilization.
2. Shunts precursors for both cortisol and aldosterone to make sex steroids.
3. Due to deficiency of enzyme needed for cortisol synthesis, leading to excess ACTH production; 21 hydroxylase deficiency responsible for 90–95%; 3/4 of these cases are "salt-wasters" as well. Remainder of CAH pts lack 11-β-hydroxylase, 3-β-hydroxydehydrogenase, or 17-hydroxylase.
4. *Prenatal* (females): Mullerian tissue (ovaries, fallopian tubes, uterus) unaffected, but have masculinized external genitalia. W/ correction of endocrine problem and reconstructive surgery, can bear children.
5. *Postnatal*:
   a. *Both*:
      i. Pts w/ 21-hydroxylase deficiency appear well immediately after birth, but after 2–3 wk decompensate due to salt loss and resulting hypovolemia (hyperkalemia also common). *Consider dx in any hypotensive infant w/ hyponatremia, hyperkalemia, and metabolic acidosis.*
      ii. Less dramatic cases may present w/ rapid somatic growth, advanced bone age, early closure of epiphyses (short stature), +/– hyperpigmentation.
   b. *Females*: virilization, hirsutism, polycystic ovaries, menstrual irregularities.
   c. *Males*: enlarged phallus, increased muscle mass, body hair by 2–3 yo; fertility may be impaired.
   d. *Note: virilizing sx in children may also be due to adrenocortical carcinoma—must consider this dx. Unlike CAH, pts usu. will have hypercortisolism.*

IX. GASTROINTESTINAL BLEEDING: most common cause in young children is Meckel's diverticulum. Other sources to consider include anal fissure from constipation, juvenile polyps, and other dx more commonly seen in adults such as ulcers (often due to NSAIDs), varices, etc.

X. PEDIATRIC ONCOLOGY

A. Most common tumor in children is leukemia.

B. Most common solid tumor in children is brain cancer.

C. Neuroblastoma: slightly less common than nephroblastoma (below) at ~ 1:10 million children.

1. Derived from neural crest cells, demonstrate wide range of behavior (benign/spontaneous regression to malignant).
2. Majority of cases present in infancy. *Site of primary tumor*: adrenal > other retroperitoneum > mediastinum > pelvis > neck > other. Most commonly metastasizes to bone. Median age at dx = 2 yo.

3. Etiology linked to proto-oncogene N-*myc* amplification; inversely assoc. w/ *TRK* expression.
4. *W/u*: imaging depends on site of primary tumor but should include chest CT scan as well as MIBG scan to r/o metastasis. Labs should include complete chemistry w/ BUN/Cr, LFTs, LDH, plasma/urine homovanillic acid and vanillylmandelic acid.
5. Early stage tx → excision alone. Mod/high risk → neoadjuvant chemotx + surgery + BM transplant +/– XRT.

D. Nephroblastoma (Wilm's tumor): most common extracranial solid tumor in childhood (~ 1:9 million children).

1. Derived from metanephric blastema, but often contains extrarenal tissue as well (cartilage, muscle, etc.).
2. *Assoc. syndromes*:
   a. *WAGR* (**W**ilm's tumor, **a**niridia, **GU** malformations, mental **r**etardation).
   b. *Beckwith-Wiedemann*: other tumors include hepatoblastoma, rhabdomyosarcoma, and adrenal cortical carcinoma. (See section XI. on syndromes below.)
   c. *Denys-Drash*: male pseudohermaphrodism a/o renal dz (nephritic syndrome or glomerulonephritis) and nephroblastoma.
3. Etiology linked to deletion of WTI (Wilm's tumor suppressor gene) at 11p13.
4. Most commonly present w/ abdominal mass, abdominal pain, HTN, hematuria, a/o fever at 3–4 yo.
5. *Tx*: transperitoneal nephrectomy (inspect contralateral kidney, bx LN, etc.); neoadjuvant chemotx given if tumor extends into IVC. Prognosis overall 85% long-term survival.

E. Rhabdomyosarcoma: < 5% of childhood malignancies.

1. Commonly presents in head/neck, GU tract, and extremities.
2. Most cases sporadic, although condition assoc. w/ Li-Fraumeni syndrome, neurofibromatosis-1, and Beckwith-Wiedemann syndrome.
3. *Tx*: multimodality (usu. surgery + chemo +/– XRT). 60% overall 5-yr survival.

F. Liver tumors: 2% childhood malignancies.

1. *Hepatoblastoma*: usu. between 1–3 yo. 70% overall long-term survival.
   a. Usu. unifocal.
   b. Assoc. w/ Beckwith-Wiedemann syndrome and hemihypertrophy, children w/ parents w/ FAP, fetal alcohol syndrome, Wilm's tumor, Fanconi's syndrome; trisomy 2, trisomy 20, 11p and β-catenin gene mutations frequently implicated. Tx similar to hepatocellular carcinoma (below); neoadjuvant chemotx can facilitate resection more frequently than for HCC (below).
2. *Hepatocellular carcinoma*: usu. ~ 12 yo or older, more often multicentric and aggressive than hepatoblastoma, same risk factors as in adult HCC in addition to hepatocyte growth factor gene (*Met*) mutations (see Chapter 12). 25% overall long-term survival.

G. Teratoma

1. Tumors that contain more than 1 embryonic germ cell layer, at least 1 of which is ectopic.
2. Most often present in infancy, often in sacrococcygeal area, particularly in females; those fitting this pattern are generally benign.
3. In older children, tumors are more likely to involve gonads and be malignant.
4. Surgery is the common principle for all teratomas (critical to resect coccyx in sacrococcygeal lesions), although some malignant varieties warrant multimodality intervention.

XI. SYNDROMES

A. Trisomy 21 (Down syndrome): neonatal hypotonia, protruding tongue, mental retardation, simian crease, assoc. also w/ duodenal atresia and cardiac lesions.

B. Trisomy 18 (Edward syndrome): low birth wt, delayed mental development, low-set ears, micrognathia, umbilical hernia, inguinal hernia, diastasis recti, cryptorchidism, VSD/ASD/PDA, horseshoe kidney, hydronephrosis, polycystic kidney, coloboma, pectus carinatum, microcephaly.

C. Trisomy 13 (Patau syndrome): severe mental retardation, seizures, microcephaly, microphthalmia, cleft lip/palate, hypotelorism, coloboma, simian crease, polydactyly, umbilical hernia, inguinal hernia, cryptorchidism, micrognathia, hypotonia, skeletal limb anomalies.

D. **Beckwith-Wiedemann syndrome:** macrosomia, macroglossia, visceromegaly, umbilical hernia/omphalocele, neonatal hypoglycemia, hemihypertrophy, various malignancies (hepatoblastoma, adrenocortical carcinoma, etc.).

E. **Pentology of Cantrell:** epigastric omphalocele, sternal cleft, Morgagni hernia, cardiac defect (usu. VSD or left ventricular diverticulum), ectopia cordis.

F. **VACTERL:** **v**ertebral, **a**nal, **c**ardiac, **t**racheo**e**sophageal, **r**enal, **r**adial **l**imb.

CHAPTER 21

IMMUNOLOGY AND TRANSPLANT

I. IMMUNOLOGY

A. Immunology and infections

1. *Role of cytokines*
    a. *IL-1*: produced by macrophage; primary pyrogen, leads to prostaglandin E in hypothalamus.
    b. *IL-2*: upregulates T-cell function, activates NK cells.
    c. *IL-4*: antiinflammatory inhibits IgG, suppresses cytokine synthesis, produced in large quantities in AIDS.
    d. *IL-6*: proinflammatory.
    e. *IL-10*: antiinflammatory.
    f. *IL-13*: antiinflammatory.
    g. *TGF-B*: antiproliferative except for fibroblast.
    h. *TNF-alpha*: activates phagocytosis, antiviral, induces inflammation.
2. *Role of cells*
    a. *Macrophage* (origin is monocyte in bloodstream): presents antigen (along w/ B lymphocytes and dendritic cells) and elaborates cytokines to both amplify and make the immune response more specific.
    b. *Leukocyte*: destroys foreign organisms via ingestion and oxidation. *Defect in neutrophil* (i.e., diabetes mellitus, Chédiak-Higashi syndrome) results in severe bacterial infections, often gram-negative as well as invasive fungal infections. Also may result in chronic granulomatous dz (no superoxide radical); may see recurrent staphylococcal infections as well.
    c. *Lymphocyte*: see below under "acquired, cell-mediated."

B. Immunology

1. *Major histocompatibility complex (MHC) genes on chromosome 6* → human leukocyte antigen (HLA).
    a. *MHC/Class I*: all nucleated cells; presents endogenous Ag; binds CD-8; killed by Tc (cytotoxic); important for viruses, cancer.
    b. *MHC/Class II*: B lymphocytes, monocytes, macrophages, activated T lymphocytes, Langerhans cells; presents exogenous/foreign Ag to Th cells; binds CD-4. Includes HLA-DR.
2. *Types of immunity*:
    a. *Innate vs acquired*
        i. *Innate/nonspecific*: complement, NK cell, NKT cell, gamma-delta cell; "pattern recognition."
            - *Complement*: directly activated by endotoxin, foreign material, or microorganisms **or** by IgG/IgM binding to foreign antigen. Also plays a supportive role in opsonization.
                - Can *directly* kill gram-negatives or viruses, generally not gram-positives—assists w/ those).
                - *Heat-labile proteins*: opsonize bacteria for phagocytosis, lyse some bacteria/foreign cells, produce chemokines, increase vascular permeability, promote mast cell degradation → smooth muscle contraction.
                - *Classical pathway*: begins w/ C1q binding to Ab (IgG or IgM) w/ bound Ag → leads to common C3 (itself helps w/ phagocytosis).
                - *Alternate pathway*: begins w/ C3 via IgA/IgE or nonimmunologic (i.e., LPS, bacterial component—most common means).
                - C5-9 = membrane attack complex = final common pathway, which forms hole in cell wall.

- Deficit in C3 usu. lethal w/ severe bacterial infections.
- Deficit in C5-9 increased risk of infection w/ *Neisseria* (*N. meningitidis, N. gonorrhoeae*).

ii. *Acquired*: antigen specific:

- *T cell*:
  - *CD4+ cells*: main role is to secrete cytokines, referred to as T helper cells.
    - *Th1*: generates IL-2, INF-gamma to stimulate Tc/IL-8 (*Example*: INF helps fight hepatitis C through Th1).
    - *Th2*: helps B cells perform class II binding via IL-10, IL-4.
  - *CD8+ cells* (cytotoxic T lymphocytes): recognize target cells by MHC Class I signature, and destroy cells via enzymatic lysis or inducing apoptosis.
- *B cell*: composed of heavy and light chains; IgM (from B lymphocytes, can activate complement) undergoes isotype switch to produce IgG (activates complement, binds macrophages, can cross placenta), IgA (secreted in mucosa, breast milk), IgE (activates mast cells and basophils to release histamine, serotonin), and IgD from plasma cells.
- *Costimulation*: signal 1 w/out signal 2 induces energy.

b. *Cell-mediated vs humoral*

i. *Cell-mediated immunity*

- *Mediated by*:
  - Phagocytosis.
  - Cytotoxic T cells (recognize/bind Ag + MHC I, release perforin, cytokines).
  - NK cells (not restricted to MHC, most directed toward tumor cells, unclear mechanism of recognition, but kills like cytotoxic T cells).
  - Killer cells (bind to Fc receptors), in ADCC.
  - Defect (SCID, immunosuppressants, DiGeorge, AIDS) susceptible to viruses, fungi, and parasites (*Pneumocystic, Cryptosporidium*), intracellular bacteria, tumors.
  - Important in transplant rejection and delayed hypersensitivity.

ii. *Humoral immunity*

- Mediated by antibodies and complement.
- Requires MHC II (antigen-presenting cells, i.e., B cells, macrophage).
- Defect (SCID, HypoGG, myeloma, catabolism) susceptible to bacteria, toxins, and viruses prior to cell entry.
  - Effects delayed after neonatal period, then manifest w/ recurrent respiratory tract infections.
  - Encapsulated bacteria (pneumococcus, *H. flu*, meningococcus) particularly problematic.
  - May result from X-linked hyperIgM syndrome, X-linked agammaglobulinemia, myeloma, CLL.

3. *Types of allergic reactions*

a. *Type I*

i. "Immediate hypersensitivity."

ii. Involves IgE and mast cells, histiocytes.

iii. Hay fever, penicillin allergy, bee stings, mold allergies are examples.

b. *Type II*

i. "Cytotoxic hypersensitivity."

ii. Involves IgG and K cells (ADCC), complement.

iii. Pemphigus, autoimmune hemolytic anemia, Goodpasture's are examples.

c. *Type III*

i. "Immune complex hypersensitivity."

ii. Rheumatoid arthritis, serum sickness are examples.

d. *Type IV*
  i. "Delayed hypersensitivity."
  ii. Mediated by T cells, macrophages.
  iii. Skin wheal is an example.

4. *Markers of immunosuppression*
  a. Absolute lymphocyte count.
  b. Delayed hypersensitivity skin testing.
  c. Nutrition parameters (i.e., albumin).

C. Immunology and cancer

1. AIDS pts at higher risk of Kaposi's sarcoma (assoc. w/ human herpes virus 8–HHV8) and anal squamous cell carcinoma.
2. *Transplant pt elevated risk*: skin cancer (esp. kidney txp); lymphoma (esp. liver txp); hepatobiliary malignancy; Kaposi's sarcoma; vulvar malignancy.

D. Immunosuppression and surgical disease

1. *HIV*
  a. *Criteria for AIDS–HIV (+) and*:
    i. CD4(+) < 200
    ii. AIDS-defining illness
      - *Infectious*: thrush, toxoplasmosis, *Pneumocystis carinii* infection, disseminated TB or MAI, HSV esophagitis/pneumonia, cryptosporidiosis, nocardiasis, extrapulmonary coccidioidomycosis/cryptococcosis/histoplasmosis, extralymphatic CMV infection, extraintestinal *Strongyloides stercoralis* infection.
      - *Neoplastic*: Kaposi's sarcoma, lymphoma (non-Hodgkin's, B-cell, or undifferentiated), invasive cervical cancer.
  b. *Surgical implications*:
    i. *GI*:
      - *Anorectal*: poor wound healing, increased risk of condylomata and anal SCCA.
      - *Appendicitis*: increased incidence from CMV, Kaposi's, etc. May lack usual findings such as leukocytosis.
      - *GI bleeding*: Kaposi's sarcoma, GI lymphoma, CMV.
      - *GI perforation*: usu. midgut, usu. from CMV, but may be from malignancies.
      - *Hepatobiliary*: cryptosporidial cholecystitis, atypical hepatic abscesses (*E. histolytica*, *C. albicans*, etc.), AIDS-associated cholangiopathy (RUQ pain, alkaline phosphatase elevation, etc.—due to opportunistic organisms infecting biliary tree).
    ii. *Vascular*: increased risk of vasculitis and mycotic aneurysms from *Salmonella*.
  c. *Malignancy*: see section C above on immunology and cancer.
2. *Steroids*
  a. Inhibit DNA and RNA synthesis as well as elaboration of IL-1, IL-2, IL-6, INF-γ, TNF-α. Also inhibit chemotaxis.
  b. *Wound healing*: administration (not topical) of vitamin A (25,000 IU/d) helps minimize the untoward effects of corticosteroids on wound healing.
3. *Neoplasms*
  a. *Leukemia*: neutropenic colitis may mimic surgical abdomen.
4. *Other immunosuppressive factors*:
  a. *Blood transfusion*: increased risk of perioperative infection and possible acceleration of malignancy.
  b. *Malnutrition*: increased risk of perioperative infection. See Chapter 1 on fluids, electrolytes, metabolism, and nutrition. Of note, diet supplementation w/ omega-3-fatty acids and arginine appears to augment T-cell function.
  c. *Trauma/shock*: impaired WBC function, impaired B-cell function, impaired CMI; worst at 24–48 h post-injury.

d. *Age*
   i. *Extreme youth*: IgM production far below adult until ~ 2 yo.
   ii. *Elderly*: impaired T-cell stimulation and reduced IgG response to immune challenge.
e. *Diabetes mellitus*
   i. Accelerated atherosclerosis results in poor perfusion.
   ii. Hyperglycemia (esp. > 180) results in impaired WBC chemotaxis, phagocytosis.
f. *Splenectomy*: see Chapter 18 on spleen.

II. TRANSPLANT

A. Post-transplant complications

1. *Rejection*:
   a. *Hyperacute*: in minutes, from preformed Ab, prevent w/ cross-match.
   b. *Acute vascular*: minutes–hours, Ab-mediated, tx w/ plasmapheresis/IVIg.
   c. *Acute cellular*: 5–7 d most common, but can happen at any time, T-cell mediated, see lymphocytic infiltration, tx w/ aggressive immunosuppression.
   d. *Chronic* (gradual): years, from Ab/B cell, see fibrosis/scarring, "vanishing bile duct syndrome" in liver; glomerular sclerosis in kidneys.
   e. W/u w/ H&P, immunosuppressant drug levels (esp. calcineurin inhibitors—cyclosporine, tacrolimus), possibly biopsy. May be also caused by infectious etiologies (i.e., CMV, polyoma virus in kidney, etc.).
2. *Malignancy*:
   a. *Most common*: cervical CA (HPV), vulvar/perineal cancer (HSV), squamous cell CA (HPV), Kaposi sarcoma (EBV), and lymphoma (HTLV-1).
   b. *Posttransplant lymphoproliferative disorder* (PTLD): related to intensity of immunosuppression, particularly of T cells. More commonly seen w/ transplantation of critical organs (heart, lung)—5–10% vs only 1% in renal transplant pts. Assoc. w/ Epstein-Barr virus. B-cell lymphomas of transplant organ, GI tract, or CNS most often. Most cases present w/in 1 yr, but may present 10–15 yr later. Treat by reducing immunosuppression if possible and giving anti-CD 20 monoclonal antibodies such as Rituximab; 80–90% survival w/ appropriate tx.
3. *Infection*:
   a. *First mo*: high risk of wound infection, UTI, pneumonia.
   b. *First 6 mo*: increased risk of viral opportunistic pathogens—CMV (esophagitis, GI ulceration/hemorrhage, pneumonia, renal insufficiency, malaise), *Candida*, *Pneumocystis carinii*.
      i. Prophylactic antibacterials, antivirals, antifungals given as appropriate.

B. Cytokines

1. *IL-2*: T lymphocytes secrete, upregulate immune system via B-cell proliferation and differentiation. Blocked by cyclosporine, tacrolimus, rapamycin.

C. Specific organs

1. In United States, transplant organs allocated/distributed by UNOS (*www.unos.org*), which also tracks outcomes. Brain death is not absolute prerequisite for donation. One-yr survival for most transplant pts is ~ 90%.
2. *Liver*:
   a. *Preop*:
      i. Cross-match not that important, too close can be harmful, just ABO.
      ii. EtOH most common of ESLD, but hepatitis C most common cause for transplant candidates; 100% reinfection, w/ variable clinical manifestations, most w/ good long-term results. One-yr survival 90% for nonhepatitis pts, 80% for pts w/ hepatitis C (vs 10–15% w/out transplant).
      iii. *Traditional contraindications for recipient*: HIV infection; active substance abuse; life-limiting comorbidities; uncontrolled psychiatric d/o; inability to comply w/ pre-/posttransplant regimes.
      iv. *Other criteria for liver transplantation*:
         - *Model of end-stage liver dz (MELD) score*:
            - *3 components*: (1) serum creatinine, (2) total bilirubin, (3) INR.

   - Score each from 1 upward (max Cr = 4); max score = 40.
   - MELD = 10 [0.957 Ln(Cr) + 0.378 Ln(Tbil) + 1.12 Ln(INR) + 0.643].
   - Average score for pt undergoing transplant in USA = 20.

  v. *Hepatorenal syndrome*: renal dysfunction seen in assoc. w/ liver failure, secondary to renal vasoconstriction (pseudo-prerenal picture not responsive to fluid). Can fully reverse w/ timely liver transplantation.

  vi. Fulminant hepatic failure. Only ~ 5% of cases of transplant. Etiologies include acetaminophen, viral dz, etc.

 b. *Intraop*:

  i. *Partial transplantation*: left lateral segment transplantation developed initially for children, but right lobe transplantation has been performed for adults as well. Major drawback is risk to donor (mortality 1 per 300, which is 10× greater than for renal donors); outcome not better than w/ cadaveric sources, but do increase total number of available organs.

3. *Heart*:

 a. *Preop*:

  i. *Survival*: > 80% at 1 yr, > 70% at 5 yr.

  ii. *Contraindications for recipient*: malignancy, recent PE, infection, fixed pulmonary resistance (unresponsive to vasodilators) > 6 Wood units.

  iii. *Contraindications for donor*: infection, extracranial malignancy, ventricular dysrhythmias, and death from CO poisoning w/ blood carboxyhemoglobin > 20%.

  iv. ABO and size (w/in 20% body wt) most important for screening; HLA done only if high PRA.

 b. *Intraop*: orthotopic placement w/ 4–6 anastomoses.

 c. *Postop*:

  i. *Early*:

   - RV dysfunction common, partly secondary to high pulmonary pressures—give inotropes and pulmonary vasodilators first several days.
   - Tachycardia (~ 100 bpm) secondary to loss of vagal innervation, unresponsive to digoxin and atropine; bradydysrhythmias, however, respond well to isoproterenol or pacing.

  ii. Acute rejection often manifests w/ fatigue and tachydysrhythmias.

  iii. Leading cause of morbidity/mortality after first year is cardiac allograft vasculopathy (CAV)—caveat, MI in transplant heart does not sense pain/angina. Only tx is retransplantation.

  iv. Other problems include susceptibility to CMV, EBV, VSV, and HSV types 1, 2, and 6, and exceptionally high rate of PTLD.

4. *Kidney*:

 a. *Preop*:

  i. Renal transplantation results in 2- to 3-fold increase in life expectancy compared w/ remaining on hemodialysis for pts w/ CRI, offers more independence, and is cheaper in the long run. 1-yr survival 90% (deceased donor) to 95% (living donor) postop.

  ii. *Contraindications for donor*: HIV, sepsis, non-CNS malignancy. Age > 65, HTN may be appropriate to bx.

  iii. *Contraindications for recipient*: cardiopulmonary insufficiency, morbid obesity, PAD, cerebrovascular dz, tobacco abuse, hepatic insufficiency.

  iv. Living donors are typically 18–55 yo, in good health, w/ 2 normal, functioning kidneys. Outcomes are better w/ living donors, even if mismatched HLA.

   - Oblique incision made to harvest usu. left kidney (longer vein); laparoscopic approach also done.

  v. *Prelude to transplant*: vascular access and dialysis.

   - *Indication*:
     - *Nondiabetic*: Cr 6–7 mg/dL, GFR 10–15 cc/min.
     - *Diabetic*: Cr 4–5 mg/dL, GFR 15–25 cc/min.
   - Wait 2+ wk before using PTFE graft and 4–6 wk before using native fistula.

b. *Intraop*:
   i. Extraperitoneal approach through LLQ or RLQ oblique incision.
   ii. Ligate lymphatics overlying iliac vessels to prevent postop lymphocele.
   iii. Usu. arterial and venous end-to-side anastomoses to EIA & V.
   iv. Donor ureter usu. sewn to recipient bladder, but recipient ureter can be sewn to donor renal pelvis.
   v. Frequently, mannitol a/o furosemide given before unclamping vessels.
c. *Postop*:
   i. *Oliguria, rising creatinine*
      - *Immediately postop*
         - Most often secondary to ATN a/o delayed graft function (~ 1/3 of cases), usu. from reperfusion injury—much less common in living donor cases. Usu. self-limited.
         - Consider duplex scan or radioisotope renal perfusion scan.
         - Gradual tapering over time suggests rejection whereas sudden anuria often represents thromboses and requires emergent reexploration. Arterial injuries and majority of venous thromboses require surgery; rarely anticoagulation may be used for venous problem.
         - *Urine leak*: manifest as fluid collection a/o rising creatinine. Generally from ureteral ischemia and may be initially treated w/ stenting and percutaneous drainage, although surgical reconstruction may become necessary.
      - *Weeks to months later may mean*:
         - Immunosuppression toxicity (nephritis not seen on bx).
         - Graft rejection (see interstitial nephritis on bx).
         - Renal vasculature thrombosis (uncommon this far out from surgery).
         - *CMV*: treatable w/ gancyclovir, rarely leads to graft loss.
         - Polyoma virus (see interstitial nephritis on bx, doesn't respond/progresses w/ medical tx/ immunosuppression). A nephrotropic slow virus not uncommon in general population, symptomatic in ~ 5% of renal transplant pts, w/ graft loss in 50% of those. Can monitor for this postop w/ urine cytology or serum PCR. Attempt to tx by *decreasing* immunosuppressants.
   ii. *Other*:
      - *Urine leak*: see entry ci. above under immediately postop.
         - Lymphocele.
         - *Renal transplant artery stenosis* (RTAS): usu. 3–24 mo postop, manifesting w/ HTN, renal insufficiency. Usu. managed w/ percutaneous stenting.
         - *Tertiary hyperparathyroidism*: indication for subtotal parathyroidectomy or total parathyroidectomy w/ implantation of part of one gland into forearm.

5. *Pancreas*
   a. Generally indicated for renal transplant pts (i.e., txp for diabetic nephropathy) w/ brittle diabetes mellitus.
   b. *Technical aspects*: pancreas is situated in pelvis, w/ vessels anastomosed to iliacs. Pancreatic duct is drained into bladder (advantages—follow urine amylase for rejection, ease of bx; disadvantage—metabolic acidosis from bicarb loss, cystitis) or bowel.
   c. *Postop*:
      i. > 70% of pts become insulin-independent, and pt survival at 1 yr > 90%.
      ii. Rejection manifests w/ exocrine insufficiency before endocrine insufficiency.

D. Tolerance and immunosuppresive drugs

1. *Steroids*: block IL-I, blunting inflammatory response. In kidney and pancreas transplants, rapidly weaning off of prednisone (i.e., after pod #5) has been achieved by administration of *thymoglobulin* + rapamycin (usu. in addition to mycophenolate and cyclosporine).

2. *OKT3*: murine Ab that reacts w/ CD-3 on T lymphocytes, blocking generation and function of T cells to Ag challenge. Side effects include fever, diarrhea, bronchospasm, pulmonary edema, meningeal irritation; profound cytokine release.
3. *Cyclosporine* (calcineurin inhibitor): nephrotoxic, hepatotoxic, HTN, gingival hypertrophy, hirsutism.
4. *FK 506/Tacrolimus* (calcineurin inhibitor): nephrotoxic, hepatotoxic, neurotoxic, hyperglycemia, hyperkalemia.
5. *Azathioprim* (antimetabolite): block purine metabolism; less bone marrow depression than mycophenolate.
6. *Mycophenolate/Cellcept* (antimetabolite): block purine metabolism; increased diarrhea than Azathioprim.
7. *Rapamycin*: hyperlipidemia, thrombocytopenia.

CHAPTER 22

WOUND HEALING AND MANAGEMENT: TECHNIQUE AND TECHNOLOGY

TABLE 22.1. Four Phases

Phase	Time	Events	Cells	Factor
Coagulation*	1st hour	Hemostasis Vasoconstriction Fibrin deposition	Platelets Endothelium	PDGF TGF-β
Inflammation	1 h to 4 d	Vasodilatation Angiogenesis Proteoglycan deposition	Neutrophils Macrophage Monocytes	PDGF TGF-β VEGF family
Proliferation	5 to 21 d	Collagen deposition Proteoglycan deposition	Fibroblast	TGF-β
Remodeling	21 d to months	Collagen cross-linking	Fibroblast Myofibroblast	TGF-β

*Coagulation:

i. Subendothelial collagen:
   - Exposure to factor VII starts extrinsic coagulation cascade.
   - Exposure to platelets activates platelets to degranulate:
     - Platelet α granules: PDGF, TGF-β, Plt factor 4.
     - Platelet dense granules: serotonin, ADP, Ca^{++}, histamine, epinephrine.

ii. Platelets:
   - Degranulate as described above.
   - Adhere to damaged endothelium via von Willebrand factor.

I. WOUND HEALING

A. Principal actors

1. *Cells*: after initial injury, fibroblast is most important cell type and helps coordinate healing response.
2. *Factors*:
   a. *PDGF*: important role in angiogenesis.
   b. *TGF-beta*: important antiproliferative factor and plays a role in Marfan syndrome.
   c. *TNF*: involved in systemic inflammation and apoptosis.
   d. *Interleukins*: IL-1, IL-6, IL-8 esp. important in wound healing.
   e. *iNOS*: involved in cell signaling and smooth muscle relaxation.
   f. *VEGF*: important stimulant of angiogenesis in both wound healing and neoplasia.
   g. *EGF*: regulates cell growth and differentiation; may be implicated in dz's such as Dupuytren's.
3. *Matrix*:
   a. *Collagen*: triple helix molecule, synthesis requires ascorbic acid, ferrous iron, alpha-ketoglutarate, and oxygen. Proline and lysine hydroxylation key step.
      i. *Types*:
         - I—90% of adult collagen.
         - II—cartilage, vitreous humor, intervertebral disk.
         - III—most common in fetal and healing tissue (skin, blood vessel, internal organs).
         - IV—basement membranes.

b. *Glycosaminoglycans*: long unbranched polysaccharides w/ wide variety of functions (heparin in blood, chondroitin in cartilage, hyaluronan in synovial fluid).

c. *Elastic fibers*: diminish w/ age.

B. Pathology assoc. w/ wound healing

1. Nutritional and metabolic derangements
   a. *Diabetes mellitus*: serum glucose > 180 impairs WBC chemotaxis and cell killing.
   b. *Vitamin C deficiency*: scurvy; abnormal bleeding and delayed wound healing.
2. Environment
   a. *Corticosteroids*: multifactorial impairment of wound healing.
   b. *Tobacco*: nicotine induces vasospasm, decreasing tissue perfusion.
   c. *Irradiation*: many effects, the most important of which is obliterative endarteritis, decreasing perfusion.
   d. *Mechanical*: any pressure that exceeds capillary pressure (~ 29–32 mm Hg) can lead to venous followed by arterial insufficiency.
3. Congenital
   a. *Ehlers-Danlos*: syndrome of variable degree of joint hypermobility, skin extensibility, skin fragility, predisposition to bruising, and other manifestations (i.e., hernias, bowel a/o arterial rupture, bladder and bowel diverticuli). Divided into types I–IX; inheritance pattern varies. Due to problems such as (depends on subtype) type III collagen, copper metabolism, and enzyme deficiency in procollagen processing. No specific tx, although pts w/ type IV should be screened for cardiovascular disorders.
   b. *Marfan's*: autosomal dominant syndrome w/ abnormalities of skeleton (i.e., hypermobile joints, kyphoscoliosis), eyes (i.e., lens dislocation), and CV system (i.e. MVP, aortic dilatation). Spontaneous PTX not uncommon. Aortic a/o mitral valve replacement may be necessary; increased risk for AAA. Close f/u of scoliosis warranted. Follow for signs of retinal detachment if have lens subluxation.

C. Options for wound coverage

1. *Primary closure*: approximating wound edges at surgery.
2. *Secondary closure*: allowing wound to "fill in" by granulating, contracting, and reepithelializing.
3. *Negative-pressure dressing*: accelerates process of secondary closure by removing excess fluids along w/ potential inflammatory mediators/cytokines, and stimulating granulation tissue formation.
4. *Dermal coverage*: placement helps decrease fluid loss, protect against infection, and premature granulation tissue formation. Most products should remain intact 2–10 d before removal and replacement w/ autograft.
   a. *Integra*: matrix of cross-linked bovine collagen and glycosaminoglycan (scaffold) and a semipermeable silicone layer to prevent water loss.
   b. *Biobrane*: collagen bonded to nylon.
   c. *TransCyte*: Biobrane + growth factors.
   d. *Xenograft* (pigskin).
   e. *Allograft* (cadaveric skin).
   f. *Autograft* (pt's own skin).
5. *Z-plasty*: increases the length along the common limb of the "Z." Use equal limbs, w/ angles 30–90°.
   a. 30° → 25% increase in length. 45° → 50% increase. 60° → 75% increase. 75° → 100% increase. 90° → 120% increase. 60° is optimal—less than this doesn't achieve optimal length, and greater than this creates undue tension.
6. *Pedicled flaps*: brings in healthy tissue still attached to original blood supply.
7. *Free flaps*: requires anastomosis to recipient site vessels using loupe (or more commonly microscope).

D. Suture style

1. *Simple*: most common. Important for needle to enter and exit at right angle to surface to achieve eversion.
2. *Horizontal mattress*: excellent for achieving eversion in difficult areas (e.g., glabrous skin).
3. *Vertical mattress*: good for eversion as well, frequently used for shorter wounds than horizontal mattress.
4. *Running locking*: hemostatic, also useful ("water tight") for ascetic abdomens prone to leak.

5. *Lembert*: used to reinforce and invert bowel anastomoses, these are interrupted seromuscular bites placed approximately 2.5 cm from edge. If done as interrupted horizontal mattress, referred to as Halstead suture. If done as running horizontal mattress, referred to as Cushing suture.
6. *Gambee*: used to appose and invert structures such as mucosa, this suture has also been utilized in closing abdominal defects. The suture is placed through the serosa, passing through the full thickness of bowel (or abdominal) wall, then back through the mucosa to exit through the submucosa on the same side/limb, before running the reverse pattern on the opposite side/limb. A variant of this entails taking full thickness of one side/limb, then turning back to enter the submucosa and exit through the mucosa (creating a loop), then reversing this on the opposite side/limb.
7. *Connell*: a continuous full-thickness suture run as a "U" in bowel anastomoses, essentially a running horizontal mattress stitch.
8. *Purse-string*: useful for helping circular wounds close.
9. *Subcuticular*: running or interrupted sutures placed in subcuticular tissue.

II. TECHNOLOGY

A. Diagnostic imaging

1. *Ultrasound*: excellent for distinguishing solid vs cystic structures. Generates impulses and interprets echoes utilizing piezoelectric effect.
2. *CT*: uses ionizing radiation to generate images of cuts through various axes of the body.
3. *MRI*: uses properties of magnetic spin of hydrogen atoms in tissue to generate images. Excellent modality for soft-tissue imaging.
4. *Nuclear medicine*:
    a. *MIGB*: involves cholesterol synthesis, good for adrenal medulla.
    b. *NP-59* (iodocholesterol scan): good for adrenal cortex.
    c. *Gallium*: Ga-67 localizes in areas of osteomyelitis or other infection via granulocyte/bacterial uptake and by binding to lactoferrin at the site of infection. Of note, Ga-67 citrate is also a bone agent and accumulates at site of increased bone remodeling, not just osteomyelitis.
    d. *Indium*: WBC can be labeled w/ In-111, or, more recently w/ Tc-99m-HMPAO. Tc-labeled leukocytes generally provide better images, however.
    e. *Tc-Sestamibi scans*:
        i. Most often used to identify parathyroid adenomas.
        ii. Specificity can be increased w/ subtraction imaging utilizing Tc-pertechnetate or I-123 to outline thyroid.
        iii. Similarly, can give thallium (uptake by thyroid and parathyroid) and pertechnetate (uptake by thyroid only), then subtract out the latter, leaving only parathyroid tissue images behind. False positives may occur w/ abnormal thyroid function.
        iv. Tc localizes in thyroid tissue, similar to iodine (also in salivary glands).
    f. *PET scans*: use fluoridated glucose to emit positrons. Cancers demonstrate accelerated glycolysis, and 18 fluorodeoxyglucose competes w/ glucose (and is trapped intracellularly).
    g. *SPECT scans*: uses single photons (not 2 as w/ PET), most often uses Tc-99.
    h. *Lung scans*:
        i. Use Tc bound to macro-aggregated albumin, which is filtered out in *perfused* lung.
        ii. Used Xe gas for *ventilation* assay, but now more commonly use aerosolized Tc-99.
    i. *Liver scans*:
        i. Actually focus on RES *phagocytes* (Kupffer cells) w/ Tc-99–labeled sulfur colloid (can also be filtered in spleen, lungs, marrow).
        ii. To focus on *hepatocytes*, iminodiacetic acid compounds are tagged w/ Tc-99; give good picture of liver/biliary tract.
    j. *Bone scans*: bisphosphonates are complexed w/ Tc-99; then wait 2–3 h; focuses on osteoblast activity.
    k. *Cardiac*:
        i. *Infarct imaging*: uses radioactive phosphate.

   ii. *Myocardial function study*: MUGA, assesses left ventricle's ability to pump blood → ejection fraction.
   iii. *Myocardial perfusion study*: uses Tl-201 or Tc-99 w/ SPECT imaging, looking at perfusion in thin planes (at rest and w/ stress—exercise or dobutamine).

B. Therapeutics

1. *Laparoscopy*
   a. *Physiology*
      i. *Pulmonary effects*: increased peak airway pressures, increased end-tidal CO_2, decreased pulmonary compliance, decreased vital capacity, possible respiratory acidosis.
      ii. *Circulatory effects*: increased CVP, SVR, and MAP, increased cardiac work; arteriolar dilation and myocardial depression secondary to increased CO_2; variable effects on BP; possible increase of sympathetics, renin-angiotensin, vasopressin.
      iii. *Renal effects*: decreased renal perfusion.
      iv. *Coagulation effects*: increased LE venous stasis.
      v. *CNS*: increased ICP.
      vi. *GI*: decreased sympathetic-induced ileus.
      vii. *Effects on pregnancy*: although alterations in fetal heart rate have been observed, effects on fetal development have not been proven to be injurious beyond standard risks of general anesthetic surgery.
2. *Electrosurgery*
   a. Relies on alternating current (electrocautery refers to use of direct current that doesn't travel through body). Tissues create impedance and resulting heat. Typically operates at 100 kHz so as to not stimulate muscle/nerves, which could be stimulated by usual 60 Hz frequency.
   b. *Bipolar*: active and return electrodes at surgical site (2 tines). No "grounding pad" required.
   c. *Monopolar*: active electrode in wound, requires return electrode ("grounding pad") as current flows through the body.
   d. *Waveforms*: different effects on tissue.
      i. *Cut*: constant waveform, vaporizes/cuts tissue by heating very rapidly. 100% "on" duty cycle.
      ii. *Coag*: actual "on time" of waveform is severely reduced, heating tissue more slowly, causing coagulation instead of vaporization. 6% "on" duty cycle. *Note*: one can cut also w/ coag (and coagulate w/ cut to lesser degree), but results in higher voltage and charring.
      iii. *Blend 1*: 50% time "on" duty cycle (balance of coagulation and cutting).
      iv. *Blend 2*: 40% time "on" duty cycle (better at coagulation than cutting).
      v. *Blend 3*: 25% time "on" duty cycle (more cutting than pure "coag" mode).
3. *CUSA* (cavitronic ultrasonic aspirator): hollow titanium tip vibrates rapidly in tissue, creating focused regions of alternately high and low pressure. Low pressure creates vacuum in cells, which lyse them. Much less collateral injury tissues than Bovie (0.5-mm vs 4-mm band of damage). Works best in moist tissue.
4. *Harmonic scalpel*: cuts/coagulates w/ minimal collateral damage. After coapting tissue, blade vibrates at 55,500 Hz, denaturing protein, resulting in coagulation. Thermal signature much lower (50–100°C compared to electrocautery 150–400°C).

CHAPTER 23

MEDICAL PROBLEMS OF SURGICAL PATIENTS

I. NEUROLOGIC

A. Delirium tremens: see section X. at the end of this chapter.

B. Myasthenia gravis

1. Autoimmune dz w/ Ab to postsynaptic nicotinic acetylcholine receptors of voluntary muscles; gen. asthenia, may first manifest w/ diplopia a/o ptosis. May have dyspnea, difficulty chewing, etc.
2. Dx w/ Tensilon test, which blocks hydrolysis of Ach in synaptic cleft, thus improving sx, EMG, and other modalities.
3. ~ 3/4 of pts have thymic disorders (85% w/ hyperplasia, 15% w/ thymomas).
4. *Tx*:
   a. *Anticholinesterase medications*: neostigmine, pyridostigmine—act like Tensilon (edrophonium). Pyridostigmine is preferred agent, usu. given as 60 mg PO q 3–6 h. Side effects include diarrhea, intestinal cramping, nausea, salivation, and lacrimation. Excessive secretion can cause airway compromise in perioperative period.
   b. *Immunotherapy*: prn short-term suppression w/ plasmapheresis a/o immunoglobulin.
   c. *Immunosuppression*: corticosteroids, azathioprine (Imuran), cyclosporine (Sandimmune) used for long-term suppression. Latter 2 meds usu. for cases refractory to steroids a/o thymectomy.
   d. Thymectomy improves sx in most pts, for reasons that are not always clear. Consideration for surgery should be entertained early in dz course for adolescents (possible developmental effects if sooner) to adults up to ~ 60 yo (diminishing effects possibly from thymic involution w/ age). Increases sensitivity to anticholinesterases. For details of operation, see Chapter 26 on key steps in key operations.

C. Seizures

1. *General* (tonic clonic, tonic, clonic, myoclonic, absence), *partial* (simple, complex, etc.).
2. *Lower threshold*: head trauma, CNS or systemic infections, hyperventilation, sleep deprivation, CVA, metabolic (alkalosis, hypoglycemia, etc.), alcohol withdrawal.
3. *Tx*:
   a. *Prophylaxis*: pts at risk for early posttraumatic seizures (acute intracranial hemorrhage/hematoma, open depressed skull fx w/ parenchymal injury, etc.) → loading dose phenytoin/fosphenytoin, 20 mg/kg, then maintain therapeutic levels for 1 wk.
   b. *General*: see Chapter 25 on common problems on call.
4. *Anticonvulsant agents*:
   a. *Phenytoin* (Dilantin®): generalized tonic-clonic sz, simple-complex partial sz, occ. absence; oral loading.
      i. *Dosage*:
         - Oral loading dose = 300–600 mg PO q 4 h to achieve 17 mg/kg
         - Oral maintenance dose = 300–600 mg/d divided 2 or 3 times per day
         - Parenteral loading dose = 18 mg/kg *slow* IV (peds = 20 mg/kg *slow* IV)—must use NS as vehicle
         - Parenteral maintenance dose = 200–500 mg/d (peds = 4–7 mg/kg/d)
      ii. *Miscellaneous*:
         - Potential side effect = *hypotension* (negative inotrope). Monitor carefully in trauma pts. Arrythmias also possible if given too quickly IV. Side effects 2/2 propylene glycol, w/ which it is marketed. Fosphenytoin (below) is preferred for parenteral use. Teratogenic. Assoc. w/ Stevens-Johnson syndrome.
   b. *Fosphenytoin* (Cerebyx®):
      i. Same indications for phenytoin, but is preferred (in adults) for parenteral administration for 5 or fewer days. May be given in dextrose solution or NS, and is less taxing to peripheral

veins. Can also be given faster than phenytoin, w/ ↓ risk hypotension. Metabolized to phenytoin. Risk of Stevens-Johnson syndrome.

ii. Dosage is in phenytoin equivalents (PE). Generally load as 1–1.5 g IV.

c. *Carbamazapine* (Tegretol®): partial seizures, trigeminal neuralgia.

i. *Dosage*: 600–2000 mg/d (peds = 20–30 mg/kg/d) PO.

ii. *Miscellaneous*: may contribute to or cause SIADH, self-limited leucopenia, Stevens-Johnson syndrome.

d. *Valproate* (Depakote®): generalized tonic-clonic sz, absence sz. (*Note*: Ethosuximide preferred for absence sz.)

i. *Dosage*: 600–3000 mg/d (peds = 15–60 mg/kg/d) PO.

ii. *Miscellaneous*: assoc. w/ pancreatitis. Teratogenic. Hepatitis risk in pts < 2 yo.

e. *Phenobarbital*: generalized tonic-clonic sz, partial sz, febrile sz.

i. *Dosage* (same for PO, IV, or IM):

- *Adults*: load w/ 20 mg/kg slow IV (< 100 mg/min), then maintain w/ 100–300 mg/d (divide 2–3 times per day).
- *Peds*: load w/ 15–20 mg/kg, then maintain w/ 2–6 mg/kg/d (divide 2 times per day).

ii. *Miscellaneous*: assoc. w/ significant cognitive impairment and paradoxical hyperactivity in children. Maternal use assoc. w/ infant hemorrhage.

f. *Levetiracetam* (Keppra®): partial sz in adults.

i. *Dosage*: 500 mg PO 2 times per day, titrate biweekly up to 3000 mg/d

D. **Delirium:** acutely altered alertness (increased or decreased), awareness, and attention due to systemic process (hypoxia, hypoglycemia, toxins, hyperammonemia, uremia) or local pathology (brain tumor or hematoma). Sleep-wake cycle generally disrupted. Sx may include hallucinations, delusions, agitation, autonomic changes.

E. **Dementia:** chronic state of impaired orientation and long-term memory. Attention and sleep-wake cycle intact.

F. **Parkinson's disease:** usu. sporadic degradation of nigrostriatal dopaminergic system; stiffness, slowness, rigidity of facial expression, and tremor (diminishes w/ voluntary motion or complete rest).

1. *Tx tremor*: may include anticholinergics (rest tremor) or propanolol/primidone (action tremor). Levodopa for akinesia, postural imbalance. Deep brain stimulation at subthalamic nucleus useful for all aspects.

G. **Neuroleptic malignant syndrome:** triad of fever, extrapyramidal dysfunction (catatonia/dystonia, tremors, rigidity, etc.), and autonomic dysfunction (tachycardia, labile BP, urinary incontinence, diaphoresis, etc.) most commonly assoc. w/ haloperidol, though other psychotropic medications have been implicated. Leukocytosis (up to 30 K) and CK elevation may be seen. Usu. in young males. Primary tx is d/c medication, but sx may last > 1 wk after cessation (offending agents not amenable to dialysis). Bromocriptine (7.5–60 mg/d in 3 divided doses); dantrolene and amantadine may also be useful. [Caroff S, et al., *Med Clin North Am.* 1993;77:185.]

H. **Malignant hyperthermia:** see Chapter 3 on anesthesia.

I. **Cerebrovascular accident:** see Chapter 25 on common problems on call.

II. CARDIOVASCULAR

A. Preoperative evaluation

1. Cardiac w/u

a. *Major clinical predictors*: unstable/severe angina, MI w/in past 4 wk, decompensated CHF, evidence of large ischemic burden by clinical sx/noninvasive testing, significant arrhythmias (high-grade AV block, symptomatic ventricular arrhythmias in setting of underlying heart dz, supraventricular arrhythmias w/ uncontrolled ventricular rate), or severe valvular dz. Identify and treat problem before elective surgery.

i. Symptomatic stenotic valve lesions may merit preop percutaneous valvotomy or valve replacement to prevent perioperative HF or shock whereas symptomatic regurgitant valve dz can generally be managed medically.

ii. Preop noninvasive evaluation of LV function indicated for current or poorly controlled HF (class I data) or prior HF or dyspnea of unknown origin (class IIa data).

iii. Preop 12-lead EKG indicated for recent chest pain or ischemic equivalent in intermediate- or high-risk pts w/ planned intermediate- or high-risk surgery (class I data) or asx pts w/ DM (class IIa). Class IIb data represent pts w/ prior coronary revascularization; asx male > 45 yo or female > 55 yo w/ 2+ atherosclerotic risk factors; prior hospital admission for cardiac causes.

iv. *Exercise/physiological stress testing indicated for*:

- *Class I* (evidence a/o general agreement is useful/effective): dx of adults w/ intermediate pretest probability of CAD; prognostic assessment of pt undergoing initial eval for suspected/proven CAD or subjects w/ significant change in clinical status; demonstration of proof of myocardial ischemia before coronary revascularization; evaluation of adequacy of medical tx or prognostic assessment after an acute coronary syndrome.
- *Class IIa* (conflicting evidence/opinion, but wt of evidence is in favor): evaluation of exercise capacity when subjective assessment is unreliable.
- *Class IIb* (similar to above, but less well-established): dx of CAD pts w/ high or low pretest probability; those w/ resting ST depression < 1 mm, those taking digitalis, or those w/ EKG criteria for LVH; detection of restenosis in high-risk asymptomatic pts w/in the initial months after percutaneous coronary intervention.

v. *Coronary angiography is indicated for*:

- *Class I*: evidence for high risk of adverse outcome based on noninvasive test results; angina unresponsive to medical tx; unstable angina (esp. if planning intermediate- or high-risk noncardiac surgery; equivocal noninvasive test results in pts for high-risk surgery).
- *Class IIa*: multiple markers of intermediate clinical risk and planned vascular surgery (noninvasive studies should be considered first); moderate/large ischemia on noninvasive testing but w/out high-risk features and lower left ventricular EF.
- *Class IIb*: perioperative MI; medically stabilized class III/IV angina and planned low-risk or minor surgery.

b. *Intermediate clinical predictors*: mild angina pectoris, prior MI (> 1 mo prior), compensated or prior CHF (esp. insulin-dependent) DM, or renal insufficiency (Cr > 2): consideration of functional capacity and surgery-specific risk identifies those who need advanced testing.

c. *Minor clinical predictors*: advanced age, abnormal EKG (LVII, LBBB, ST-T abn.), rhythm other than sinus (i.e., Afib), low functional capacity (inability to climb 1 flight of stairs w/ bag of groceries), hx of stroke, or uncontrolled systemic hypertension:

i. HTN of SBP ≥ 180, DBP ≥ 110 definitely requires control; beta-blockade is particularly protective.

ii. Frequent premature beats a/o asx nonsustained v-tach not assoc. w/ increased risk of nonfatal MI/cardiac death and generally do not require aggressive perioperative monitoring or tx.

d. If s/p CABG in past 5 yr and has had no clinical change w/out recurrent ischemic sx, no further cardiac w/u is required.

e. If pt has had a favorable coronary evaluation in past 2 yr and has not had a change in clinical status, repeat testing usu. not necessary.

f. Implantable pacemakers or ICDs should be turned off immediately before surgery and then back on postop.

g. *High-risk surgery is defined as*: emergency major operations, aortic/major vascular, peripheral vascular; anticipated prolonged surgery w/ large fluid shifts/blood loss.

h. *Intermediate risk surgery is defined as*: CEA, major head/neck, intraperitoneal/intrathoracic, orthopedic, prostate.

i. *Low-risk surgery is defined as*: endoscopic, superficial, cataract, breast. [Eagle KA, et al., ACC/AHA guideline update for perioperative cardiovascular evaluation for noncardiac surgery–executive summary. *Circulation*. 2002;105:1257–67.]

2. Coronary-artery revascularization before elective vascular surgery does not appear to significantly alter long-term outcome—it merely transfers the operative mortality risk to the cardiac surgeon instead of the vascular surgeon. No preop CABG unless pt has stand-alone indications for it. [McFalls EO, et al., Coronary-artery revascularization before elective major vascular surgery. *N Engl J Med*. 2004;351(27)2795–804.]

B. Hypertension

1. *Medical tx*: (*Note*: significant HTN should not be lowered too rapidly—a reasonable goal is to decrease by 25% in the first h, then to ~ 160/100 w/in 6 h.
   a. *Benign*
   b. *Urgent*: require ↓ w/in several hours. SBP > 200 or DBP > 125 (or any HTN + optic disk edema—asymptomatic). Parenteral tx not generally needed.
      i. *Oral tx*:
         - *Captopril*: 12.5–25 mg, effective in 15–30 min.
         - *Clonidine*: 0.2 mg (then 0.1 mg q h to total of 0.8 mg), effective w/in hours. *Caveat*: rebound HTN, sedation.
         - *Nifedipine*: sublingual (10 mg) is rapidly acting, but should be used w/ beta blocker to prevent reflex tachycardia (MI has been reported). Hypotension significant risk, assoc. w/ CVA.
      ii. *Emergent*: require ↓ w/in 1 h to decrease morbidity/mortality. Diastolic BP usu. > 130 mm Hg. Sx may include encephalopathy (HA, confusion, etc.), nephropathy (hematuria, proteineuria, etc.), incracranial hemorrhage, preeclampsia, angina, pulmonary edema, or MI.
         - *Parenteral therapy often indicated*: see Chapter 7 on cardiac, for specific agents.
      iii. *Malignant*: HTN + encephalopathy or nephropathy + papilledema.
         - *Parenteral therapy indicated*: see Chapter 7 on cardiac for specific agents.
   c. *Surgical causes* (5% of all cases of HTN):
      i. *Pheochromocytoma*: see Chapter 13 on endocrine.
      ii. *Conn's dz*: see Chapter 13 on endocrine.
      iii. *Cushing's syndrome*: see Chapter 13 on endocrine.
      iv. *Coarctation of aorta*: see Chapter 11 on vascular.
      v. *Renal artery stenosis*: see Chapter 11 on vascular.
      vi. *Hyperthyroidism*: see Chapter 13 on endocrine.

III. PULMONARY

A. Asthma: inflammatory obstructive process causing wheezing, cough, etc.

1. *Tx*: gauge response by clinical appearance, pulse oximetry, and peak expiratory flow (PEF). Supplemental oxygen important for all exacerbations.
   a. *Mild* (PEF > 80%):
      i. *Short-acting β_2-agonist inhaler*: albuterol (MDI 0.09 mg/puff given 2–12 puffs q 30–60 min vs inhaler 2.5 mg) is standard. Terbutaline also commonly used.
      ii. *Inhaled corticosteroid*: if already taking one, double the dose; o/w, consider initiating tx. Beclomethasone, budesonide, fluticasone, and triamcinolone most common MDIs.
      iii. *Oral corticosteroids*: 3–10 d of tx (i.e., 5–60 mg prednisone daily) may be appropriate for cases refractory to above.
   b. *Moderate–severe* (severe = < 200 L/min):
      i. Oxygen, short-acting β_2-agonist inhaler, and systemic corticosteroids (IV or PO) are key.
      ii. Rarely, severe cases (i.e., FEV < 25%) may gain small additional benefit from IV magnesium SO_4.

B. COPD

1. Broadly classified into types A ("pink puffer"/emphysema dominant) and B ("blue bloater"/bronchitis dominant).
   a. *Type A*: usu. dyspneic, thin, w/ hyperinflated lungs on CXR.
   b. *Type B*: usu. w/ cough, often overweight, w/ rhonchi. CXR usu. normal volume lungs. Pulmonary artery pressures elevated c/w type A pts. OSA frequently present.
2. *Tx*:
   a. *Medical*: smoking cessation, oxygen therapy are important nonpharmacologic adjuncts.
      i. *Anticholinergics*: ipratropium bromide (drug of choice)—2–4 puffs q 6 h.

ii. *β_2-agonists* (short-acting): albuterol (more rapid onset, but shorter duration, more side effects).

iii. *Theophylline*: occasionally used for sx refractory to the above.

iv. *Corticosteroids*: only ~ 10% of pts respond, rarely used.

v. *Antibiotics*: exacerbations in type B pts may benefit from tx w/ TMP-SMX, Augmentin®, or doxycycline.

b. *Surgical*: bullectomy, lung volume reduction surgery, or bilateral lung transplantation may be appropriate in select pts.

C. **OSA**: upper airway obstruction during sleep from loss of muscle tone.

1. *Risk factors*: obesity, micrognathia, macroglossia, alcohol or sedative usage, smoking, hypothyroidism.
2. *Complications*: hypoxia can result in bradyarrhythmias or even arrest, w/ risk of tachyarrhythmias (atrial fibrillation, etc.) after resumption of breathing.
3. *Tx*:
   a. *Nonsurgical*: wt loss, avoidance of sedatives/alcohol, CPAP.
   b. *Surgical*: uvulopalatopharyngoplasty, septoplasty. Wt loss surgery should be considered.

D. **Pulmonary embolism:** see Chapter 8 on thoracic and esophagus.

E. **Pulmonary hypertension**

1. *Etiologies*: multiple, including HIV, portal HTN, toxins, glycogen storage dz's, left-sided heart dz, COPD, sleep apnea, chronic high-altitude exposure, PE, sarcoidosis, histiocytosis-X, SLE, scleroderma, etc.
2. *Dx*: may present w/ dyspnea, chest pain, syncope. EKG (RVH, RAE), CXR (central PA enlargement w/ peripheral pruning), echocardiography may suggest dx.
   a. Gold standard is PA catheter w/ mean pulmonary artery pressure > 25 mm Hg at rest or > 30 mm Hg w/ exercise and pulmonary artery wedge pressure of < 15 mm Hg.
3. *Tx*:
   a. Oxygen supplementation to reverse hypoxic vasoconstriction.
   b. Warfarin w/ goal of INR of 2.0 (benefit thought decrease small thromboses in pulm vasculature).
   c. Calcium channel blockers decreasing in popularity.
   d. *Prostanoids*: vasodilators w/ antiplatelet effects (epoprostenol).
   e. Endothelin-receptor antagonists (bosentan).
   f. Phosphodiesterase inhibitors (i.e., sildenafil [Viagra]).
   g. HMG-CoA reductase inhibitors (i.e., simvastatin)—research still preliminary.
   h. *Surgery*: atrial septotomy may improve sx; lung transplantation last resort.

IV. GASTROINTESTINAL

A. **Irritable bowel syndrome**

1. *Dx criteria* (Rome II consensus statement of Am. Gastroenterol. Assoc.):
   a. At least 12 total wk (not nec. consecutive) in past year of abd. pain/discomfort w/ 2 of the following 3:
      i. Relieved w/ defecation, *a/o*. . .
      ii. Onset assoc. w/ change in frequency of stool, *a/o*. . .
      iii. Onset assoc. w/ change in form/appearance of stool.
   b. *In general, suggested by*: abnormal stool frequency (> 3 BM/d or < 3 BM/wk), abnormal stool form (unusually hard/soft, etc.), passage of mucus, a/o bloating or subjective distension.
2. *Tx*:
   a. *Depending on sx*: loperamide, stool softeners, psychotherapy/antidepressants.
   b. Avoid red meat, fried/fatty foods, dairy, chocolate, coffee, EtOH, carbonated beverages.
   c. Increase fiber, fresh fruits/vegetables.

B. **Cirrhosis and ascites:** see Chapter 16 on hepatobiliary.

C. **Hepatitis:** see Table 23.1. [Information below in part from: Kim AI, Saab SS, Interpretation of laboratory tests for diagnosing viral hepatitis. *Hospital Physician*. Sept 2004;15–9.]

TABLE 23.1. Summary of Hepatitides

Hep.	Type	Trans.	Incub.	Dx	Other
A	RNA	Fecal-oral	2–7 wk	IgM anti-HAV	– Most common hep. worldwide – 2/3 cases asymptomatic – IgM detectable w/ sx and for 4–6 mo – IgG = immune – Natural infection = lifetime immunity – Vaccination good 10–20 yr – No chronic dz
B	Double-shelled DNA	Blood/sex	8–24 wk	IgM anti-HBc HBsAg	– 9th cause of death worldwide – 10% develop chronic dz – Infectivity correlate w/ HBeAg (+) – * See below for details of serology – Tx: protease inhibitors (Epivir, Adefovir), interferon, transplant
C	RNA	Blood/sex	2–13 wk	HCV EIA HCV RNA	– 6 genotypes (type 1 seen most in United States, relatively poor responder to tx) – Acute dz very mild, often rarely dx'd – 80% develop chronic dz – #1 indication for liver transplant – Tx: interferon, transplant
D	Defective RNA	Blood/sex	3–7 wk	IgM anti-HDV	– Requires HBV infection to establish – Uncommon in W. Europe, N. America, E. Asia – May potentiate HBV to fulminant liver dz
E	RNA	Fecal-oral	2–9 wk	IgM/G anti-HEV	– Uncommon in N. America – No chronic dz – IgM, IgG serology ~ 50%, 90% sensitive, detectable once symptomatic

*HBsAg detectable by ELISA at 6 wk of infection, and should be cleared 4–6 mo after infection, w/ gradual appearance of anti-HBs Ab, which results in immunity. During this period, the only identifiable markers may be IgM and IgG anti-HBc (which can also be noted w/ onset of sx). IgM anti-HBc suggests recent infection (new or reactivation). Vaccination produces HBs only, the titers of which wane w/ time.

10% of cases develop chronic HBV (usu. infants, immunocompromised, and hemodialysis pts); dx by HBsAg in serum > 6 mo. Infectivity correlates w/ presence of serum HBeAg. Active chronic dz has, among other things, HBeAg (+), elevated transaminases, and liver bx w/ characteristic changes. Inactive chronic dz has HBeAg (–), anti-HBe (+), HBV DNA < 105 copies/mL, normal transaminase levels, and unremarkable liver bx.

1. *Other causes of acute liver dysfunction/failure include*: acetaminophen (#1—tx = acetylcysteine), INH, tricyclic antidepressants, volatile anesthetics (esp. halothane), NSAIDs, *Amanita phylloides*, carbon tetrachloride, aflatoxin, hepatitis A and B, shock, Budd-Chiari syndrome, Wilson dz, hyperthermia, hepatectomy, Reye syndrome, rarely other viruses.

D. Peptic ulcers

1. *Non-H. pylori, non-NSAID ulcer tx*:
   a. *Duodenal*: omeprazole 20 mg or lansoprazole 15 mg PO q d × 4 wk *or* ranitidine 300 mg or famotidine 40 mg PO at bedtime × 6 wk *or* sucralfate 1 g PO 4 times per day.
   b. *Gastric* (or complicated duodenal): omeprazole 20 mg PO 2 times per day or lansoprazole 30 mg PO q d × 6–8 wk *or* ranitidine 150 mg PO 2 times per day or famotidine 20 mg PO 2 times per day × 8–12 wk.
   c. *NSAID-related ulcer prophylaxis* (if prior ulcers, on steroids/anticoagulants, a/o > 70 yo):
      i. Misoprostol 100–200 μg PO 3 times per day or 4 times per day *or* (if intolerant of misoprostol) PPI PO q d.
   d. *H. pylori-related ulcer*:
      i. Omeprazole 20 mg PO 2 times per day or lansoprazole 30 mg PO 2 times per day (before meals) *plus* (all other meds w/ meals):
         - Metronidazole 500 mg PO 2 times per day + clarithromycin 500 mg PO 2 times per day *or*
         - Amoxicillin 1 g PO 2 times per day + clarithromycin 500 mg PO 2 times per day *or*

- Bismuth subsalicylate 2 tabs PO 4 times per day + tetracycline 500 mg PO 3 times per day + metronidazole 250 mg PO 4 times per day

ii. After 2 wk of one of the above regimens, continue another 4–8 wk w/ PPI/H_2 blocker tx as outlined under "non-*H. pylori*, non-NSAID ulcer tx."

V. RENAL

A. **End-stage renal diseases:** see Chapter 5 on renal.

VI. HEMOTOLOGIC

A. **Sickle cell anemia**

1. AR gene in 8% of African Americans.
2. Manifestations may include jaundice, calcium bilirubinate gallstones, splenomegaly, pretibial ulceration, etc. Severe pain (i.e., abdomen, long bones, chest) from vaso-occlusive ischemic events may last for days, possibly accompanied by fever, mimicking a "surgical abdomen." May also cause CVA, priapism, bone ischemia (predisposed to osteomyelitis w/ *Staphylococcus* > *Salmonella*), hematuria, and retinopathy. Lab findings may include hemolytic anemia, reticulocytosis, Howell-Jolly bodies, target cells, WBC up to 15 K, thrombocytosis, and indirect hyperbilirubinemia.
3. *Tx*:
   a. *Chronic*: folate supplementation, pneumococcal vaccination. Hydroxyurea is given to some pts w/ frequent debilitating pain to stimulate erythropoiesis.
   b. *Acute*: IV hydration, supplemental oxygen, analgesia. Exchange transfusions indicated for CVA, priapism and refractory pain.

B. **G6PD deficiency:** X-linked dz usu. in black males (10%) resulting in episodic hemolytic anemia from relative RBC ability to handle oxidative stresses; *precipitating agents include*: fava beans, primaquine, dapsone, quinine, sulfonamides, and nitrofurantoin.

C. **Leukemia**

1. *Acute*
   a. Generally present w/ pancytopenia +/– circulating blasts in labs (often hyperuricemia, occ. DIC), clinically may have bleeding diathesis, infectious complication, bone pain, gum hypertrophy, etc.
   b. *Acute myelogenous leukemia* (AML): usu. age at dx ~ 60 yo. Tx w/ anthracycline + cytarabine → complete remission in majority of pts.
   c. *Acute lymphoblastic leukemia* (ALL): usu. age at dx ~ 5 yo. Adults tx'd w/ combination chemotx results in complete remission in up to 90%.
2. *Chronic lymphocytic leukemia* (CLL): clonal malignancy of B lymphocytes, most often dx'd ~ 65 yo. Generally present w/ WBC > 20 K due to lymphocytosis. Tx may not be needed for early or mild dz; anemia, thrombocytopenia, symptomatic LAD, or profound fatigue may be tx'd w/ Fludarabine + rituximab. Age 2 yo survival > 90%.
3. *Hairy-cell leukemia*: rare, usu. occurs in males ~ 55 yo. Relatively indolent, presents w/ pancytopenia, marked splenomegaly, frequent hepatomegaly, fatigue, occasionally recurrent infections. Drug of choice is cladribine—excellent prognosis. Splenectomy rarely performed as palliative measure in refractory cases.

D. **Methemoglobinemia:** a state of hgb oxidized to the ferric state, which does not carry oxygen.

1. *Associated agents*: benzocaine, lidocaine, aniline, nitrites/nitrates (NTG, nitroprusside, silver nitrate, amyl nitrite), NO, dapsone (subacute onset), phenazopyridine (Pyridium®), sulfonamides, phenacetin, chlorate.
2. *Tx*:
   a. R/o cyanosis from lung pathology or right → left cardiac shunt.
   b. *Methylene blue*: 2 mg/kg IVP for acute toxicity, or 100–300 mg/d for chronic toxicity.
   c. *Ascorbic acid*: 300–500 mg/d for chronic toxicity.

E. **Deep venous thrombosis:** see Chapters 2 and 11.

VII. ENDOCRINE

A. **Diabetes mellitus**

1. *Perioperative management*
   a. Above blood glucose of 180, neutrophil chemotaxis and cell-killing is impaired.

b. Check glucose immediately postop, on arrival to ward, and q 6 h thereafter.
c. Place on basal insulin dose, w/ following sliding scale (glucose [mg/dL]):
   i. 0–70: give juice, a/o $^1/_2$ amp D50, call house officer.
   ii. 71–150: no additional insulin.
   iii. 151–200: 2 U regular insulin SQ.
   iv. 201–250: 4 U regular insulin SQ.
   v. 251–300: 6 U regular insulin SQ.
   vi. 301–350: 8 U regular insulin SQ.
   vii. 351–400: 10 U regular insulin SQ.
   viii. 400: 12 U regular insulin SQ; call house officer.

2. In critically ill pts, tight glucose control (80–110) assoc. w/ better outcomes.
   a. In ICU environment can do insulin drip, initially checking glucose q 1 h. Sample *initial* infusion rate:
      i. < 60 → 25 cc D50% IV.
      ii. 60–80 → 0, recheck in 1 h.
      iii. 81–110 → do nothing.
      iv. 111–150 → bolus 2 U insulin, then run at 1 U/h.
      v. 151–200 → bolus 2 U insulin, then run at 2 U/h.
      vi. 201–250 → bolus 4 U insulin, then run at 2 U/h.
      vii. 251–300 → bolus 6 U insulin, then run at 4 U/h.
      viii. 301–350 → bolus 8 U insulin, then run at 4 U/h.
      ix. 350 → bolus 10 U insulin, then run at 4 U/h.

3. *Diabetic ketoacidosis*
   a. In 20%, no antecedent h/o DM. In 50%, concomitant or precipitating condition, usu. infection.
   b. *Dx*: hyperglycemia (usu. > 250 mg/dL), and bicarbonate < 20 mEq/L. Ketone (+) blood, urine. *Note*: anion gap can be normal w/ DKA secondary to renal tubular reabsorption of Cl^-.
   c. *Tx* ("I fix patient's problems"):
      i. *Insulin*: 0.1 U/kg IVP, then 0.1 U/kg/h drip.
         - If serum glucose doesn't drop by 10% in first h, double the dose.
         - Decrease dose by 50% once serum bicarbonate > 16 mEq/L.
      ii. *Fluid* (pts usu. several liters dehydrated, 50–100 cc/kg):
         - NSat 1 L/h × 2 h.
         - Follow w/ $^1/_2$ NS at 250–500 cc/h.
         - Dextrose can be added to IVF when serum glucose < 250 mg/dL.
      iii. *Potassium* (although often not immediately apparent, usu. 3–5 mEq/kg deficit exists):
         - Serum levels will fall w/ commencement of insulin therapy and resolution of acidosis.
         - Early replacement and initially hourly monitoring essential.
      iv. *Phosphate*:
         - Check level 4 h after beginning therapy and replete as indicated.

B. Diabetes insipidus

1. Deficit in secretion or action of antidiuretic hormone (ADH).
2. *Presentation/dx*: hypotonic polyuria w/ hypernatremia, hyperosmolality, hypovolema. Check urine osmolality and serum sodium to narrow differential dx.
3. *Central/neurogenic*: may occur w/ variety of hypothalamic/pituitary lesions (trauma, tumors, infarction, surgery, infiltrative dz).
4. *Nephrogenic*: kidneys do not respond to ADH. Management more difficult; rehydrate w/ isotonic fluids.
5. *Electrolytes*: follow closely, esp. K^+, replacing as necessary. Replace Na^+ slowly in cases longer than 48 h, at 1–2 mEq/L/h. If seizing, replace quickly until stops seizing (usu. ~ 165 MEq/L).

C. **Thyroid:** see Chapter 13 on endocrine.

D. **Parathyroid:** see Chapter 13 on endocrine.

E. **Adrenal**

1. *Excess*

a. Only 2.5–7.5 mg PO q d of prednisone, can, over time (i.e., > 1 mo), lead to significant osteopenia and increased fracture risk.

b. *Delayed wound healing*: tx w/ vitamin A (20,000 PO daily for 5–20 d). See Chapter 22 on wound healing and management.

d. Hypertension.

e. Hyperglycemia.

f. *Insufficiency* (Addison's dz): see Chapter 13 on endocrine.

VIII. RHEUMATOLOGIC

A. **Rheumatoid arthritis:** for the nonorthopaedic surgeon, the 2 main complications of rheumatoid arthritis of concern are cervical spine subluxation (caution when intubating) and Felty's syndrome (immune neutropenia and splenomegaly in a pt w/ seropositive nodular RA—splenectomy can be therapeutic in cases refractory to methotrexate or infliximab).

B. **Gout**

1. Exquisitely painful arthropathy caused by precipitation of uric acids in joint. *Can present w/*: first MTP pain (podagra)—1/2 of first attacks, remarkably tender erythematous joint, fever/chills.

2. *Dx*: differential dx = septic joint, pseudogout (deposition of calcium pyrophosphate crystals).

a. Leukocytosis common.

b. Hyperuricemia, increased urinary uric acid (24 h).

c. Joint aspiration (gold standard) → polarizing microscopy demonstrates negatively birefringent needle-shaped crystals. Should also do Cx/gram stain.

3. *Tx*: acute → *indomethacin*, 50 mg PO 3 times per day × 2–3 d, then 25 mg PO 3 times per day × 4–10 d. *Alternate* agent = colchicine 0.5–1.2 mg PO q 2 h until relief or side effects (N, diarrhea); prednisone 40–60 mg PO q d × 5 d; intraarticular triamcinolone (20 mg); ACTH sc 40 U q 8–12 h.

a. *Avoid*: ASA, phenylbutazone. Acetaminophen not useful.

b. Prophylaxis (recurrent dz, uric acid urolithiasis, tophaceous gout) → see sections e. and f. below.

c. Check 24-h uric acid level in urine.

d. Low-dose indomethacin and colchicine may be started concurrently.

e. *Overproducer or overexcreter*:

i. Allopurinol 100–300 mg PO/d (adjust for chronic kidney dz).

f. *Underexcreter*:

i. Allopurinol as above, Probenecid 250–1500 mg PO 2 times per day, Sulfapyrazine 50–100 mg PO 2 times per day.

ii. *Avoid* purine-rich foods (liver, kidney, sardines, trout, scallops, bacon, turkey, venison, veal the highest, followed by beef, chicken, pork, crab, lobster, shrimp, asparagus, mushrooms, spinach, etc.), EtOH, and thiazide diuretics.

C. **Systemic lupus erythematosus**

1. Can cause mesenteric vasculitis and present as an acute abdomen, "lupus enteritis."

a. *Assoc. lab findings*: elevated ESR, low complement, anemia, thrombocytopenia, anti-ds DNA, anti-Smith antibody, anti-RNP antibody.

b. *Dx*: polyarteritis nodosa, Churg-Strauss syndrome, Henoch-Schonlein purpura, Behçet's syndrome, and Takayasu's arteritis.

c. *Tx*: limited evidence exists for tx w/ prednisone and cyclophosphamide.

D. **Sarcoidosis**

1. Multiorgan granulomatous dz of unknown etiology. Frequently involves lung, skin, and eyes, followed by liver/spleen, heart, and brain.

a. *Lung*: 90% of cases, from adenopathy to fibrosis and restrictive lung dz.

b. *Skin*: hyper/hypopigmentation, keloid rxn.

c. *Eye*: 20%—usu. uveitis, lacrimal gland dysfunction.
d. *Neuro*: Bell's palsy, lymphocytic meningitis, DI secondary to hypothalamic involvement possible.
e. *Liver/spleen*: > 50% of cases, usu. asymptomatic. LFTs may be mildly elevated. Hyperbilirubinemia indicates significant dz. Marked splenomegaly can result in splenic rupture—splenectomy may be indicated.
f. *Heart*: heart block occurs less frequently than cardiomyopathy.

2. *Dx*:
   a. Bx of involved organ w/ noncaseating granuloma diagnostic, although pulmonary berylliosis hard to distinguish (get occupational hx). Serum angiotensin-converting enzyme (ACE) levels are usu. elevated. BAL ↑ lymphocytes and ↑ CD4:CD8 ratio suggestive. Serum Ca^{++} ↑ 10% of cases (along w/ low–normal phosphorus)—secondary to granuloma effect on vitamin D_3.
3. *Tx*:
   a. Spontaneous resolution may occur in first few years.
      i. *Acute dz*: erythema nodosum, anterior uveitis, hypercalcemia, CN VII palsy.
      ii. *Chronic dz*: lupus pernio, posterior uveitis, pars planitis, bone cysts, renal stones, cardiomyopathy, CNS mass.
   b. *Indications for tx*: symptoms or hypercalcemia.
   c. *Topical tx* (i.e., corticosteroid creams, etc.) are first-line. Systemic corticosteroids mainstay. Chloroquine, methotrexate, azathioprine, cyclophosphamide, thalidomide may be useful alternatives.

E. Scleroderma (systemic sclerosis)

1. Pathologic overproduction of collagen and other matrix proteins w/ fibrosis and vascular injury. Affects all races, predominantly in women; uncertain etiology.
2. *Dx*: generally clinical, w/ constellation of Raynaud's phenomenon plus typical skin and visceral findings described below. CREST (cutaneous calcinosis, Raynaud's phenomenon, esophageal dysmotility, sclerodactyly, telangectasia) syndrome pts generally have dz localized to face and hands and have better prognosis than those w/ diffuse dz. *Lab values*: ESR usu. *not* elevated, whereas antibodies (antinuclear, anticentromere, etc.) usu. are.
3. *Clinical pathology and tx* (*Note:* corticosteroids *not* effective in scleroderma):
   a. *General*: fever, malaise common.
   b. *Raynaud's phenomenon*: common, early finding (calcium channel blockers; IV iloprost for digital ulcers).
   c. *Skin*: subcutaneous edema, thickening, hyper-/depigmentation, digital ulceration.
   d. *Musculoskeletal*: arthralgias—common, early finding.
   e. *GI*: esophageal dysmotility, GERD (PPI).
   f. *Cardiac*: HTN (ACEi); pericarditis, heart block.
   g. *Renal*: renal crisis (ACEi).
   h. *Pulmonary*: interstitial/fibrotic lung dz (cyclophosphamide), pulmonary HTN.

IX. INFECTIOUS

A. Tuberculosis (Mycobacterium tuberculosis)

1. Latent TB is clinically and radiographically undetectable, limited by intact cell-mediated immunity.
   a. *Dx*: tuberculin skin test (Mantoux method)—0.1 cc of PPD (5 U) injected intradermallly in volar forearm w/ 27-g needle, then induration width measured 48–72 h later. *Note*: up to 10 wk may be necessary to develop immune response after exposure. *Criteria for (+) PPD*: no risk factors → 15+ mm; recent immigrants from endemic countries, various moderate-risk conditions/living situations → 10+ mm; HIV (+) pts, recent contacts of those w/ active TB, CXR w/ fibrotic changes suggestive of dz, and immunosuppressed (organ transplant or > 15 mg/d of prednisone × 1+ mo) → 5+ mm.
   b. *Tx*: 6–9 mo of isoniazid.
2. Progressive TB occurs in 5% of primary cases, presenting w/ cough, malaise, and possibly anorexia, fever, night sweats, a/o mild hemoptysis, etc.
   a. *Dx*:

i. *Radiographic*: in CXR, only minority of pts demonstrate cavitation (more common in reactivation cases), Ghon complexes (calcified 1° focus), or Ranke (calcified 1° focus + calcified hilar LNs) complexes. Most commonly, relatively nonspecific findings such as small homogeneous infiltrates, hilar LAD, and limited atelectasis.

ii. *Microbiologic*: sputum cx should be obtained (not just staining for AFB).

b. *Tx*: Common regimen → isoniazid, rifampin, pyrazinamide, and ethambutol × 2 mo, then isoniazide and rifampin × 4 more mo.

i. *Isoniazid*: side effects—hepatitis, peripheral neuropathy.

ii. *Rifampin*: side effects—hepatitis, fever, renal dysfunction, GI upset.

iii. *Ethambutol*: side effects—reversible optic neuritis, rash.

iv. *Streptomycin*: side effects—CN VIII toxicity, renal dysfunction.

v. *Pyrazinamide*: side effects—hepatotoxic, GI upset, hyperuricemia, arthralgias.

B. HIV/AIDS

1. Seroconversion usu. w/in 6–12 wk.
2. If exposed, AZT + lamivudine may decrease incidence of exposure if given early (1–2 h).
3. AIDS dx if CD4+ count < 200 or if HIV w/ defining opportunistic infection.
4. *Indications for operation*:

a. *Infectious complications most common*:

i. CMV intestinal dz (usu. colon)—bleeding, perforation, or pain/peritonitis.

ii. Lower GI bleeds can also be caused by bacteria or HSV.

b. *Neoplastic dz next most common indication for OR*:

i. Non-Hodgkin's lymphoma (usu. B-cell) most common offender.

- Most often involves stomach, followed by rectum; tx w/ chemotx.

ii. Kaposi's sarcoma actually more common in AIDS, but less commonly causes surgical lesions.

- Upper GI bleeds usu. from Kaposi's, followed by lymphoma.

X. ALCOHOL AND DRUG USE

A. Alcohol

1. *Metabolic*

a. Chronic alcoholism often presents w/ electrolyte derangements such as hyponatremia, hypokalemia, hypophosphatemia, and hypomagnesemia in addition to hypoglycemia.

b. Lactate acidosis and hyperchloremic acidosis are commonly seen.

c. *Alcoholic ketoacidosis*: presents w/ AG acidosis and (+) ketones in blood/urine after acute binge.

i. Results from hepatic metabolism of ethanol, yielding NADH and pressuring conversion of acetoacetate to β-hydroxybutyrate (acetoacetate test in blood, urine may resultantly *not* test positive for this ketone).

ii. Treat w/ dextrose-containing saline infusion to diminish liver production of ketones and aid renal perfusion and filtration of ketones.

2. *Neurologic* (delirium tremens)

a. Overactivity of central nervous system, largely mediated by GABA receptor, and manifesting w/ hyperthermia, tachycardia, hypertension, and potentially hallucinations. Tremulousness, hyperreflexia, nausea, vomiting, sz possible.

i. May present w/in 8 h and generally end w/in 1 wk after last alcohol intake in medical pts. In surgical pts, onset may be delayed up to 14 d because of anesthetic and narcotic effects.

b. Prophylaxis is warranted if have evidence of abuse (positive answers to "CAGE" questions or significantly elevated BAC).

i. Thiamine, 100 mg IV q d × 3 d. Some recommend continuing thiamine as 50 mg PO/d for several wk.

ii. MVI, I amp IV q d × 3 d. Again, oral MVI for several wk is likely appropriate.

iii. Folate, 1 mg IV/PO q d × 3 d.

iv. Benzodiazepines act specifically on GABA receptor and are most effective, although clonidine may be used w/ some success as well.

- *Asymptomatic*: consider observation q 6 h or prophylaxis w/ lorazepam (Ativan) as 2 mg q 8 h × 24 h followed by continued physical exam q 6 h.
- *Mildly symptomatic*: begin w/ lorazepam as 2–4 mg q 6 h × 24–48 h, followed by tapering over 72 h.
- *Moderately/severely symptomatic*: place in critical care setting, give lorazepam 4 mg IV initially, then 4 mg IV q 2–4 h × 24 h or until sx have stabilized, then 2 mg IV/PO q 6 h × 48 h; then 2 mg IV/PO q 12 h × 48 h, then discontinue. Alternately, give as much lorazepam or chlordiazepoxide/Librium (baseline dose is 25–100 mg PO/IV q 6 h) as needed to control sx the first 24 h, then cut in half subsequent days, w/ goal to be off w/in 72 h (to avoid inducing BZD withdrawals from longer therapy).

B. Cocaine

1. Half-life of 90 min[2]. Withdrawal may present as depression, fatigue, chills, muscular pain, involuntary motor activity.
2. Manage withdrawal w/ quiet environment and possibly bromocriptine or tricyclic antidepressants.
3. Preoperatively, get EKG at high risk for arrhythmias and ischemic dz.
4. *Other complications may include*: asthma, seizures, intestinal ischemia, hepatic necrosis, fever, rhabdomyolysis, and thrombocytopenia.

CHAPTER 24

PHARMACOLOGY AND SURGICAL PHARMACOPOEIA

I. PHARMACOLOGY

A. Pharmacokinetics

1. pK = pH at which 50% of molecule is ionized.
   a. Ionized substances do not tend to diffuse well across cell membranes—phenomenon of "ion-trapping" dictates how much of a "ionizable" substance will diffuse or remain in one compartment.
   b. The ratio of final concentrations between two compartments is a direct function of the ratio of the pK of the two compartments (difference of pK of 1 results in a 10-fold [10^1] difference in concentration).
   c. Weak acids tend to accumulate where there is a high pH (i.e., weak acids are well absorbed through the stomach into the more alkaline blood and tend to stay on the "blood side" where they are ionized).
   d. Weak bases tend to accumulate where there is a low pH (i.e., weak bases tend to not diffuse across an acidic stomach, but rather stay ionized on the stomach side).
2. *Inhibition*
   a. *Competitive*: shifts concentration/effect curve to right (more drug required to get same effect), results from binding at same side, can ultimately still achieve same effect w/ enough drug.
   b. *Noncompetitive*: shifts concentration/effect curve downwards, results from antagonist binding at different side, decreases the maximum effect of the drug regardless of concentration.
   c. *Partition coefficient* = K_p = ability of substance to diffuse across membrane, increases w/ lipid solubility.
   d. *Diffusion coefficient* = $K_d = [(d)(r)]/(d-r)$.
   e. *Therapeutic index* = LD_{50} / ED_{50}.
3. *Pharmacokinetics and interactions*
   a. Cytochrome p450
      i. Series of reactions broadly classified into redox and organification. Hundreds of medications are metabolized through this pathway. *Those w/ the lowest therapeutic index include*: antiarrhythmics, anticonvulsants, antineoplastic drugs, immunosuppressive drugs, oral anticoagulants, and theophylline.
      ii. *Induced* by phenobarbital/anticonvulsants, Rifampin, chronic EtOH, cigarette smoking: Decrease serum levels of drugs metabolized through this route.
      iii. *Inhibited* by ketoconazole, fluconazole, itraconazole, isoniazid, amiodarone, cimetidine, acute EtOH intoxication, erythromycin, neuroleptics, SSRIs, tricyclic antidepressants, OCPs, quinidine, clarithromycin, protease inhibitors, 1 quart grapefruit juice: increase serum levels of drugs metabolized through this route.
4. *Important side effects*
   a. *Antibiotics*
      i. *Doxycycline*: tooth discoloration if under 8 yo. Photosensitivity.
      ii. *Fluoroquinolones*: may affect cartilage development if under 18 yo. p450 inhibitor.
      iii. *Sulfonamides*: Stevens-Johnson syndrome, TEN, hepatic necrosis, agranulocytosis, anaphylaxis.
      iv. *Amphotericin*: hypotension, nephrotoxicity, RTA, pulmonary reactions.
      v. *Aminoglycosides*: ototoxicity, nephrotoxicity.
      vi. *Metronidazole*: peripheral neuropathy, seizures (caution if CNS dz), Antabuse-effect.
   b. *Antitumor*
      i. *Doxorubicin*: myelosuppression, cardiotoxicity.
      ii. *Methotrexate*: myelosuppression, hepatotoxicity, nephrotoxicity, pulmonary toxicity.

iii. *Bleomycin*: pneumonitis progressing to pulmonary fibrosis (10%).

iv. *Cyclophosphamide*: hemorrhagic cystitis, jaundice.

c. *Cardiac*

i. *Digoxin*: sinus bradycardia, ventricular fibrillation.

ii. *Beta blockers*: exacerbation of bronchospasm in nonselective agents.

d. *Anti-inflammatory*

i. *Infliximab*: activation/reactivation of TB, invasive fungal infection.

ii. *Xigris*: hemorrhage.

B. Antibiotics: beta-lactams include both penicillins and cephalosporins. Bacteriocidal, they bind to a variety of penicillin-binding proteins to inhibit cell wall synthesis. Resistance can be from induction of chromosomal beta-lactamase, or plasmid-derived enzymatic binding/degradation.

1. *Penicillins*—bacteriocidal, beta-lactam inhibitors, discovered by Alexander Fleming (surgeon).

a. *1st gen*: Benzathine penicillin (**Bicillin L-A**) 1.2 M U IM (peds < 27 kg 0.3–0.6 M U IM, > 27 kg 0.9 M U IM).

i. Syphilis; lasts 2–4 wk.

ii. **Penicillin G**: 250,000–400,000 kg/d (8–24 M U in adult) IV divided q 4–6 h.

iii. Pneumococcus, severe clostridial infections.

iv. Penicillin V (**Pen-Vee K**) 250–500 mg PO 4 times per day (peds 25–50 mg/kg/d divided 2–3 times per day).

v. Good choice for "strep throat."

- *Note:* all 1st-gen penicillin covers most streptococcus, oral anaerobes.

b. *2nd gen*: **Dicloxacillin** (Dynapen) 125–500 mg PO 4 times per day.

i. **Nafcillin** (Nallpen) 1–2 g IM/IV q 4 h.

ii. **Oxacillin** (Bactocill) 1–2 g IM/IV q 4–6 h.

- *Note*: all 2nd-gen penicillin are for penicillinase resistant; most streptococcus, *S. aureus*.

c. *3rd gen*: **Amoxicillin** (Amoxil, Trimox) 250–500 mg PO 3 times per day *or* 500–875 PO 2 times per day.

i. Popular choice for uncomplicated otitis media and acute sinusitis amoxicillin-clavulanate (**Augmentin**) 500–875 mg PO 2 times per day *or* 250–500 mg PO 3 times per day (Augmentin XR) 2 tabs PO q 12 h w/ meals.

ii. Popular for recurrent otitis media, sinusitis, and community-acquired pneumonia ampicillin-sulbactam (**Unasyn**) 1.5–3 g IM/IV q 6 h.

iii. Reasonable choice for intraabdominal prophylaxis in biliary, appendix surgery.

- *Note*: all 3rd-gen penicillin are for most streptococcus, some gram-negative rods.

d. *4th gen*: Piperacillin-tazobactam (**Zosyn**) 3.375–4.5 IV q 6 h.

i. Excellent GPC, GNR, and anaerobe coverage; good for wet gangrene ticarcillin-clavulanate (**Timentin**) 3.1 g IV q 4–6 h.

- *Note*: all 4th-gen penicillin have some *Pseudomonas* coverage.

2. *Cephalosporins* 10–15% cross-rxn w/ penicillin allergic pts.

a. *1st gen*: GPC (incl. *S. aureus*), basic GNR.

i. Cefazolin (**Ancef**) 0.5–1.5 g IM/IV q 6–9 h.

ii. Cephalexin (**Keflex**) 250–500 mg PO 4 times per day.

b. *2nd gen*: diminished *S. aureus*, better GNR, some w/ anaerobic activity.

i. **Cefotetan** (Cefotan) 1–2 g IM/IV q 12 h (renal and *biliary* excretion).

ii. **Cefoxitin** (Mefoxin) 1–2 g IM/IV q 6–8 h (renal excretion only).

iii. **Cefuroxime** (Zinacef) 750–1500 mg IM/IV q 8 h.

iv. Loracarbef (**Lorabid**) 200–400 mg PO 2 times per day.

v. **Cefaclor** (Ceclor) 250–500 mg PO 3 times per day.

c. *3rd gen*: even less *S. aureus*, even better GNR, some w/ *Pseudomonas* activity.

i. Cefixime (**Suprax**) 400 mg PO q d.

ii. **Cefotaxime** (Claforan) 1–2 g IV/IM q 6–8 h.

iii. **Ceftazidime** (Fortaz) 1–2 g IV q 8–12 h.

iv. Ceftriaxone (**Rocephin**) 1–2 g IM/IV q 24 h (use 2 g if meningitis); single 125–250 mg for gonorrhea.

d. *4th gen*: extended antipseudomonal activity.

i. **Cefepime** (Maxipime) 0.5–2 g IM/IV q 12 h.

3. *Fluoroquinolones* (similar parenteral and enteral bioavailability; avoid if less than 12 yo; act by inhibiting DNA gyrase).

a. *1st gen*: **Nalidixic acid** (NegGram) 1 g PO 4 times per day—GNR except *Pseudomonas*, for UTI only.

b. *2nd gen*: **Ciprofloxacin** (Cipro) 200–400 mg IV q 8–12 h *or* 250–750 PO 2 times per day—GNR some *Pseudomonas*, some *S. aureus* and atypicals, not pneumococcus.

c. *3rd gen*: **Levofloxacin** (Levaquin) 250–500 mg IV/PO q d—GNR more *Pseudomonas*, *S. aureus*, pneumococcus, more atypicals.

d. *4th gen*: **Gatifloxacin** (Tequin) 400 mg IV/PO q d—same as 3rd gen w/ broad anaerobe coverage.

4. *Aminoglycosides*: require entry into cell, thus are generally given w/ a beta-lactam drug to facilitate entry. Irreversibly bind to 30s ribosomal subunit (bacteriocidal); active-transport into bacterial cell as well as into cochlear and proximal renal tubule cells.

a. **Gentamicin** (Garamycin) 3–5 mg/kg/d IM/IV divided q 8 h *or* 5–7 mg/kg IV q 24 h 1 time per day dosing less nephrotoxic.

b. **Tobramycin** (Nebcin) 3–5 mg/kg/d IM/IV divided q 8 h *or* 5–7 mg/kg IV q 24 h.

c. **Neomycin:** PO administration w/out absorption; for hepatic encephalopathy 4–12 g PO/d, divided q 6–8 h.

5. *Anaerobic*

a. **Clindamycin** (Cleocin) 600–900 mg IV q 8 h *or* 150–450 mg PO 4 times per day—reversibly binds to 50s subunit. Good G+ and anaerobe coverage, excellent choice for head/neck/upper pharyngeal surgery. IV form excellent for clostridial infections as decreases elaboration of toxin.

b. Metronidazole (**Flagyl**)—*bacterial infections*: load 1 g IV then 500 mg IV/PO q 6 h—*bacterial vaginosis*: 500 mg PO 2 times per day × 7 d; wide spectrum against all anaerobes, works by toxic intermediate degrading DNA and other macromolecules, disulfiram-like effect, should give PO instead of IV for *C. difficile* colitis.

6. *Carbapenems* good for necrotizing pancreatitis, life-threatening cholecystitis.

a. **Imipenem-cilastatin** (Primaxin) 250–1000 mg IV q 6–8 h.

b. **Meropenem** (Merrem IV) 1 g IV q 8 h.

7. *Tetracyclines*: avoid if less than 8 yo, discolors teeth. Reversible binding to 50s subunit.

a. **Doxycycline** (Vibramycin) 100 mg PO 2 times per day (after 1st day, may change to 100 PO q d); IV form available for severe infections.

b. **Tetracycline** (Sumycin) 250–500 mg PO 4 times per day.

8. *Macrolides* reversibly bind to 50s subunit of ribosome. Erythromycin prokinetic via stimulating motilin receptors in gut.

a. **Erythromycin base** (E-mycin) 400 mg PO 4 times per day.

b. **Clarithromycin** (Biaxin) 250–500 mg PO 2 times per day; (Biaxin XL) 1000 mg PO q d.

c. **Azithromycin** (Zithromax) 500 mg IV q d; (Z-pak) 500 mg PO day 1, then 250 mg PO q d for 4 more days.

9. *Miscellaneous*

a. **Rifampin** (Rimactane) 600 mg PO 2 times per day. (*Note*: may turn urine a/o contact lenses orange.)

b. **Vancomycin** (Vancocin) 1 g IV q 12 h.

i. *C. diff*: 40 mg/kg up to 2000 mg/d PO divided 3–4 times per day × 7–10 d.

ii. Binds to non-PBP to inhibit polymerization of peptidoglycan.

iii. First choice for *S. epidermidis*, MRSA, *C. difficile* not responsive to metronidazole.

c. **Linezolid** (Zyvox): good for MRSA; 400–600 mg IV/PO q 12 h.

d. Tigecycline (**Tygacil**): good for MRSA (w/ addit. anaerobe, most GNR coverage) 100 mg IV once, then 50 mg IV q 12 h.

e. Trimethoprim-sulfamethoxazole (**Bactrim**, **Septra**) 1 tab PO 2 times per day (available as single-strength or double-strength).

C. **Antifungals**

1. **Amphotericin B:** binds ergosterol in fungal cell wall. Test dosing recommended.
   a. Amphotericin B deoxycholate (Fungizone): 0.25–1.5 mg/kg/d IV.
   b. Amphotericin B lipid (AmBisome): 3–5 mg/kg/d IV.
2. *Imidazoles*: inhibit synthesis of steroid precursors of ergosterol.
   a. **Fluconazole** (Diflucan): 400 mg IV q d, good for *C. albicans*, but not for *C. torulopsis* or *C. glabrata* (need ampho).
   b. **Ketoconazole** (Nizoral): 200–400 mg PO q d (significant hepatoxicity risk; don't give w/ PPI, H_2 blockers, or BZDs).
   c. **Itraconazole** (Sporanox): pulse dosing for onychomycosis 200 mg PO 2 times per day × 1 wk, then 3 wk off (1 mo for fingernails, up to 4 mo for toenails). For thrush, 100–200 mg PO q d.
3. **Griseolfulvin:** (tinea capitis) 500 mg PO q d × 4–6 wk.

D. **Antivirals**: typically nucleoside analogues, may inhibit DNA synthetase.

1. **Acyclovir** (Zovirax)—anti-HSV: symptomatic genital herpes—400 mg PO 3 times per day × 5–10 d. Shingles/oster—800 mg PO 5 times per day × 10 d.
2. **Valganciclovir** (Valcyte)—anti-CMV: prophylaxis in transplant pts—900 mg PO q d postop d 10–100.

E. **Cardiac meds**

1. **Atropine** 0.5–1.0 mg IV.
2. **Epinephrine** 1 mg IV.
3. **Vasopressin** 40 U IV.
4. **Lidocaine** 1–1.5 mg/kg IV.
5. **Adenosine** (Adenocard) 6 mg rapid IVP, then 12 mg IVP.
6. **Digoxin** 0.125–0.5 mg IV.
7. **Diltiazim** (Cardizem) 0.25 mg/kg over 2 min.
8. **Hydralazine** 20–40 mg IV.
9. **Labetalol** (Normadyne) 10–20 mg IV over 2 min, may repeat in 20 min as needed (max 300 mg).
10. **Verapamil** (Calan) 5–10 mg IV over 2 min.

F. **Paralytics**

1. **Succinylcholine** 1–1.5 mg/kg IV (usu. give 100–120 mg).
2. Pancuronium (**Pavulon**) 0.1 mg/kg IV.
3. **Vecuronium** (Norcuron) 0.1 mg/kg IV.

G. **Neuro meds (sedatives and anticonvulsants)**

1. Diazepam (**Valium**) 5 mg IV prn.
2. Lorazepam (**Ativan**) 2 mg IV q 1 h prn.
3. Midazolam (**Versed**) 1–2 mg IV prn (0.1 mg/kg).
4. Phenobarbital 15–20 mg/kg IV.
5. Phenytoin (**Dilantin**) 15–20 mg/kg IV (max 50 mg/min).
   a. For seizure prophylaxis in head-injured pts (see Chapter 9, head section). Random phenytoin levels should be drawn 18 h after loading. High-risk pts should have level 15–20 mg/dL; if < 15, bolus 300 mg phenytoin slow IVP, if < 10, give 500 mg. Low-risk pts should be 10–20 mg/dL; if < 10, bolus 500 mg slow IVP. Give daily as 100 mg IV/PO 3 times per day or as 5–6 mg/kg IV

or PO q d, holding tube feeds 2 h before and after dosing. If repeatedly out of range, calculate corrected phenytoin level = (phenytoin level)/[0.2 × (albumin level) + 0.1].

6. Fosphenytoin (**Cerebyx**): load as 1 g IV or 10–20 mg/kg of phentoin equivalent IV.
7. Propofol: for induction—40 mg IV q 10 sec; for ventilator sedation—5–50 mcg/kg/min.
8. Haloperidol (**Haldol**) 2–5 mg IV/IM 3 times per day prn.

H. Analgesics

1. Acetaminophen (**Tylenol**): 325–650 mg PO/PR q 4–6 h prn, up to 4 g/d. Avoid in hepatic insufficiency.
2. Acetaminophen/hydrocodone (**Vicodin**): available as 5/500, 7.5/750, usu. 1–2 tabs PO q 4–6 h prn.
3. Morphine: usu. given 1–4 mg IV q 15–30 min prn. Watch respiratory depression.
4. Meperidine (**Demerol**): usu. given as 100 mg IV q 3 h.
5. Fentanyl: usu. given as 0.1 mg IV q 1 h.
6. Hydromorphone (**Dilaudid**): usu. given as 1–4 mg PO q 4–6 h (0.5–2 mg IV q 4–6 h).

I. Overdose (adult doses listed)

1. *Ingested poison* (general—not alcohols, acids/bases, petroleum products, or inorganic minerals):
   a. Activated charcoal 1–2 gm/kg PO/NGT.
   b. Ipecac syrup, 15–30 mL (not for acids/bases, petroleum, etc., or if altered mental status).
2. *Beta blockers*: glucagon 2–5 mg IV, then 2–5 mg/h IV.
3. *Benzodiazepines*: flumazenil 0.2 mg IV, then 0.2–0.5 mg IV q 1–3 min to max of 3 mg.
4. *Digoxin*: digoxin immune Fab, # vials IV = (serum dig level ng/mL × kg)/100.
5. *Opioid narcotics*: naloxone 0.4–2 mg q 2–3 min prn.
6. *Cyanide*: amyl nitrite (inhaled) 0.3 mL → Na^+ nitrite 300 mg IV → Na^+ thiosulfate 12.5 mg IV.
7. *Methemoglobinemia*: methylene blue, 1–2 mg/K IV over 5 min.
8. *Lidocaine*: Provides airway support as needed and treats seizures w/ benzodiazepines, not phenytoin.
9. *Tricyclics* (or severe metabolic acidosis): sodium bicarbonate, 1 mEq/kg IV up to 100 mEq per dose.

J. Gastrointestinal

1. Dicyclomine (**Bentyl**): intestinal spasm → 10–20 mg PO/IM 4 times per day prn.
2. **Milk of Magnesia** (magnesium hydroxide): 30–60 mL PO for constipation.
3. **"Black & white:"** 30 mL of Milk of Magnesia and 5 mL of cascara fluid extract.
4. **Bubble gum enema**: 240 mL of 1:1 mixture of mineral oil and docusate (Colace).
5. **SMOG enema**: 240 mL of 1:1:1 mixture of normal saline, mineral oil, and glycerin.
6. **GI cocktail**: 2% viscous lidocaine (10 mL) + Donnatal (10 mL) + Maalox/Mylanta (30 mL).
7. **Imodium** (loperamide): 4 mg PO once, then 2 mg PO after each loose/unformed BM up to 16 mg/d.
8. **Neostigmine** (for Ogilvie's syndrome): 1–2 mg IV over 3–5 min. Monitor for symptomatic bradycardia (tx w/ atropine or glycopyrrolate).
9. **Lactulose**: 15–45 mL of syrup 1–4 times per day (higher doses for hepatic encephalopathy, not for constipation).

K. Commonly used medicines in pediatrics

1. *Analgesics*
   a. Acetaminophen (**Tylenol**) liquid: 10–15 mg/kg/dose PO/PR q 4–6 h prn.
   b. Acetaminophen w/ codeine (**Tylenol #3**) elixir: (12/120 per 5 mL): 3–6 yo → 5 mL/dose; age 7–12 yo → 10 mL/dose.
   c. Ibuprofen (**Motrin**): 5–10 mg/kg PO q 6–8 h.
   d. **Morphine** sulfate: 0.1 mg/kg IV/IM/SC q 3–4 h.
2. *Sedatives, other neurotropic agents*
   a. Midazolam (**Versed**): 0.5–1.0 mg/kg up to 20 mg (PO); 0.1–0.15 mg/kg (IM). IV administration:
      i. *Age 6 mo–5 yo*: 0.05–0.1 mg/kg, then titrated up to 0.6 mg/kg.
      ii. *Age 5 yo–12 yo*: 0.025–0.05 mg/kg, then titrated up to 0.4 mg/kg.

3. *GI*
   a. Promethazine (**Phenergan**): 0.25–1 mg/kg PO/IM/PR q 4–6 h. (Contraindicated under 2 yo.)
   b. Ondansetron (**Zofran**): infants → 0.1 mg/kg IV (under 40 kg) or 4 mg IV if > 40 kg (give over 2–5 min).
4. *Abx* (*Note*: below doses are for children > 28 d old and 50 kg or less)
   a. *Oral*
      i. Amoxicillin (**Amoxil**): 45–80 mg/kg/d divided 2 times per day (higher dose is for otitis media).
      ii. Amoxicillin/clavulanic acid (**Augmentin**): 45 mg/kg/d divided 2 times per day.
      iii. Cephalexin (**Keflex**): 25–50 mg/kg/d divided 4 times per day.
      iv. **Clindamycin** (Cleocin): susp. 8–25 mg/kg/d PO divided 2–3 times per day.
      v. Metronidazole (**Flagyl**): 10–15 mg/kg/dose 3 times per day.
      vi. TMP-SMX (**Bactrim**): susp. 5 mL/10 kg/dose PO 2 times per day.
   b. *Parenteral*
      i. Ampicillin: 25 mg/kg/dose q 6 h up to 12 g/d.
      ii. Ampicillin/sulbatam (**Unasyn**):
         - *Infants*: 25–37.5 mg ampicillin/kg/dose IV/IM q 6 h.
         - *Children*: 25–50 mg ampicillin kg/dose IV/IM q 6 h.
      iii. Cefazolin (**Ancef**): 25–50 mg/kg/d IV/IM divided q 6–8 h.
      iv. **Cefoxitin** (Mefoxin): 80–160 mg/kg/d IV divided q 4–8 h.
      v. Ceftriaxone (**Rocephin**): 50–75 mg/kg/d divided 2 times per day or q d (do not exceed 2 g).
      vi. **Clindamycin** (Cleocin): 20–40 mg/kg/d IV divided q 6–8 h.
      vii. **Gentamicin** (Garamycin): 2–2.5 mg/kg IV q 8 h.
      viii. Metronidazole (**Flagyl**): 7.5–15 mg/kg IV q 6 h (higher dose for *C. difficile*).
      ix. Piperacillin/tazobactam (**Zosyn**): 240 mg/kg/d IV of piperacillin divided q 8 h.
      x. **Vancomycin** (Vancocin): 10–15 mg/kg IV q 6 h.

L. Side effects of commonly used oral supplements

1. *Aloe vera*: abdominal cramps, hypokalemia.
2. *Bitter melon*: hypoglycemia.
3. *Bitter orange*: tachycardia, arrhythmia.
4. *Black cohosh*: GI upset; uncertain effect on breast cancer.
5. *Comfrey*: hepatotoxicity.
6. *Dong quai*: photosensitivity, variable effects on warfarin.
7. *Echinacea*: not recommended if autoimmune dz, MS, TB, AIDS, leukemia; possible hepatotoxicity.
8. *Ephedra* (ma huang): HTN, arrhythmia, tremor, MI, CVA.
9. *Fish oil*: *in vitro* increase in bleeding time not consistently reported as hemorrhage risk in clinical series.
10. *Garlic*: possibly increases warfarin effects; hypoglycemia and hypothyroidism in large doses.
11. *Gingko biloba*: possibly increases bleeding time.
12. *Ginseng*: decreases warfarin effects (lowers INR); hypoglycemia in large doses.
13. *Guaraná*: tachycardia, hypertension (caffeine-like).
14. *Kava*: potentiates sedative effects of anticonvulsants; torticollis; oral dyskinesia, poss. hepatotoxic.
15. *St. John's wort*: decreases levels of anti-viral Indinavine®, decreases efficacy of digoxin and cyclosporine, phototoxicity, uncertain interaction w/ SSRIs.

CHAPTER 25

COMMON PROBLEMS ON CALL AND BLS/ACLS

I. **AIRWAY/BREATHING** (*note*: have low threshold for arranging urgent transport to ICU while addressing primary problem)

   A. **Hx**

      1. *Surgical*

         a. Recent neck surgery may result in a compressive hematoma and airway compromise secondary to laryngeal edema; difficult to intubate. Tx is emergency evacuation of hematoma/clot, often followed by cricothyroidotomy or tracheostomy.

         b. Tracheostomy. Check for obstruction, mechanical problems. Place ETT or tracheostomy for emergent control.

      2. *Medical*

         a. H/o anaphylaxis? Asthma? COPD?

   B. **Physical exam**

      1. *Dysphonia*: suggests problems w/ vocal cords (i.e., edema, nerve injury, etc.).
      2. *Wheezing*: suggests lower airway obstruction (i.e., asthma).
      3. *Stridor*: suggests upper airway obstruction (i.e., foreign body).
      4. *Look at trachea, jugular veins*: may be displaced (trachea) or distended (veins) due to mass, tension PTX. Vein distension also suggests pericardial tamponade.
      5. *Listen to breath sounds and percuss*: absent or decreased breath sounds and hyperresonance suggests PTX; absent or decreased breath sounds w/ dullness suggests hemothorax or empyema—any absent or decreased breath sounds in an unstable pt merits an emergent chest tube.

   C. **Other**

      1. *Pulse oximetry* ("pulse ox"):

         a. May not be accurate in cold extremities or in room w/ bright lights.

         b. *Hypoxia may be due to*:

            i. Carbon monoxide poisoning
            ii. Methemoglobinemia
            iii. *Poisoning*: cyanide, nitroprusside

      2. *Arterial blood gas* (ABG): always obtain for breathing sx; analyze as described in Chapter 6.

II. **CIRCULATION** (as w/ airway problems, have low threshold for transfer to ICU as problem is being addressed and make sure adequate IV access is obtained).

   A. **Tachycardia**

      1. *Hx*

         a. *Surgical* (thoracic—tamponade [?]; orthopaedic—fat embolism [?]; postop fluid overload—Afib [?])

         b. *Medical* (medications, caffeine)

      2. *Physical exam*: anxious? in pain? rate? arrhythmia? strong or thready pulse? fever?

   B. **Hypotension**

      1. *Hx*

         a. *Surgical*: bleeding, anesthetic/narcotic, etc.

         b. *Medical*: medication, cardiac hx, etc.

      2. *Physical exam*

      3. *Etiology*

         a. Hypovolemia (flat jugular veins, dry mucosa, skin turgor?)

         b. Anaphylaxis (wheezing? angioedema? rash? etc.)

C. **Bleeding**
1. *Hx*
   a. *Surgical.*
   b. *Medical*: renal, liver dz, lupus, medications (including herbals).
2. *Physical exam*
   a. Where is bleeding coming from? Surgical wound, rectal exam, IV or arteriogram puncture site, epistaxis.
3. *Other*
   a. *Labs*: CBC (*thrombocytopenia ddx*: see Chapter 2), PT/PTT (*Elevation ddx*: see Chapter 2).

III. **DISABILITY (NEUROLOGIC)**

A. **Altered mental status**
1. *Hx*
2. *Physical exam*
3. *Other*
   a. Pulse oximetry to evaluate for hypoxia.
   b. Capillary blood glucose (CBG) to evaluate for hypoglycemia.
   c. Thorough neuro exam, particular attention to symmetric reflexes and papillary size/response.

B. **Pain**
1. *Hx and physical*
2. *Headache*
3. *Abdomen*
4. *Extremity*

C. **Seizures**
1. *Hx*
2. *Ensure ABCs controlled*
   a. Supplemental oxygen, airway control.
3. *Pharmacologic control*: diazepam (Valium) 5 mg IV q 5–10 min prn; phenytoin and phenobarbital are backup agents.

IV. **OTHER**

A. **Cardiovascular**
1. *Chest pain*
   a. *Hx* (acute, chronic, postprandial, etc.)
   b. *Character* (crushing, radiating, burning, etc.)
   c. *Etiology*
      i. *Cardiac*: see section V. below on acute coronary syndrome.
      ii. *Pulmonary embolism*: see Chapter 8.
      iii. *Pneumothorax*: place chest tube.
      iv. *GERD*: usu. by hx or response to GI meds.
2. *Vascular insufficiency or pulse change*

B. **Pulmonary:** see section I. above on airway/breathing.

C. **Gastrointestinal**
1. *Constipation* (may need disimpaction a/o laxatives).
2. *Diarrhea* (*etiology*: meds, infectious [need stool WBC, Cx, etc.], postsurgical changes).
3. *Nausea/emesis*: Zofran usu. better tolerated, less sedating than phenergan.
4. *Singultus* (hiccups): usu. innocuous, but diaphragmatic irritation (e.g., subphrenic abscess) important.

D. **Genitourinary**
1. *Urinary retention*: place Foley (flush Foley if one already placed).
2. *Dysuria*: check urinalysis and UCx (cx may still be positive w/ negative urinalysis).

3. *Bloody or other unusual appearance to urine*: urology consult for hematuria (may ultimately require cytology, cx, cystoscopy, etc.).
4. *Oliguria/anuria*: place Foley if haven't done so, eval hemodynamics, UA, Chem 7 for starters.

E. Metabolic

1. *Hyperglycemic/hypoglycemic* → see Chapter 1.
2. *Electrolyte abnormality* → see Chapter 1.

V. ACUTE CORONARY SYNDROME (derived from American Heart Association, 2010)

A. Support ABCs, prepare for CPR/code.

B. Give: O_2 at 4 L/min (SaO_2 > 90%); ASA at 160–325 mg; NTG SL/IV; morphine IV if NTG not adequate.

C. Obtain: IV access; 12-lead EKG; portable CXR; electrolytes/CBC/troponin/CK-MB; targeted hx w/ focus on fibrinolytic checklist/contraindications.

D. Results of 12-lead EKG:

1. *ST elevation or (presumably) new LBBB*:
   a. *Begin adjunctive tx*: beta blockers, heparin (LMWH or UFH), clopidogrel.
   b. If < 12 h or high-risk (refractory ischemic chest pain, recurrent/persistent ST deviation, VT, sx of heart failure) → consult cardiology for PCI or fibrinolysis.
   c. Otherwise, admit to monitored bed, continue ASA, heparin, and start ACEi/ARB and statin w/in 24 h.
2. *ST depression or dynamic T wave inversion*:
   a. *Begin adjunctive tx*: beta blockers, heparin (LMWH or UFH), clopidogrel, NTG, glycoprotein IIb/IIIa inhib.
   b. Admit to monitored bed, continue ASA, heparin, and start ACEi/ARB and statin w/in 24 h.
3. *Normal or nondiagnostic ST/T wave changes*:
   a. If develops high-risk criteria (see above) or becomes troponin-positive, tx as sections D1. or D2. above. Immediately above as appropriate.
   b. Otherwise, observe w/ serial cardiac markers, EKG/telemetry, etc., until resolves. Consider stress test before d/c.

VI. BASIC LIFE SUPPORT (derived from American Heart Association, 2010)

A. Obstructed airway

1. Do not interfere if pt can speak or effectively cough.
2. *If conscious*:
   a. *Adult/child*: Heimlich maneuver (or chest thrusts if obese/pregnant) until cleared or unresponsive.
   b. *Infant*: place pt prone over arm w/ head lower than feet and give 5 back blows, then turn over for 5 chest thrusts in lower sternum. Repeat until cleared or unresponsive.
3. *If unconscious*:
   a. *Adult*: call for EMS/defibrillator, then initiate CPR (after removing any visible object in mouth).
   b. *Child/infant*: initiate CPR (after removing any visible object in mouth), then call EMS after 2 min.

B. No movement or response → call code/help, then get defibrillator/AED.

C. Open airway, check breathing.

1. *If not breathing, give 2 breaths.*
2. *If no response, check pulse.*
   a. If pulse w/in 10 sec, give 1 breath q 5–6 sec and recheck pulse every 2 min.
   b. If no pulse w/in 10 sec, give 30 compressions (100/min), then open airway, give 2 breaths, and resume compression/breath cycles. Continue until defibrillator arrives, other providers take over, or pulse is regained.
      i. For *2-rescuer CPR in children*, the ratio of breaths to compressions is 15:2.

D. Defibrillator arrives—rhythm possibly amenable to shock?

1. *Yes*: give 1 shock, then resume CPR for 5 cycles.
2. *No*: resume CPR for 5 cycles and check rhythm every 5 cycles, continuing until others take over or pt moves.

VII. **ADVANCED CARDIAC LIFE SUPPORT** (derived from American Heart Association, 2010)

A. **General** (apneic, pulseless, unresponsive)

1. Call code, start CPR—ABCs, attach defibrillator/monitor rhythm.
    a. Open airway, check breathing—if not breathing, begin chest compressions, then breaths at ratio of 30:2 if by self.
2. Check rhythm and pulse regularly, give 100% oxygen, get bed board.
3. *Simultaneous w/ resuscitation, attempt to rectify any underlying causes*:
    a. *H*: hypovolemia, hypoxia, hypo-/hyperkalemia, hypothermia, hydrogen ion (acidosis).
    b. *T*: trauma (hypovolemia, ICP), thrombosis (MI, PE), tamponade (pericardial), tension PTX, toxins.

B. **Tachyarrhythmias**

1. *VFib/pulseless VTach*
    a. CPR until defib available.
    b. Defib, biphasic (unsynch) 200 J → 200–300 J → 360 J (start w/ 360 if monophasic).
    c. Intubate, IV access, CPR prn.
    d. *Epinephrine* 1 mg IVP → 360 J **or** *Vasopressin* 40 U IVP → 360 J.
        i. May give epinephrine 1 mg IVP q 3–5 min.
    e. Immediately resume CPR, then check rhythm/shock again in 2 min (5 CPR cycles), and consider:
        i. *Amiodarone* (300 mg IVP—can repeat w/ 150 mg)→ 360 J **or**
        ii. If stable or converts can start w/ 150 mg over 10 min, then gtt 1 mg/min × 6 h, then 0.5 mg min × 18 h.
        iii. *Lidocaine* (1.0–1.5 mg/kg IVP—can repeat as 1/2 dose up to 3 mg/kg) → 360 J **and/or,**
        iv. *Magnesium* (1–2 g if torsades de pointes, hypomagnesemic, or refractory) → 360 J.
    f. Immediately resume CPR for 2 min (5 cycles) before checking rhythm/shocking again.
2. *Unstable tachycardia w/ pulses* (monomorphic VT, PSVT, AFib, AFlutter)
    a. Oxygen, IV, pulse ox.
    b. Have intubation/code cart nearby.
    c. Consider premedication (midazolam, etc.).
    d. *Synchronized cardioversion*:
        i. 50 J (PSVT or AFlutter only) → 100 J → 200 J → 300 J → 360 J.
        ii. 100 J for all other rhythms.
3. *Narrow complex SVT* (stable)
    a. Vagal maneuvers (carotid massage if no carotid dz/bruits, or Valsalva).
    b. Adenosine (6 mg push, then 12 mg; may repeat 12 mg once).
    c. If rhythm converts, monitor for recurrence (tx w/ adenosine, diltiazem, or beta antagonist).
    d. If does not convert, control rate (diltiazim, beta antagonist, etc.), w/u cause.
4. *Stable AFib, AFlutter*
    a. *< 48 h*:
        i. First control rate w/ beta blocker (esmolol) or calcium channel blocker (diltiazim).
        ii. Next control rhythm w/ amiodarone or DC CV as above; can also load w/ digoxin.
    b. *> 48 h*:
        i. Do not DC CV unless embolic precautions/anticoagulated; use antiarrhythmics w/ caution.
        ii. Ideally AC × 3 wk, then CV, then 4 more wk AC.
        iii. More rapidly, use heparin and TEE, CV w/in 24 h, then AC × 4 wk.
5. *Stable wide complex tachycardia*
    a. 12-lead EKG.
    b. Amiodarone (150 mg IV over 10 min, repeat to max of 2.2 g per 24 h) or DC cardioversion.

c. If AFib w/ preexcitation (i.e., WPW), avoid AV blocking (digoxing, diltiazim, adenosine).
d. Torsades de pointes → magnesium sulfate, 1–2 g loaded IV over 5–60 min, then infused.

C. Asystole/PEA/bradycardia

1. *PEA/asystole* (confirm in 2 leads; note if only have defib pads, should shock, as only have 2 leads and could actually be fine VFib) *or PEA*
   a. Continue CPR (see section VI. above), intubate, 100% O_2, IV access.
   b. *Consider causes*:
      i. *Hypoxemia/respiratory arrest* → mechanical ventilation.
      ii. *Hyperkalemia* → 10% Ca^{++} chloride 10 cc IVP; 1 ampule D_{50} w/ 10 U reg insulin IVP; albuterol nebs 20–40 mg in 4 cc NS; Kayexalate 50 g w/ 200 cc 70% sorbitol PO. Consider sodium bicarbonate 50 mEq IV over 1–5 min; consider dialysis.
      iii. *Hypokalemia* → give potassium.
      iv. *Acidosis* → sodium bicarbonate 1 mEq/kg IV.
      v. *Hypothermia* → undertake active/passive rewarming.
      vi. *Overdose*:
         - *Narcotics* → naloxone (0.4–2.0 mg q 2 min up to 10 mg).
         - *Benzodiazepines* → flumazenil (0.2 mg IV over 15 sec, then 0.3 IV over 30 sec. Repeat up to total of 3 mg).
         - *Cyclic antidepressants* → sodium bicarbonate 1 mEq/kg (50 mEq fine for most adults). Can create gtt w/ 3 amps bicarb: 1 L D_5W (150 mEq); run at 100 mL/h, titrated to pH of 7.5.
         - *Digitalis* → digibind (chronic intox 3–5 vials IV 120–200 mg; acute intox dosage varies but average is 10 vials 400 mg, up to 20 vials [800 mg may be required]).
         - *Calcium channel blockers* → Ca^{++} chloride (10 cc of 10% soln) + glucagon (1–5 mg IV/IM over 2–5 min).
         - *Beta blockers* → glucagon (1–5 mg IV/IM over 2–5 min).
   c. Epinephrine 1 mg IVP, repeat q 3–5 min *or* vasopressin, 40 U IV once.
   d. Atropine 1 mg IVP, may repeat once or twice every 3–5 min.
2. *Unstable bradycardia*
   a. Oxygen, IV access, EKG.
   b. Prepare for transcutaneous pacing (particularly if Mobitz type II 2nd-degree block or 3rd-degree block).
   c. Atropine 0.5 mg IV, may repeat up to total of 3 mg (pace if not effective).
   d. Consider dopamine IV 2–10 mcg/kg/min or epinephrine IV 2–10 mcg/min while awaiting pacer (or if pacer ineffective).

VIII. SUSPECTED CVA/STROKE (derived from American Heart Association, 2010)

A. Immediately

1. *Assess vital signs, SaO_2* (give O_2 if needed) *and glucose* (give glucose if needed).
2. *Assure good IV access.*
3. *Perform neurologic screening assessment.*
   a. Review hx, establish time of sx onset, and perform neuro exam.
      i. Have pt smile, check for pronator drift (10 sec), and have pt say, "You can't teach a dog new tricks."
      ii. Acute asymmetry/abnormalities in any 1 of the above is sufficient for clinical dx.
4. *Activate stroke team.*
5. *Obtain emergent 12-lead EKG and noncontrast head CT.*

B. CT scan w/ evidence of hemorrhage?

1. *Yes* → consult neurologist/neurosurgeon; go to section 3. below.
2. *No* → check for fibrinolytic exclusions and repeat neuro exam.

a. *Absolute contraindications*: h/o intracranial hemorrhage; anatomic cerebral vascular lesion such as AVM; intracranial malignancy; ischemic CVA w/in 3 mo (except ischemic CVA w/in 3 h); suspected aortic dissection; significant closed head or facial trauma w/in 3 mo.

b. *Relative contraindications*: h/o poorly controlled HTN or acute uncontrolled HTN (SBP > 180, DBP > 110); > 10 min of CPR or major surgery w/in 3 wk; noncompressible vascular punctures; pregnancy; active peptic ulcer; current use of anticoagulants; prior allergic rxn to streptokinase (if that agent is used).

c. *If no contraindication*, consider tPA (no anticoagulants or ASA × 24 h), go to section 3. below. *Note*: must administer tPA w/in 3 h of sx onset.

d. If either of above questions are positive, give aspirin and go to section 3. below.

3. *For all*: begin stroke pathway, admit to stroke unit if possible, monitor tx BP/glucose, monitor neuro status, and re-image if acute deterioration.

CHAPTER 26

KEY STEPS IN KEY OPERATIONS

I. NONVASCULAR

A. Proximal gut

1. *Stomach*
   a. *Nissen fundoplication* (laparoscopic)
      i. *Indications*: GERD refractory to medical tx or in pts unable to tolerate medical tx.
      ii. *Instruments*: Nathanson liver retractor.
         - Place on split-leg OR table that can airplane.
         - Initial trocar (10 mm) 12 cm inferior to xiphoid (or $^2/_3$ the distance from xiphoid to umbilicus).
         - Surgeon stands between legs w/ assistant to right of surgeon and camera operator to left of surgeon.
         - Veress needle or Hasson method used to achieve pneumoperitoneum. Place camera through 10-mm port.
         - Retract liver w/ self-retaining device (i.e., Nathanson liver retractor)—use 5 mm trocar just below and to left of xiphoid to create tract (remove trocar before placing liver retractor).
         - Place 2 additional 10-mm ports, each about $^1/_2$ the distance from xiphoid to camera port, 1 under each subcostal margin by several finger breadths (these ports plus the liver retractor and camera port make a diamond or square shape). Also place a 5-mm port further laterally along the left anterior axillary line.
         - Using harmonic scalpel, divide gastrohepatic omentum beginning inferior to hepatic branch of vagus nerve followed by division of phrenoesophageal membrane. Next, divide gastrophrenic ligament w/ ultrasonic shears to mobilize GE junction. Dissect adjacent to crura and diaphragm to avoid injury to vessels and nerves.
         - Grasp and elevate right crus of diaphragm to bluntly develop plane between this and right wall of esophagus. Sweep posterior vagus toward esophagus. Hands move opposite one another in "breaststroke" fashion.
         - Grasp and elevate left crus of diaphragm, then sweep tissue downward, exposing anterior vagus before continuing blunt dissection cephalad along anterior aorta.
         - Continue blunt paraesophageal dissection bilaterally into mediastinum.
         - Take down short gastric vessels 10–15 cm along cephalad aspect of greater curvature of stomach. (Assistant grasps greater curvature, pulling it cephalad and to pt's right.)
         - Surgeon then crosses hands to elevate greater curvature and access lesser sac. Once in lesser sac, assistant pulls stomach toward camera as well as pt's right. Using harmonic shears, divide short gastric vessels from inferior to GE junction (free fundus entirely from left crus of diaphragm).
         - In retroesophageal space, further bluntly dissect to develop window and achieve at least 4 cm of intraabdominal esophagus.
         - Place atraumatic/Babcock clamp through window and grasp fundus; pull left → right posterior to esophagus to deliver to other Babcock clamp. Then position above hepatic branch of vagus nerve.
         - Perform "shoeshine" maneuver to evaluate tension while holding epiphrenic fat pad inferiorly.
         - Approximate crura w/ large braided polyester sutures posterior to esophagus.
         - Dilate esophagus and place 60 Fr Maloney dilator for wrap.
         - Perform wrap w/ large braided polyester sutures. First (most inferior) suture grabs partial-thickness fundus on both sides of esophagus, but not esophagus itself.

- Place 2 additional sutures cephalad to this, incorporating partial-thickness anterior esophagus to create a loose fundoplication 2 cm long.

b. *Total gastrectomy*

i. *Indications*: proximal gastric adenocarcinoma, Z-E syndrome.

- Frequently extends in submucosa further than grossly appreciated, warranting 6-cm proximal and distal resection margins. Total gastrectomy should be avoided due to its morbidity but is often necessary for extensive proximal gastric cancers; when performed, a jejunal reservoir should be added (i.e., Roux-en-Y esophagojejunostomy w/ J-pouch).
- Body and antral adenocarcinoma traditionally tx'd w/ radical subtotal gastrectomy: ~ 80% distal gastrectomy; ligation of right gastric, right gastroepiploic, and left gastric arteries at origin w/ resection of associated LNs; excision of lesser and greater omentum.
- Cardia and fundus adenocarcinoma tx'd w/ total gastrectomy or proximal subtotal gastrectomy: high ligation of left gastric artery; removal of gastrosplenic ligament and lesser omentum; removal of crural LNs. If close to GE junction, resect distal esophagus.
- Billroth II reconstruction can be achieved if at least 30% of proximal stomach remains. If less remains, consider Roux limb or Billroth II w/ Braun enteroenterostomy. Billroth I reconstruction usu. avoided from concern for local recurrence.
- *R1 versus R2 dissection*: Latter has not consistently translated into improved survival in U.S. reports.

ii. *Procedure*:

- Pt supine. If GE junction is involved, thoracic approach may also be required. Long upper midline or bilateral subcostal incisions are equally appropriate. Laparoscopy sometimes done first to exclude metastatic dz.
- Greater omentum removed from the colon. The right gastroepiploic vessel is ligated. Dissection continues laterally along the greater curvature until the distal splenic vessel is skeletonized, allowing ligation of the short gastric vessels close to the spleen, if the spleen is to be preserved. The left gastroepiploic vessel is ligated.
- Division of the duodenum just distal to the pylorus is then done, allowing the stomach to be mobilized to the left. The right gastric artery is ligated close to its origin. The porta, hepatic artery, and celiac axis are able to be skeletonized. This is where the node bearing tissue is located.
- Division of the left gastric artery close to its origin. This allows completion of the splenic vessel skeletonization.
- The esophageal hiatus is mobilized by dividing the peritoneum at the hiatus, which allows clearing of the right crus and paracardial nodes and the left crus, w/ subsequent division of the esophagus.
- A Roux-en-Y reconstruction is normally done. The jejunum is divided distal the ligament of Treitz. The loop is 40–50 cm in length to minimize reflux. A retrocolic passage is commonly used. Hand-sewn or EEA anastomosis of the jejunum to the esophagus is appropriate. The duodenojejunostomy can also be hand-sewn or stapled.

2. *Vagotomy*

a. *Truncal vagotomy*

i. *Indications*: duodenal ulcers, type II and III gastric ulcers.

ii. *Instruments*: nerve hook, clips, Babcock forceps, upper hand retractor.

- Incise from xiphoid to 5 cm below umbilicus. Place upper hand retractor and place in reverse Trendelenburg. May need to incise triangular ligament and retract left lobe of liver to pt's right.
- Pick up peritoneum overlying abdominal esophagus w/ Debakey forceps and incise w/ Metzenbaums. Use Kuttner to develop groove between esophagus and adjacent crura (expose anterior $^2/_3$ of esophagus). Encircle esophagus w/ right index finger.
- Left (anterior) vagus often branches into 2 or more trunks w/ main one going along anterior wall of lower esophagus and other branches intimate w/ the longitudinal musculature; can place gentle caudal traction on stomach to bring these into relief. Divide nerves between clips.

- Right (posterior) vagus often 2–3 cm lateral and posterior to right esophageal wall. Run right index finger behind esophagus from right to left (just anterior to aorta), then flex to touch the right crus—nerve should be w/in this grasp. Gentle caudad traction on left gastric artery may help nerve stand out w/ tension. Handling trunk facilitated w/ Mixter clamp.
- Esophagus should have distal 5 cm cleared of nerve at end of procedure.

b. *Highly selective vagotomy*

i. *Indications*: duodenal ulcers, type II and III gastric ulcers.

ii. *Instruments*: nerve hook, clips, Babcock forceps, upper hand retractor.

iii. *Insights*: only in stable pts, must include drainage procedure (pyloroplasty most common).

- Incise from xiphoid to 5 cm below umbilicus. Place upper hand retractor and place in reverse Trendelenburg. May need to incise triangular ligament and retract left lobe of liver to pt's right.
- Pick up peritoneum overlying abdominal esophagus w/ Debakey forceps and incise w/ Metzenbaums. Use Kuttner to develop groove between esophagus and adjacent crura (expose anterior $^2/_3$ of esophagus). Encircle esophagus w/ right index finger.
- Left (anterior) vagus identified by retracting the greater curvature to the left and palpating the nerve. It is encircled w/ a vessel loop. The hepatic vagal branch is also isolated. This allows visualization and preservation of the hepatic branch. The tissue between this branch and the lesser curvature is ligated, dividing the gastric vagal nerves.
- Right (posterior) vagus often 2–3 cm lateral and posterior to right esophageal wall. Run right index finger behind esophagus from right to left (just anterior to aorta), then flex to touch the right crus—nerve should be w/in this grasp. Gentle caudad traction on left gastric artery may help nerve stand out w/ tension. Trunk encircled w/ a vessel loop. The celiac branch is preserved. The tissue between these trunks and the lesser curvature is divided, including the left gastric artery.
- The criminal nerve of Grassi is a branch of the posterior trunk that enters the stomach to the left of the esophagus cephalad to the short gastric vessels.

3. *Antrectomy and reconstruction options*

a. *Antrectomy*

i. *Indications*: option for type II, III gastric ulcers.

ii. *Instruments*: upper hand retractor.

- Incise from xiphoid to 5 cm below umbilicus. Place upper hand retractor.
- Evaluate pathology in duodenum. Excessive scarring or edema in pylorus/pancreas/hepatoduodenal ligament is relative contraindication to gastrectomy (leaves difficult duodenal stump, etc.)—vagotomy and drainage procedure may be safer or more appropriate.
- Incise avascular portion of gastrohepatic ligament to the right of lesser curvature, pass left hand behind lesser curvature and up around greater curvature (deep to gastroepiploic arcade)—lifts tissue away from middle colic artery. Divide in continuity the branches from gastroepiploic to greater curvature along the stomach from pylorus halfway up to diaphragm. Free avascular attachments from posterior antrum and pancreas.
- Once halfway from pylorus and esophagogastric junction, insert a large hemostat between lesser curvature and adjacent vascular bundle (contains left gastric artery) which is in turn divided between hemostats and ligated w/ 0 silk.
- Apply Allen clamps for 3–4 cm (if plan B-II; use ~ 2–3 cm if plan B-I) at 90° angle to greater curvature at upper limit of gastroepiploic division. Divide stomach between clamps. Apply 2nd set of Allen clamps from endpoint of prior division to point of division of left gastric artery. Divide stomach between clamps.
- Close last clamped area (not to be involved in anastomosis) w/ 3-0 Vicryl beginning on lesser curvature just under the Allen clamp, running it under clamp as a horizontal mattress (basting stitch), w/out tying at end. Trim off excess tissue, then remove clamp and run back to beginning as running locking, then tie to self. Lembert over this section.
- Identify, ligate, and divide right gastric artery lateral to distal antrum along w/ smaller unnamed vessels around pylorus.

- Apply Allen clamp just distal to pylorus and divide duodenum against clamp. Before handing off specimen, take off clamp to look for rim of duodenal mucosa (to avoid retained antrum).
- Place finger in duodenal lumen to palpate ampulla of Vater (posteromedial). Decide on reconstruction method.

b. *Gastroduodenostomy—Billroth I anastomosis*

i. *Indications*: distal gastrectomy indicated as option w/ least recurrence for type II or type III gastric ulcers, early distal gastric cancer.

ii. *Instruments*: upper hand retractor, Allen clamps.

iii. *Insights*: main risks involve outlet obstruction and anastomotic leakage (both technical issues). Splenic tear may be avoided by limiting (gentle) traction on stomach to lesser curvature, in caudad direction. Gentle dissection around antrum should avoid pancreatitis.

- Perform antrectomy as described in procedure above. Will need at least 1 cm of healthy posterior duodenal wall for Billroth I. Should also have the clamped, unsutured area of stomach approximately same width as duodenal stump.
- Place corner seromuscular guy sutures, but do not tie. Place posterior Lembert sutures.
- Remove Allen clamps, use double-armed 4-0 Vicryl or PDS for running locking posterior full-thickness bites, come around sides w/ Connell suture, then complete anterior wall.
- Place anterior Lembert sutures, then crown stitch at the *Jammerecke* or "angle of sorrow" (place where Hofmeister shelf of the gastric pouch meets the duodenal anastomosis line perpendicularly)—w/ seromuscular bites of anterior gastric pouch, then posterior gastric pouch, then duodenum (similar to a purse string). U-stitch does not approximate as well.
- If available, loosely suture omentum over anastomosis.

c. *Gastrojejunostomy—Billroth II anastomosis*

i. *Indications*: proximal gastric ulcer precluding Billroth I gastrectomy, bleeding posterior duodenal ulcer (again precluding a Billroth I anastomosis).

ii. *Insights*: more ulcerogenic than B-I anastomosis.

- Perform gastrectomy as above.
- Reconstruction can be retrocolic or antecolic and can be a loop gastrojejunostomy or a Roux-en-Y.

4. *Small bowel*

a. *Resection and anastomosis*: hand-sewn end-to-end.

i. *Indications*: trauma, tumor, stricture, Crohn's.

ii. *Instruments*: noncrushing bowel clamps (Doyan, Glassman), Allen clamps, 3-0 silk, 4-0 double-armed Vicryl, 3-0 Vicryl.

iii. *Insights*: single-layer closure as good as double-layer closure. No clinical difference in outcomes in running versus interrupted sutures. Two layers will be described below. If do just one layer, do the seromuscular one. Relative contraindication (controversial) for stapled anastomosis is trauma pt w/ significant anticipated 3rd-spacing/edematous bowel; leak rate *may* be higher in this population w/ stapled anastomosis.

- Lay out involved bowel on clean pads. Score a V-shaped incision w/ scalpel or Bovie to define mesentery to be resected between clamps and tied w/ 2-0 Vicryl.
- After resecting mesentery, apply Allen clamps on specimen side of bowel, then noncrushing intestinal clamps on the "staying-in" sides, 10 cm away. Divide bowel between clamps w/ scalpel. Ensure mesenteric side clear of fat for 1 cm each margin.
- W/ 3-0 silk, place seromuscular (Lembert) stitches to antimesenteric and mesenteric edges. Tie, but do not cut (will use as guys). Next rotate slightly to one side (will refer to this as "anterior" side), and place row of Lembert stitches by successive bisection.
- Rotate bowel w/ guy sutures to expose mucosal surface of "anterior" side. In midsection, place double-armed 4-0 Vicryl; tie, and run w/ locking sutures in opposite directions. Transition at edges to Connell stitching, run to each other, then tie off.
- Place row of Lembert sutures on "posterior" row to finish. Cut all sutures.
- Close mesenteric defect w/ running 2-0 Vicryl, taking care not to injure vessels.

b. *Resection and anastomosis*: hand-sewn side-to-side.
   i. Mesenteric and bowel division as above.
   ii. Align the divided ends and place a seromuscular (Lembert) 3-0 silk to maintain alignment. Place a 2nd Lembert about 5–6 cm back from the divided ends. Place hemostats on both of these to serve as guys. The space between these stitches will become the anastomosis. Place a row of Lembert stitches by successive bisection.
   iii. Perform the enterotomies w/ cut cautery on both sides just above the Lembert row. Do not injure the opposite wall of the bowel.
   iv. Create the anastomosis w/ a 4-0 Vicryl or chromic suture, starting in the middle of the Lembert row and working in opposite directions. This can be done w/ either a double-armed suture or 2 separate sutures. The Connell stitch is used to transition at the corner to the anterior surface.
   v. Place another row of Lembert sutures anteriorly to finish. Cut all sutures.
   vi. Close mesenteric defect w/ running 2-0 Vicryl, taking care not to injure vessel.

c. *Resection and anastomosis*: stapled side-to-side.
   i. Mesenteric division as above.
   ii. Apply Allen clamps on specimen side of bowel, then noncrushing intestinal clamps on the "staying-in" sides, 10 cm away from the division point. Fire the linear stapler on either side of the division point. Ensure mesenteric side clear of fat for 1 cm each margin.
   iii. Align the divided stapled ends and place a seromuscular (Lembert) 3-0 silk to maintain alignment. Place a 2nd Lembert about 5–6 cm back from the divided ends. Place hemostats on both of these to serve as guys. The space between these stitches will become the anastomosis.
   iv. Open a small corner of each limb at the staple line. Insert one leg of the linear stapler into each leg of the anastomosis. Align the stapler and fire.
   v. The enterotomy at the end can be closed by an additional firing of the linear stapler, effectively removing the stapled ends or by closing the defect in a hand-sewn fashion, as above. Lembert sutures are sometimes placed to invert the staple lines, esp. at the corners, but are not mandatory.

d. *Pyloroplasty/strictureplasty*
   i. *Indications*: for pyloric stenosis reconstruction or to facilitate postvagotomy emptying, Crohn's dz, radiation enteritis, etc.
      - Diffuse involvement of small bowel w/ multiple strictures.
      - Stricture in pt w/ prior resection of > 100 cm small bowel or short gut syndrome.
      - Rapid recurrence of Crohn's w/ obstruction.
      - Noninflamed fibrotic stricture.
   ii. *Contraindications*:
      - Perforation.
      - Multiple strictures in short segment.
      - Stricture close to planned resection.
      - Colonic strictures.
      - Mesenteric marginal ulceration, bleeding, or friability.
      - Suspicion of cancer w/in stricture.
   iii. *Heineke-Mikulicz* (pyloroplasty or stricture)
      - Good for short strictures (< 10 cm long).
      - Can hand-sew or staple.
      - Make longitudinal incision the length of the stricture, then close transversely w/ interrupted sutures as above.
   iv. *Finney* (pyloroplasty or stricture)
      - Appropriate for 10- to 20-cm long strictures.
      - Potential complication is bacterial overgrowth in resulting pouch/"diverticulum."
      - Incise distal stomach and proximal duodenum in continuity, appose edges, and sew together.

v. *Jaboulay* (pyloroplasty)
   - Appropriate for 10- to 20-cm long strictures w/ indurated or difficult pylorus/D1.
   - Technically similar to Finney, but the pylorus is not incised. (Think **J**aboulay = **J**ump over pylorus/D1.)

vi. *Side-to-side isoperistaltic strictureplasty* (stricture)
   - First described by Michelazzi, this is reserved for Crohn's pts w/ long or multiple strictures of small intestines in whom adequate resection is prohibitive due to total length of involved segments.
   - Perform by laying long segments of small intestine over each other in isoperistaltic orientation, then creating enterotomies for entire length and sewing as side-to-side for entire length.

B. Colon

1. *Open right hemicolectomy*
   a. *End-to-side ileocolic anastomosis hand-sewn*
      i. Divide lateral attachments from cecum to hepatocolic ligament. (*Note*: may need to divide, ligate small vessels in latter.) Retract right colon medially, bluntly pull down areolar tissue in plane lateral to colon w/ right index finger wrapped in moist gauze. Identify, preserve ureter.
      ii. Divide, ligate right omentum between clamps.
      iii. Using Mixter clamp to isolate, divide, ligate right branch of middle colic (cecal tumor) or trunk of middle colic (hepatic flexure tumor).
      iv. Identify mesenteric wedge, divide between successive clamps. *Note*, clearing mesentery at bowel edges and lifting bowel w/ umbilical tapes or towels may be useful for exposure.
      v. Place straight clamps at limits of bowel margins, then noncrushing bowel clamps on "staying in" sides, 10 cm away. Divide bowel w/ scalpel.
      vi. Oversew transverse colon w/ whip stitch, then remove clamp. Lembert the end. Place bowel clamp along anterior taenia to evert a lip.
      vii. Bring ileum up perpendicular to transverse colon and Lembert posterior row, leaving outer stitches long as guides.
      viii. Sharply open the lip of colon, and open clamp on ileum. Use double-armed 4-0 Vicryl in running, locking suture for posterior mucosa, then transition anteriorly as Connell stitching (see "end-to-end small bowel anastomosis," above).
      ix. Palpate to ensure adequate lumen. Close mesenteric defect w/ running 3-0 Vicryl.
   b. *End-to-end ileocolic anastomosis*
      i. Perform initial steps as for bowel resection, described in section A4a. above, including ileum and colon.
      ii. Bring ileum up to transverse colon end-on w/ mesenteries aligned. On antimesenteric border of small bowel, make a "Cheatle slit" for 1–2 cm to accommodate the differences in diameter.
      iii. Place antimesenteric, then mesenteric Lembert sutures to serve as guys w/ 3-0 or 4-0 silk. Place hemostats on these.
      iv. Rotate bowel slightly, and complete "anterior" layer of Lembert sutures.
      v. Flip bowel over using guy sutures, and use double-armed 4-0 Vicryl in middle of mucosa to begin running locking sutures in opposite directions. At edges, transition to Connell stitches, then tie together in middle.
      vi. Place "posterior" row of Lembert sutures.
   c. *Laparoscopic right hemicolectomy*
      i. *Setup*: 2 surgeons on pt's left side. *Ports*: three 5-mm ports (subxiphoid, suprapubic, LUQ) and one 12-mm port (left mid-abdomen for stapler). Extraction site on right mid-abdomen. Begin w/ camera in suprapubic midline port.
      ii. Explore abdomen by lifting greater omentum to view right/transverse colon/mesocolon.
      iii. Lift up TI/cecum to identify ileocolic artery pedicle. Duodenum is located just cephalad to the ileocolic artery. Skeletonize ileocolic trunk w/ harmonic scalpel, avoiding duodenum. Bluntly dissect posteriorly/circumferentially around trunk.

iv. Divide ileocolic trunk w/ linear cutting stapler proximally, close to duodenum.
v. Dissect along right lateral gutter (white line of Toldt) to mobilize cecum and ascending colon, from lateral to medial. Look for ureter crossing over iliac artery. Bluntly dissect ascending mesocolon away from retroperitoneum, working laterally.
vi. Move from inferior to superior; once at hepatic flexure, move camera to left mid-abdomen to better view right transverse colon. Moving medially along right transverse colon, duodenum encountered again.
vii. Divide small bowel mesentery w/ ultrasonic shears. Begin at site of division of ileocolic trunk and end at site of planned TI resection several cm proximal to ileocecal valve.
viii. Divide mesocolon w/ ultrasonic shears up to right branch of middle colic artery, which is divided w/ linear cutting stapler.
ix. Divide TI w/ linear cutting stapler.
x. Incise for a "mini-celiotomy" in RLQ or right mid-abdomen and place wound protector inside incision.
xi. Bring specimen out through incision, beginning w/ the divided TI.
xii. Fashion a stapled functional end-to-end anastomosis.
xiii. Return bowel to peritoneal cavity, and close mesenteric defect if desired/able.

d. *Low anterior resection*
   i. *Indications*: rectal lesions that may be resected and still leave enough distal rectum for anastomosis.
   ii. *Instruments*: Allen stirrups, Mixter clamp, long Metzenbaum scissors, vessel loop, Balfour w/ bladder blade, 3-0 popoff silk, double-armed 4-0 PDS or Vicryl, Keith needle w/ 3-0 or 4-0 PDS or Vicryl.
      - Pt in modified lithotomy position (hips flexed 15°, abducted 45° w/ Lloyd-Davies or Allen stirrups). Surgeon on left.
      - Midline incision from 6 cm below xiphoid to pubis.
      - Inspect/palpate liver, then eviscerate small bowel.
      - Expose left lateral peritoneal gutter, retracting sigmoid skyward and medially w/ left hand and dividing attachments w/ Metzenbaums in right hand along white line of Toldt. Use sponge stick to sweep down areolar tissue.
      - Identify left ureter, encircling it w/ vessel loop, then continue division along lateral rectum down to rectovesical pouch. Reexamine ureter, tracing it into pelvis.
      - Retract sigmoid to pt's left and incise along right side of sigmoid mesocolon base beginning at aortic bifurcation, continuing caudad along fusion of mesosigmoid and right lateral leaf of peritoneum in presacral space. Stay medial to right ureter, continuing incision to rectovesical (male) or rectovaginal (female) pouch.
      - *If able, incise peritoneum of rectovesical/uterine (female) pouch—can do this step later if unable to sufficiently visualize/expose at this point.*
      - Lift sigmoid skyward and gently mobilize gonadal vein from lateral mesocolon. Palpate IMA between deep margin of mesosigmoid and aortic bifurcation. If pt not obese, identify and ligate branches of IMA distal to left colic artery w/ 2-0 silk and divide mesentery. Bluntly sweep divided mesosigmoid off anterior surface of aorta/iliacs, leaving hypogastric (sympathetic) nerves intact.
      - Lift sigmoid again and use long Metzenbaum scissors to bluntly dissect presacral tissue/mesorectum, first on right of midline, then left. Bovie electrocautery is then used to divide the midline tissue, which contains middle sacral artery.
      - Use hand to bluntly extend presacral dissection bilaterally down to level of lateral ligaments. Gently apply traction on rectum to the right, stretching the left lateral ligament and facilitating division (use Bovie w/ ligament over a Mixter clamp). Repeat on other side to divide right lateral ligament. (Before dividing each, recheck ureter and hypogastric nerve on each side.)
      - Divide Waldeyer's fascia (from coccyx to posterior rectal wall).
      - Use bladder retractor to pull bladder/uterus anteriorly and caudally. Complete division of anterior peritoneum circumferentially.

- Mobilize proximal colon as necessary, dividing paracolic gutter peritoneum and "renocolic" ligament. Divide splenic flexure.
- Prepare rectal stump by first finding point 4–5 cm distal to tumor, and place large right-angle clamp there.
- *Anastomosis*:
    - *Baker (side-to-end colorectal) anastomosis, hand-sewn*:
        - Doubly clamp proximal colon. Divide and oversew the proximal end only w/ basting stitch + running locking/Connell + Lembert.
        - Singly clamp rectum distal to tumor, but proximal to planned level of division. Bring side of proximal colon down distal to angled clamp on rectum. Place guy sutures on both sides laterally, followed by posterior row of Lemberts by sequential bisection.
        - Incise enterotomies on both sides, then place running locking sutures (full-thickness) posteriorly; when come to sides, transect back wall of rectum and remove clamp. Transition to Connell sutures, then anterior row of Lemberts. Remove clamp on rectum and place anterior Lemberts.

e. *Laparoscopic-assisted sigmoid colectomy*

i. *Setup*: pt on split-leg table or in stirrups in modified lithotomy position, w/ hips, knees flexed. Surgeon on pt's right, one assistant between legs, other assistant on pt's left.

ii. Camera placed through 12-mm periumbilical port. Two additional right-sided 12-mm ports placed in mid-clavicular line to form isosceles triangle.

iii. W/ blunt instruments (i.e., 10-mm Babcock), take down any left-sided adhesions. W/ pt in Trendelenburg and right-side down, gently move left colon medially.

iv. Dissect up (caudad to cephalad) white line of Toldt w/ harmonic scalpel, simultaneously dissecting lateral to medial to avoid injuring ureter. Use traction and positioning to provide exposure.

v. Bring colon down to anterior peritoneal reflection and mark proximal end w/ clips to indicate site of subsequent division.

vi. W/ electrocautery, score medial aspect of left mesocolon to expose vessels, which are divided w/ linear cutting stapler.

vii. Score remaining mesocolon down to transition of left colon to sigmoid (indicated by confluence of taeniae, as well as relation to sacral promontory and proctoscopic measurement of ~ 15 cm).

viii. Make a posterior window at lower limit of dissection of rectum. Use window to staple across rectal stump.

ix. Create additional port at left paraumbilical space and enlarge until able to insert 3-cm wound drape. Divide colon at previously clipped site and place anvil into distal end.

x. Return bowel to abdomen, close left side port site. Reestablish pneumoperitoneum.

xi. Insert stapler w/ trocar through anus to rectal staple line w/ goal to penetrate through line or in antimesenteric area.

xii. Once orange band is exposed on trocar base (use Babcock to assist in telescoping tissue to achieve this), slide anvil over receptacle trocar. Fire stapler once bowel aligned.

xiii. Clamp bowel proximal to anastomosis, perform endoscopy from below to examine and air-test anastomosis w/ saline in pelvis. Examine doughnuts. Close incisions.

f. *Abdominoperineal resection*

i. *Indication*: distal rectal/anal lesions not amenable to therapy that would preserve sphincters/continence.

- Pt position, incision, and initial mobilization of rectum identical as for low anterior resection (see section d. above).
- *Perineal dissection*:
    - Close anus w/ purse-string suture.
    - Make longitudinal elliptical incision over perineum centered over anus, continuing through perirectal fat to levators (control hemorrhoidal vessel bleeding w/ electrocautery).

- Divide anococcygeal ligament w/ electrocautery. Posterior to rectum *sharply* divide Waldeyer's fascia just deep to anococcygeal ligament. Circumferentially connect perineal dissection space w/ pelvic dissection space.
- Divide levator muscles bilaterally from posteriorly to anteriorly, leaving some diaphragm tissue attached to specimen. After carefully dissecting anteriorly (avoid urethral injury) and dividing remaining attachments to prostate (in men), deliver specimen off the field. In women, dissection will follow just posterior to vagina. If concerned about vaginal wall viability from close dissection, remove that portion of vaginal wall rather than allow it to necrose postop.

- *Closure of pelvic floor*:
  - Place drain(s) through stab incisions to lie along coccyx/presacral space.
  - If able, reapproximate levators w/ 2-0 absorbable suture (if portion of posterior vagina was excised, suture vaginal edges to levator and perineal fat if unable to close primarily w/ ease). The remainder of perineum is closed in layers w/ absorbable suture and immediately place drains on suction.
  - If able, close the pelvic peritoneum w/ absorbable suture.
- Colostomy is fashioned as usual. If able to primarily close pelvic peritoneum, the colon segment can be tunneled under peritoneum of left paracolic gutter to anterolateral abdominal wall.

g. *Appendectomy*

i. Consider laparoscopic if obese, female of reproductive age, or anticipate heavy contamination.

ii. *Open*

- Transverse incision either at McBurney point, or about 1–2 cm cephalad of point of maximal tenderness.
- Score external oblique in direction of fibers, then divide; appendiceal retractors or small Richardson retractors are useful. Next, using Pean clamps in alternating orientation w/ assistant, divide internal oblique and transversus abdominus muscles bluntly (muscle-splitting technique) until encounter peritoneum.
- Pick up peritoneum w/ DeBakey forceps along w/ assistant, release, regrasp, then sharply incise peritoneum before exploring w/ finger. Spread wound w/ appendiceal retractors. Palpate w/ index finger for indurated appendix, being careful to pause and feel for pulsation (ensure not iliac artery) before attempting to bring to wound. Alternately, can use Raytec traction on cecum to trace down to appendix by following taenia. Babcock clamps placed around base of appendix help maintain traction.
- Place Pean clamp at base of appendix for several seconds, then move 1 cm distal. Ligate at crimped section w/ 2-0 chromic gut. Divide appendix at proximal edge of clamp w/ #15 blade, then touch tip of blade to exposed luminal mucosa and apply electrocautery to knife to cauterize mucosa (to prevent mucocele).
- Close peritoneum w/ 3-0 Vicryl (controversial), then posterior and anterior fascia w/ 1-0 PDS. If appendix ruptured, consider leaving skin open for delayed primary repair or to heal by secondary intent.

iii. *Laparoscopic*

- Tuck left arm. Place Foley. Trendelenburg w/ right side up if desired.
- 12-mm trocar at umbilicus for camera (initially) and stapler (later). 5-mm working ports in the LLQ and suprapubic position.
- Maryland dissector to open space between appendiceal base and mesoappendix.
- Change to 5-mm camera in LLQ and fire linear stapler w/ tissue load across the base of the appendix, then use vascular load for the mesoappendix.
- Place appendix in an endoscopic retrieval bag through the 12-mm umbilical port.

h. *Ostomies*

i. *Gastrostomy*

- Make transverse incision in RUQ. Bring stomach up to wound w/ Babcock forceps. Create 2 concentric purse-string sutures w/ 2-0 silk and incise in the middle w/ Bovie. Place G-tube, then tighten inner purse-string while holding tube down to invert the stomach.

Tighten, tie outer purse-string. Suture stomach to anterior abdominal wall in 4 locations, then close abdomen.

- Can also be done laparoscopically w/ an umbilical port. The stomach is insufflated via a NG tube. An appropriate position on the anterior stomach wall is identified. A kit w/ T-fasteners and dilators is used. 3 to 4 T-fasteners are passed through the abdominal wall into the stomach around the planned gastrotomy site. A needle is used to puncture the stomach and a wire is then passed. A Seldinger technique is used to pass the dilators over the wire until the gastrostomy tube can be placed percutaneously. The balloon is inflated and the stomach wall is brought up snug against the anterior abdominal wall. The T-fasteners are secured. The insufflation of the stomach and the peritoneum is released and the umbilical incision is closed.

ii. *Jejunostomy*

- Mobilize appropriate length of jejunum. Select site for enterotomy. Place a purse-string suture. Create small enterotomy in center of purse-string. Place the feeding catheter (can be a red rubber catheter or specially fabricated tube). Secure the purse-string suture. Create a tunnel, using the end of the purse-string suture. The tunnel is run 5–7 cm over the tube. This is secured using a final purse-string at the proximal end of the tube. The tube is brought out via a stab incision on the abdominal wall and secured. A few Lembert-type seromuscular stitches are used to secure the bowel to the abdominal wall over a fair distance to prevent volvulus at the jejunostomy site. This procedure can also be done laparoscopically in a fashion similar to the laparoscopic gastrostomy. It is more challenging, however, because the small bowel cannot be insufflated and placing the T-fasteners and tube into the bowel lumen is more difficult.

iii. *End ileostomy*

- After dividing ileum at appropriate level, create skin defect approximately the size of a nickel w/ Bovie, then core out the fat down to level of fascia. Use Bovie to create cruciate incision in abdominal fascia, then spread w/ Pean clamps to penetrate abdominal wall. Dilate tract w/ fingers, then deliver ileum through wound w/ Babcock forceps. After closing and dressing the laparotomy wound, the ostomy is matured. The bowel is opened by removing the staple line or sutures. Stitches (3-0 or 4-0 Vicryl or chromic) placed at 12:00, 3:00, 6:00, and 9:00 incorporate the cut end of the bowel, and a seromuscular bite at the level of the anterior rectus fascia and the skin edge create the mucocutaneous junction ("Brooke" stitches). The rest of the bowel edge is simply secured to the skin edge w/ interrupted seromuscular bites to the skin edge (w/out the deeper bite on the bowel wall).

iv. *Loop ileostomy*

- Create abdominal wall defect as described above (make slightly larger to accommodate for loop of bowel). Bring loop of small bowel up through the hole w/ Babcocks into wound. W/ tonsil clamps, create defect in avascular area of mesentery adjacent to bowel and pass red rubber catheter through. Bring up to skin, and suture red rubber catheter to skin on both sides of wound. Next make transverse enterotomy w/ cut cautery, and suture edges to skin w/ 3-0 Vicryl. The red rubber catheter prevents slippage of the bowel back into the abdomen and is removed in 2–3 wk, once the mucocutaneous junction is healed.

v. *Loop colostomy*

- Under fluoro guidance w/ radiopaque marker, locate skin overlying colon. Make transverse 6-cm incision down to anterior rectus fascia. Score w/ Bovie a cruciate incision over rectus, then muscle split down to posterior fascia. Pick up posterior fascia w/ clamps then cut w/ Metzenbaums to enter peritoneum. Pull up loop of colon w/ Babcocks, most gauze, etc., into wound. W/ tonsil clamps, create defect in avascular area of mesentery adjacent to colon and pass red rubber catheter through. Bring up to skin, and suture red rubber catheter to skin on both sides of wound. Suture serosa to posterior fascia. Next make transverse colotomy w/ Bovie, and suture edges to skin w/ 3-0 Vicryl. The red rubber catheter prevents slippage of the bowel back into the abdomen and is removed in 2–3 wk, once the mucocutaneous junction is healed.

vi. *End colostomy*

- Essentially the same operation as for end ileostomy except that it is not critical to place the "Brooke" stitches for maturation. Only the mucocutaneous stitches are necessary.

II. HEPATOBILIARY AND PANCREAS

A. Open cholecystectomy

1. *Indications*: removal of gallbladder when laparoscopic technique impeded by lack of visualization or other technical problems, concern for malignancy, or as salvage for complications from laparoscopic technique.
2. *Instruments*: sponge stick, Kuttner dissector, Kocher clamp or large hemostat, Mixter clamp, Metzenbaums.
   a. *Retrograde:*
      i. Open w/ preferably a subcostal incision beginning 1 cm beyond linea alba, and running parallel and 4 cm caudad to inferior costal margin. After sharply incising peritoneum, grasp each side w/ ratcheted forceps or clamps to hold up for remainder of incision.
      ii. Grasp falciform ligament w/ hemostat, and gently pull liver edge down if needed. Otherwise clamp, divide, and ligate w/ 2-0 silk.
      iii. Retract liver edge w/ Deaver retractor. Place lap pad against medial lobe of liver to keep out of way. Grasp gallbladder fundus and infundibulum w/ 6" curved hemostat, pull Hartmann's pouch caudad to stretch peritoneum over cystic duct/CBD.
      iv. Incise this local peritoneum w/ Metzenbaum, dissect out junction of cystic duct/CBD. Tie off cystic duct close to GB w/ 2-0 silk. More caudad, dissect cystic artery, tie off in continuity w/ 2-0 silk and divide. Recheck cystic duct, tie again, and divide (if not planning IOC). Many authorities, however, recommend dividing artery first, dissecting out gallbladder, and then returning to divide cystic duct.
      v. Mixter/right-angle clamp useful for dissecting out duct and artery. For cystic duct, follow inferior GB edge. For artery, many times can trace back from anterior wall of GB.
      vi. If encounter bleeding, control hepatoduodenal ligament by passing index finger into foramen of Winslow, and compress against thumb.
   b. *Antegrade*:
      i. Expose as for retrograde operation.
      ii. W/ right angle clamp, doubly loop 2-0 silk around cystic duct to prevent intraoperative stone passage into CBD.
      iii. Isolate cystic artery, divide in continuity, ligating w/ 2-0 silk.
      iv. Dissect gallbladder off bed by incising serosa at fundus w/ blade, then exposing serosa w/ tonsil clamp for the Metzenbaum or Bovie, leaving submucosa on GB.
         - *Note*: may also dissect from dome down, and only approach cystic artery/duct when gallbladder is dissected off of liver.

B. Laparoscopic cholecystectomy

1. Multiple port options available. W/ a 5-mm clip applier, the procedure can easily be done w/ a 10-/12-mm port at umbilicus and three 5-mm ports in the subxiphoid and right subcostal positions.
   a. *4 ports*: (1) infraumbilical, (2) epigastric (on 3rd distance from xiphoid to umbilicus), (3) right subcostal midclavicular, (4) right subcostal lateral. Surgeon on left, works through subxiphoid and midsubcostal ports.
   b. Retract fundus superiorly and take down adhesions from GB body bluntly—grab adhesions close to GB wall to stay in relatively avascular plane. Proceed w/ dissection from lateral to medial to expose GB neck.
   c. Retract Hartmann's pouch laterally and inferiorly to expose triangle of Calot.
   d. Identify cystic artery and cystic duct before dividing any structures. Use the Maryland dissector to bluntly create the window behind the artery and between the artery and the duct. The node of Calot often lies in the space between the artery and the duct. It can be pulled down (gently), but will sometimes bleed a bit. The infundibulum/Hartmann's pouch often needs to be flipped medially as the posterolateral dissection helps delineate the cystic structures. Stay close to the gallbladder to avoid CBD injury.
   e. Once the cystic duct and artery are identified, clips can be applied.
      i. *If planning to perform cholangiography*, place clip at junction of cystic duct and infundibulum. Cut anterior cystic duct w/ scissors. Pass cholangiogram catheter through #14

angiocatheter lumen. Clip catheter in place. Shoot IOC to demonstrate dye passage into duodenum and intrahepatic biliary tree. Remove clip securing catheter and catheter. Apply 2 clips to distal cystic duct and divide.

ii. If no cholangiogram, place 2 clips on pt's side and 1 clip on gallbladder side of the cystic duct and the cystic artery and then divide.

iii. *Short cystic duct*:

- Flipping GB neck medially helpful to identify junction of cystic duct and GB.
- Primary dissection is posterolateral, then medially.
- Using a silk tie around Hartmann's pouch instead of clip preserves length for ductotomy.

f. *Significant adhesions to liver, GB*:

i. Take down by sharp dissection w/ electrocautery on low power setting.

ii. Be cognizant of location of duodenum and use traction/countertraction to dissect.

- Hydrodissection may be a useful adjunct to separating duodenum from adjacent structures.

iii. Developing window at GB neck may be easier than first dividing cystic artery.

g. *Midline intraabdominal adhesions*:

i. Use open (Hasson) technique to achieve pneumoperitoneum.

ii. Bluntly open window w/ laparoscope to allow directly visualize port placement. Subxiphoid port placed right of midline.

h. *GB bed dissection*:

i. After division of cystic duct and artery, begin dissection close to GB, away from hilar structures. Check w/ Maryland for posterior branch of the cystic artery. Can use cautery to remove the serosal attachments of the gallbladder to the liver. Reposition GB as necessary to expose lateral/medial aspects of GB attachments. Inspect GB bed for hemostasis before removal of GB.

2. *Laparoscopic entry* (for pneumoperitoneum)

a. *Veress needle* ("closed" method): make 3-mm incision just inferior to umbilicus. Grasp on both sides w/ towel clamps and lift up. Grasp Veress needle on shaft and insert through umbilical stalk at steep (i.e., 60° angle), listening/feeling for 2 clicks. W/ 10 cc syringe, aspirate back to check for succus or blood, then inject saline. If no resistance, remove syringe and watch for saline to rapidly empty hub of needle. Connect to insufflator.

b. *Hasson trocar* ("open" method): make a 10- to 11-mm incision just inferior to the umbilicus. Use cautery to dissect down to the fascia. Grasping the umbilical stalk w/ a towel clamp helps elevate the fascia. Once the fascia is cleared, it can be divided to the peritoneum. The peritoneum is elevated w/ hemostats and sharply divided w/ scissors. The peritoneal surface is swept w/ the surgeon's finger. A stay suture is placed (this can be a figure-of-eight stitch, later used to close the fascial defect) and used to secure the Hassan trochar.

c. *Common to all*: w/ lateral-most port, assistant uses 5-mm grasper to retract fundus cephalad over liver margin. W/ more medial port, retract infundibulum laterally to facilitate visualization of "critical angle." Serrated dissector or Maryland grasper in epigastric port is used to strip peritoneum of infundibulum and cystic structures parallel w/ GB. Utilization of endo shears or hook w/ electrocautery can achieve rapid dissection of GB out of fossa, but care must be taken to ensure no cautery at the hilar structures.

3. *Open common bile duct exploration*

a. *Indications*: retained stone in CBD.

b. *Instruments*: T-tube, Randall stone forceps, spoons/scoops.

i. Incise peritoneum lateral to duodenum, and mobilize duodenum medially to expose distal CBD—palpate CBD.

ii. Make 1-cm longitudinal ductotomy distal to cystic duct. Place stitch of 4-0 chromic catgut (or PDS) on each side of the opening and attach mosquito hemostats. Alternately, can place sutures first for traction.

iii. Attempt to flush proximally and distally w/ small rubber catheter and 20 cc syringe w/ saline.

iv. Pass small (#10 Foley) catheter proximally, inflate, and gently withdraw.

v. Pass Foley into duodenum, inflate, pull until holds up on sphincter, deflate just enough to pull back through sphincter, then reinflate and pull back, attempting to retrieve stones.

vi. Stone forceps can be used to retrieve stones/debris as well.

vii. *At completion of exploration, place T-tube*:

- Back cut tapers on T (away from stem), then horizontally cut off top of T as well w/ a triangle/wedge at the middle to create a hinge.
- Grasp T-tube w/ Mixter clamp at junction, w/ jaws parallel to top of T. Insert proximal limb first as far as possible, then insert distal limb.
- Place multiple interrupted sutures of 3-0 chromic gut to hub T-tube against distal margin of ductotomy. Shoot cholangiogram; place closed drain in the area.

4. *Common bile duct exploration* (alternate techniques)

a. *Removal of retained common bile duct stones*

i. Place 2 traction sutures of 4-0 chromic on anterolateral CBD, then longitudinal choledochotomy w/ 11-Blade and Pott's scissors.

ii. CBD stone < 6 mm → transcystic scope and basket retrieval.

iii. Distal impacted CBD stone → Fogarty, grasper.

iv. Retained CBD stone → post-op ERCP or transcystic/T-tube/CBD stent.

v. CBD stone > 6 mm → choledochotomy stent/basket/T-tube.

vi. Multiple CBD stones → choledochoduodenostomy/choledochojejunostomy, other biliary bypass.

vii. Can also attempt "vacuuming" out stones by truncating the flange of a #8 or #10 Fr red rubber catheter, placing the nonflanged end onto a pipette tip, and placing the large end of the pipette tip into suction tubing. Advance truncated flanged end w/ fingers or Debakey forceps. Once in, apply suction. Release suction as necessary to pull back tubing.

b. *Laparoscopic common bile duct exploration*

i. *Need*: 3-mm flexible choledochoscope w/ 2.1-mm working port; 4-mm, 12 Fr introducer sheath w/ introducer dilator; 6 Fr cholangiogram catheter; 0.035" hydrophilic guide wire w/ flexible tip; 5 Fr angioplasty catheter w/ 6-mm balloon; endoscopic wire retrieval baskets.

ii. *Steps*:

- Use 6 Fr cholangiogram catheter inserted into cystic duct to pass 0.035" wire into CBD.
- Remove catheter, leaving wire in place.
- Use 4-mm, 12 Fr introducer sheath over wire, then remove introducer dilator.
- Dilate cystic duct w/ 5 Fr angioplasty catheter and 6-mm balloon w/ 1/3 of balloon out of duct.
- Inflate to 3–6 ATM for 5 min.
- Deflate, remove, leave guide wire in place.
- Advance 3-mm choledochoscope over wire through sheath into duct.
- Use endoscopic basket/graspers to retrieve stone.
- Holding catheter in place, withdraw scope and basket together.
- Place stones on omentum for later removal from abdomen.
- Repeat cholangiogram until clear.

iii. *If unsuccessful* (i.e., stones in proximal hepatic ducts):

- ERCP.
- Laparoscopic choledochotomy and stone removal.
  - Dissect soft tissue off CBD, then sharply incise w/ scissors.
  - Place choledochoscope proximally or distally w/ padded graspers.
  - Remove stones w/ wire baskets/graspers.
  - Place 10–14 Fr T-tube (fashion appropriately) into choledochotomy and bring out through port incision.

        - Close w/ absorbable suture (i.e., PDS).
        - Shoot completion T-tube cholangiogram.
        - Place drain.
    - Open CBD exploration.

c. *Open sphincteroplasty*
   i. After removing gallbladder, perform extended Kocher maneuver to expose down to 3rd portion of duodenum.
   ii. Localization of papilla assisted by passing #4–6 Fr Fogarty catheter through cystic duct stump into duodenum.
   iii. Perform longitudinal duodenotomy and localize ampulla. Place traction sutures next to (but not into) ampullary complex. Exposure may be facilitated w/ small Richardson retractors in the duodenum.
   iv. Considering cephalad/proximal 12 o'clock, make 5-mm incision at 11 o'clock in sphincter over Fogarty catheter. Place 1–2 4-0/5-0 Vicryl sutures on each side of incised ampulla. Make figure-of-eight suture at apex of sphincterotomy. Locate pancreatic duct orifice near 5 o'clock; extend sphincterotomy 3–4 mm if necessary for exposure.

d. *Whipple procedure* (partial pancreaticoduodenectomy)
   i. *Indications*: carcinoma of ampulla, head of pancreas, distal bile duct, or duodenum.
   ii. *Contraindications*: gross invasion of IVC or SMA/SMV, distant metastases (liver, peritoneal, or celiac LNs).
    - Midline vertical incision, or in stocky persons, a chevron incision is acceptable.
    - *If malignancy not confirmed yet, divide greater omentum beneath greater curvature of stomach for access to FNA lesion.*
    - *Determine resectability*:
        - Perform extended Kocher and divide lateral duodenal ligament to expose point where SMV crosses 3rd portion of duodenum inferiorly and foramen of Winslow superiorly. (Can also find SMV by looking through a division in the infragastric greater omentum and tracing the middle colic vein down.)
        - Incise avascular gastrohepatic ligament and identify hepatic artery, then gastroduodenal artery. Divide and doubly ligate gastroduodenal artery. Portal vein should be posterior.
        - Using Kuttner, gently separate portal vein from overlying pancreas. Gently insinuate index finger between portal vein (is SMV inferiorly before the splenic vein joins behind the pancreas) and pancreas coming from above or below to determine if has invaded superior mesenteric vessels.
        - Divide and ligate right gastric artery. Skeletonize hepatic artery and CBD.
    - Perform cholecystectomy. Ligate and divide common hepatic duct just proximal to cystic duct junction.
    - Perform antrectomy (w/ vagotomy if desired), then retract stomach to pt's right to expose pancreas.
    - Divide pancreas 3 cm left of the superior mesenteric vessels w/ 35/3.5 mm linear stapler after gingerly separating pancreas from underlying splenic vein from above and below. Transect pancreas to the left of the stapler. If necessary, suture ligate superior and inferior pancreatic arteries in the stump. Insert plastic catheter into pancreatic duct.
    - Retract the resected head of pancreas stomach to pt's right to expose SMV/portal veins. Divide and ligate the multiple small branches of SMA/SMV involved w/ head of pancreas. Retract SMV to pt's left to expose underlying SMA. Divide uncinate process. Now, the antrum, duodenum, and pancreatic head only connected via duodenojejunal segment.
    - Free duodenojejunal section from ligament of Treitz, divide the mesentery, and divide jejunum just beyond LOT.
        - *Pancreaticojejunostomy*: pass 12–13 cm of proximal jejunum through defect in transverse mesocolon.
            - *Pancreaticojejunostomy* (duct to mucosa method): start along antimesenteric jejunum, about 3 cm from proximal jejunal end. Use 4-0 Prolene interrupted

sutures to bring together posterior capsule of pancreas to seromuscular layer of jejunum. Make jejunostomy incision slightly larger than diameter of pancreatic duct. Approximate pancreatic duct to full thickness of jejunal wall w/ interrupted 6-0 Prolene or PDS (posterior row). Insert 8–10 Fr pediatric feeding tube into the pancreatic duct—threadong end into jejunum and bring out from jejunum 10 cm distal to anastomosis through stab wound inabdominal wall—purse-string jejunal defect w/ 4-0 silk. Complete anterior row of anastomosis w/ 6-0 suture. Appose anterior pancreas to anterior jejunum w/ additional 4-0 sutures.

- *Pancreaticojejunostomy* (invagination method): place catheter into duct as above, secure w/ fine Vicryl. Pass 3 cm of pancreas into open end of jejunum using 4-0 Prolene guide sutures at superior and inferior poles (U-stitch w/ ends emerging 3 cm away from jejunal edge)—1 mg glucagon IV can be given to relax jejunum if diameter is initially unaccommodating.
  - If pancreas is still too wide, can fashion a true end-to-end anastomosis w/ posterior Lemberts followed by full thickness interrupted posterior, interrupted anterior, followed by anterior Lemberts. Alternately, end-to-side anastomosis can be made.
- *Hepaticojejunostomy*: make small ductotomy in hepatic duct ~ 3 cm proximal to divided end, and insert fine-tipped Mixter clamp through the defect to emerge through divided end. Grasp long arm of 16 or 18 Fr T-tube and draw into place (will divert bile while anastomosis is healing). Next, incise antimesenteric jejunum15–20 cm distal to pancreaticojejunostomy to the diameter of the hepatic duct. W/ interrupted 5-0 PDS or Vicryl, bring together full-thickness duct to full-thickness jejunum. Posterior row knots go inside lumen, anterior go outside; the latter may be seromuscular. Use Cheatle slit or differential size bites to accommodate for any size discrepancy.
- *Gastrojejunostomy*: bring proximal jejunum to stomach in antecolic route. 10–20 cm distal to hepaticojejunostomy, begin anastomosis w/ guide sutures from antimesenteric jejunum to greater curvature, approximately 3 cm proximal and posterior to gastric division. Fashion standard double-layered enteroenterostomy as described elsewhere along length of apposed surfaces.
  - *Drains*: bring T-tube through anterior wall stab wound. Bring pancreatic catheter through abdominal wall if not already done. Insert separate closed-suction drain through separate wound near hepaticojejunostomy. Separate JP drains should be placed near pancreaticojejunostomy and subhepatic spaces.

e. *Hepatic resection*
   i. *General*:
      - Maintain low CVP for elective cases (CVP 5 mm Hg).
      - Consider use of Trendelenburg to minimize risk of air embolism.
      - *Techniques for parenchymal division* (after division of capsule w/ electrocautery) *include*: finger fracture, crush w/ clamp (i.e., Kelly), stapler w/ vascular load, control of vessels/ducts w/ clips, ligatures (*Note*: some surgeons take large bites through periphery of parenchyma w/ heavy chromic suture before attempting division), ultrasonic/argon beam/electrocautery dissection, etc.
   ii. Anatomic resections (limit use of wedge resections to small [< 2 cm] peripheral lesions).
f. *Right lobectomy*
   i. Fully mobilize liver and perform cholecystectomy.
   ii. Incise right lateral aspect of hepatoduodenal ligament longitudinally, just posterior to bile duct. Just lateral to common hepatic duct, locate hepatic arteries. Ligate right hepatic artery and excise pericholedochal LNs (palpate left hepatic artery first to ensure its patency). May need to retract right hepatic duct cephalad to expose artery.
   iii. Continued retraction of right hepatic duct should now expose the bifurcation of the portal vein. Right portal vein may actually present as anterior and posterior branches leading to a trifurcation. Isolate, divide, and oversew right portal vein. Isolate, divide, and ligate right hepatic duct. The devascularized right lobe should now be grossly demarcated.

iv. Retract liver anteriorly and to pt's left, then ligate multiple small short hepatic veins between IVC and segments 1, 6, and 7, beginning caudad and working cephalad.

v. W/ continued retraction as above, divide the retrocaval ligament bridging segments 1 and 7 to expose main right hepatic vein going into IVC. Doubly clamp, divide, and oversew the "staying in side" of the right hepatic vein.

vi. Divide parenchyma on perfused side of demarcation w/ finger fracture, electrocautery, or CUSA. May clip vessels on nonperfused side, but must ligate those on perfused side. Ligate middle hepatic vein when encountered. (Use inflow vascular occlusion to stem bleeding during this phase.)

vii. Divide caudate process (between posterior portal vein and the IVC), exposing IVC.

viii. Place suction drain and bring out through dependent area of abdominal wall.

III. ENDOCRINE

A. Parathyroidectomy

1. *Indications*: hyperparathyroidism (even if asymptomatic—long-term complications in ~ 20%).
   a. If adenoma (80%), excise, but bx at least 1–2 other glands.
   b. *If hyperplasia* (15%, assoc. w/ secondary hyperparathyroidism, MEN I, MEN IIa): remove 3.5 glands or all w/ reimplantation in arm.
   c. *If carcinoma* (~ 5%): perform en bloc resection w/ thyroid lobe and regional lymph nodes.
   d. *Calciphylaxis*: perform 3.5 gland parathyroidectomy (reimplant in arm) and amputation.
2. *Incidentals and insights*: rapid drop in intraop PTH key to identifying problematic gland. Postop hypocalcemia is usu. self-limited.
3. *Incision, exposure*: place roll behind shoulders to extend the neck. Incise 2 finger breadths above sternal notch horizontally. Divide subcutaneous tissue and platysma, then elevate subplatysmal skin flaps to the thyroid cartilage notch down to the sternal notch. Divide investing fascia midline, and retract strap muscles laterally.
4. *Identify crossing of inferior thyroid artery and recurrent laryngeal nerve*: mobilize the thyroid medially, and locate the recurrent laryngeal nerve caudally.
5. *Identify inferior and superior parathyroids*:
   a. Superior parathyroid glands are superior, posterior to recurrent laryngeal nerve, usu. near cricoid.
   b. Inferior parathyroid glands are inferior, anterior to recurrent laryngeal nerve, usu. w/in 2 cm of inferior thyroid pole.
6. *Resection*: mobilize adenoma, but do not heavily manipulate the gland. Clamp and ligate pedicle, and remove gland. Identify all remaining glands and bx suspicious ones. Closure should be entertained once an appropriate drop in rapid PTH test (intraop) has been observed.
7. *Total parathyroidectomy w/ autotransplantation*:
   a. When removing parathyroid for primarily parathyroid problem, if need to reimplant, do so in arm. If removing for other reason (i.e., vascular compromise from thyroidectomy), implant in SCM.
8. *"Missing" parathyroid*:
   a. Search for hidden superior parathyroid gland in tracheoesophageal groove along carotid sheath.
   b. Search for hidden inferior parathyroid gland in thymus.
   c. U/S useful adjunct intraop. in the above.
   d. Gently pulling on an enlarged branch of inferior thyroid artery may lead to a pathologic gland.
   e. Incise thyroid capsule over discolored or enlarged areas; lobectomy is rarely indicated.
9. *Closure*: irrigate and achieve meticulous hemostasis. Reapproximate platysma w/ 3-0 absorbable sutures and close skin in subcutaneous fashion.

B. Total thyroidectomy

1. *Indications*: goiter, hyperthyroidism, thyroid carcinoma.
2. *Instruments*: skin rakes, small Richardson retractor, Kuttner/peanut dissectors, tonsil clamps.
3. *Incidentals*: postop hematoma, recurrent laryngeal nerve injury, superior laryngeal nerve injury, hypoparathyroidism, thyroid storm, hypocalcemia, or hypothyroidism.

a. Pt supine w/ head in mild extension, table in mild reverse Trendelenberg.

b. Make gently curved transverse *incision* 2–3 finger breadths above sternal notch, just beyond anterior border of SCM on each side, and down through but not beyond platysma. Dissect cephalad on undersurface of platysma until w/in 1–2 cm of thyroid cartilage notch. Similarly, elevate inferior *flap* ~ 2 cm.

c. Make vertical midline incision through *cervical fascia*, extending it cephalad and caudad for the length of the exposure. Elevate *sternohyoid* in the midline, then elevate sternothyroid and dissect away thyroid capsule bilaterally. If necessary, may divide these muscles in their upper thirds for adequate exposure in large glands.

d. Retract strap muscles laterally w/ small Richardson while *drawing thyroid medially* w/ Kuttner or Raytec sponge. Areolar tissue may be divided w/ sharp/blunt dissection. Divide and *ligate middle thyroid vein* to facilitate further exposure.

e. Identify carotid artery, and dissect through fibrous tissue medial to that vessel down to prevertebral fascia. *Retract carotid artery laterally* and dissect further medially to demonstrate *inferior thyroid artery*, which should be encircled w/ vessel loop. Gently retract the artery and follow to thyroid; it will cross the *recurrent laryngeal nerve* before reaching the gland. (*Note*: if have difficulty identifying recurrent laryngeal nerve, inferior thyroid artery, or inferior thyroids, go directly to step h. below and dissect out superior lobe first to provide better exposure.)

f. Locate *inferior parathyroid gland*, usu. situated near branching of inferior thyroid artery. Divide and ligate these branches anterior to parathyroid so as to preserve its blood supply. Also divide and ligate any branches of inferior thyroid vein.

g. Using a small hemostat, define a plane superficial to the recurrent laryngeal nerve and follow cephalad to its entry into the thyroid (some branching of the nerve may be observed). Fully dissect out lower pole of thyroid.

h. Find upper aspect of thyroid isthmus—if *pyramidal lobe* is identified extending cephalad, divide and ligate it.

i. Retract caudad and laterally the strap muscles and use Kuttner to sweep upper pole of gland away from larynx to highlight the *superior laryngeal nerve*, which is generally apposed to cricothyroid here. Also sweep lateral gland of thyroid away bluntly, ligating veins as encountered. Identify and doubly *ligate superior thyroid artery and vein*. Fully mobilize upper lobe now, attempting to identify, preserve, and dissect the parathyroid gland away from the thyroid.

j. Ensure identification of recurrent laryngeal nerve and superior and inferior parathyroid glands before proceeding to lobectomy.

k. Thyroid attached to upper 2 tracheal rings by ligament of Berry, the upper extent of which is approached by the recurrent laryngeal nerve. Carefully *divide ligament of Berry*, identifying and ligating any vessels, which pass through, and avoiding the recurrent laryngeal nerve.

l. The isthmus may be divided serially between hemostats or w/ 55/3.5 mm stapler if desire to maintain contralateral lobe. Otherwise, perform the above steps for the other side.

m. *Closure*: reapproximate strap muscles (if divided) w/ horizontal mattress sutures of 2-0 Vicryl. Loosely bring together right and left strap muscles w/ interrupted 4-0 Vicryl. Reexamine to ensure absolute hemostasis, then approximate anterior SCM and cervical fascia w/ running 3-0 Vicryl. Reapproximate platysma w/ running 4-0 Vicryl, and skin w/ running subcuticular 4-0 Monocryl.

C. Adrenalectomy

1. Laparoscopic

   a. *Contraindications*: locally invasive tumor; tumor > 10 cm; primary adrenal malignancy; prior nephrectomy, splenectomy, or liver resection.

   b. *Laparoscopic approaches*:

      i. Transabdominal lateral flank (most common—details below).

      ii. Retroperitoneal endoscopic.

      iii. Anterior transabdominal.

   c. *Right adrenalectomy*

      i. Pt in lateral/semilateral decubitus (affected side up) w/ table flexed, in reverse Trendelenburg.

      ii. Mark ant/post axillary lines, costal margin, and iliac crest before prepping.

iii. Veress needle used for pneumoperitoneum medial to anterior axillary line, 2 finger breadths below costal margin. Use optical trocar for initial entry into abdomen after pneumoperitoneum achieved.
iv. *4 ports used:*
   - 3 are 5 mm, and 1 is 11 mm (for clip applier).
   - Surgeon stands on pt's right and works through the 2 more dorsal ports.
v. Divide right triangular ligament w/ hook electrocautery (caution: IVC) and retract liver medially.
vi. Divide connective tissue between adrenal superomedial border and IVC w/ shallow passes of hook electrocautery.
vii. Push adrenal gently laterally to facilitate dissection.
viii. Isolate, clip, and divide branches of adrenal artery.
ix. Isolate, clip (adrenal side first), and divide right adrenal vein.
x. Use electrocautery to further define medial edge of adrenal.
xi. Divide peritoneum between right kidney and adrenal w/ electrocautery.
xii. Divide fat between right kidney and adrenal w/ ultrasonic coagulator or hook electrocautery.
xiii. Remove adrenal in endobag through 11-mm port site.

d. *Left adrenalectomy*
   i. Analogous positioning and port sites.
   ii. Mobilize splenic flexure of colon w/ electrocautery.
   iii. Do NOT dissect posterior to kidney at this point—will cause it to fall forward.
   iv. Place dorsal 4th port if needed.
   v. Divide splenocolic ligament at inferior pole of spleen.
   vi. Retract spleen medially and divide splenorenal ligament fully, allowing spleen and tail of pancreas to roll medially away from adrenal.
   vii. Develop plane between kidney and tail of pancreas by dividing areolar attachments to gain access to inferior adrenal and adrenal vein.
   viii. At this point, laparoscopic U/S may be useful to identify/locate adrenal in difficult cases.
   ix. Diligently work to define medial and lateral aspects of gland w/ electrocautery dissection.
   x. Identify the adrenal vein at inferomedial adrenal border, then free the border w/ hook cautery.
   xi. Divide remaining adrenal arteries w/ ultrasonic coagulator.
   xii. Divide remaining adrenal attachments medially, taking care to remain extracapsular.
   xiii. Isolate, clip, and divide the relatively long left adrenal vein.
   xiv. Elevate and divide inferior attachments of adrenal.
   xv. Place adrenal in endobag for removal through 11-mm port site.

2. Open adrenalectomy
   a. *Indications*: large (> 10 cm) mass or significant concern for malignancy.
   b. *Approaches*:
      i. *Transabdominal*:
         - *Left transabdominal adrenalectomy*:
            - Make left subcostal incision.
            - Mobilize spleen, tail of pancreas.
            - Incise Gerota's fascia along its medial and superior aspect.
            - Open tissues overlying left renal vein. Left adrenal vein usu. empties into superior aspect of left renal vein just medial to left gonadal vein.
            - Clip and divide inferior phrenic vessels as they enter the adrenal gland. Then ligate and divide left adrenal vein.
            - Clip and divide small branches of left suprarenal arteries (middle and inferior) as they enter the gland.

- *Right transabdominal adrenalectomy*:
  - Make right subcostal incision.
  - Perform Kocher maneuver to widely expose duodenum and IVC. Retract right lobe of liver cephalad.
  - Adrenal located between superomedial kidney and IVC. Incise peritoneum overlying the gland.
  - Isolate the short right adrenal vein and divide it in continuity. The remaining adrenal vessels can be divided between clips.

ii. *Posterolateral* (flank): not described here, but provides good exposure.

iii. *Thoracoabdominal*: not described here, but provides wide exposure useful for large tumors.

iv. *Posterior*: usu. reserved for bilateral dz.

- Place pt in prone position.
- Incise just above 11th rib, then divide latissimus dorsi, followed by serratus posterior along length of rib.
- Perform subperiosteal resection of 11th rib, then divide pleura and diaphragm.

IV. THORACIC

A. Esophagus

1. *Heller myotomy*

a. *Indications*: Achalasia—rarely diffuse esophageal spasm.

b. *Instruments*: Finochietto retractor, long Mayo scissors, long Metzenbaum scissors.

c. *Incidental*:

i. *Preop*: get barium swallow, EGD, manometry, NGT.

ii. *Postop*: watch for persistent/recurrent dysphagia, GERD, diaphragmatic hernia, and empyema.

- *Transthoracic approach*:
  - Pt in left lateral position. Incise along 7th intercostal space, divide serratus and latissimus w/ Bovie, then incise along upper border along upper border 8th rib, open pleura along 8th rib, then place Finochietto retractor.
  - Divide inferior pulmonary ligament, then retract left lung cephalad and anterior w/ large moist gauze pads and Harrington retractor.
  - Incise mediastinal pleura overlying distal esophagus. Gently encircle esophagus w/ index finger (feel for NGT), carefully preserving vagus nerves. Free esophagus circumferentially down to diaphragm.
  - *Achalasia*:
    - Place left index finger under distal esophagus. Longitudinally incise both longitudinal and circular muscular layers until mucosa is exposed. Continue this cephalad 2 cm above area where esophagus begins to dilate (at least 5 cm) and caudad to the esophagogastric junction (1–2 veins usu. cross transversely over the mucosa at this point). Do not go > 1 cm onto stomach (may need fundoplication if this occurs).
    - Ensure that at least 50% of mucosal circumference is freed from overlying muscular layer. Running edge of Metzenbaum under muscular layer can help accomplish this. Repair any mucosal laceration w/ interrupted 5-0 nonabsorbable sutures—luminal injection of methylene blue by anesthesiologist can help evaluate for perforation.
  - *Diffuse esophageal spasm*:
    - Perform steps above as for achalasia, but if pt has normal GE junction relaxation, do not extend down to terminal esophagus.
  - *Closure*: bring 30 Fr chest tube through stab wound in 9th intercostal space in anterior axillary line. Approximate ribs w/ 2–3 pericostal sutures of 2-0 Vicryl, then as for standard thoracotomy.

- *Transabdominal approach*:
    - Make upper vertical midline incision to or beyond xiphoid. Dissect to esophagus but do not disrupt hiatus.
    - Resect anterior fat pad. Place caudad traction on abdominal esophagus w/ left hand, and perform 5- to 6-cm anterior vertical esophagomyotomy to the left of the anterior vagus (divide both muscular layers, but not mucosa). W/ fine Pean pinzette, gently separate muscle away from underlying mucosa.
    - Next perform partial fundoplication (i.e., Dor or Toupet).

2. *Esophageal perforation*
    a. *Indications*: any demonstrated esophageal perforation unless clinically asymptomatic, and contrast swallow confirms locally confined leak (no free extravasation to other planes or cavities).
    b. *Incidentals*: broad-spectrum abx begun immediately.
        i. *Cervical*
            - Incise along *left* anterior SCM as for carotid surgery. Close in single layer w/ absorbable monofilament suture if able to find perforation. Reinforce w/ strap muscle flap if questionable viability of repair. Drain w/ closed-suction system whether or not find/repair perforation.

        ii. *Thoracic* (classically have left pleural effusion)
            - *Upper $^2/_3$ lesions*: approach w/ *right* thoracotomy in 5th/6th interspace.
            - *Lower $^1/_3$ lesions*: approach w/ *left* thoracotomy in 6th/7th interspace.
            - If treat w/in 24 h, debride and primarily close in 2 layers (inner absorbable, outer nonabsorbable).
            - *Reinforce repair w/ patch of*: mediastinal pleura flap, strip of diaphragm, stomach wall (Thal patch), or intercostal muscle.
            - Drain mediastinum and pleural space w/ 2 large-bore chest tubes.

        iii. *Abdominal*
            - Once under anesthesia, use flexible endoscopy to evaluate perforation. Make vertical midline incision. Divide left triangular ligament, and gently retract left lobe to the right.
            - Extend muscular defect w/ vertical incision as far as necessary to fully define mucosal lesion. Repair mucosal defect w/ interrupted 4-0 Vicryl, then muscle w/ interrupted 4-0 silk. Insufflate to check for leak. If pt has achalasia, perform esophagomyotomy on opposite side.
            - Buttress repair w/ partial fundic wrap or, if unable to do so, omentum.

3. *Esophagectomy*
    a. *Indications*: cancer of esophagus or gastric cardia.
    b. *Incidentals*: unresectable if there is local invasion to surrounding structures, diffuse peritoneal carcinomatosis, or liver mets.
        i. *Ivor-Lewis esophagectomy—upper abdominal and thoracic approach*:
            - Usu. for tumors in the middle to lower third of the esophagus.
            - Stomach, small bowel, or colon can be used as the replacement conduit.
                - The stomach is prepared leaving the right gastroepiploic and right gastric arteries for blood supply.
                    - The greater curve is mobilized from the spleen medially by dividing the omentum outside the gastroepiploic arcade to preserve the flow to the greater curvature.
                    - The gastrohepatic ligament must be divided and the left gastric artery is ligated.
                    - Pyloroplasty must be done to prevent gastric outlet obstruction (since the vagus nerves are divided).
                - The colon is used if the stomach is not suitable or available. Preop colonoscopy and bowel prep is necessary. Any segment of the colon can be used.
                    - The colon is mobilized as per a colectomy.

        - The greater omentum requires detachment. The vascular pedicles must be preserved and appropriate orientation maintained.
        - Restoration of continuity is a Roux-en-Y.
    - The proximal jejunum is also an option.
        - The vascular arcade must be closely inspected for adequacy and 4 sets of jejunal vessels usu. have to be divided for adequate length.
        - Restoration of continuity is a Roux-en-Y.
- The abdominal portion of the case is completed first.
    - Mobilization of the stomach and intraabdominal esophagus.
    - Preparation of the conduit.
    - Closure of the abdomen.
- The pt is repositioned for the thoracic portion. Dual-lumen endotracheal tube is essential so that single lung ventilation can occur.
    - Thoracotomy via the right 5th intercostal space.
        - The azygous vein must be divided and the mediastinal pleura is opened.
        - The left recurrent laryngeal nerve must be avoided under the arch of the aorta.
        - Sharp dissection to free the esophagus from the aorta.
        - The thoracic duct is ligated in front of the aorta just above the diaphragm.
        - The areolar tissue and the para-aortic lymph nodes are removed w/ the esophagus.
    - Intraabdominal esophagus and conduit are brought up into the chest. Should lie tension free w/in the abdomen.
    - The stomach is divided from the angle of His toward the site on the lesser curvature where the gastric arcade was divided. A linear stapler is used, and multiple firings are often necessary.
    - Esophagus is divided w/ a Satinsky clamp on the proximal portion.
    - End-to-end anastomosis performed, either hand-sewn or w/ a circular stapler.
        - For the stapled method, the anvil is placed in the proximal esophagus. Stay sutures placed circumferentially aid in the anvil insertion.
        - The handle portion is placed through the stomach through a gastrotomy, which is subsequently closed.
    - Thoracotomy closure w/ chest tube drainage.

B. Pulmonary

1. *Instruments*: long pean clamps, Finochietto retractor, lung clamps, Kocher clamps, pledgets, paracostal sutures (2-0 Vicryl w/ large needle), long right-angle clamps/bronchial clamps, long dissecting hemostat, rib approximator, scapular elevator.
    a. *Thoracotomy incision/closure* (Estrera, Johnson's):
        i. *Opening*: mark 2 finger breadths below scapular tip. Incise along this line parallel to ribs w/ knife, anteriorly along inframammary fold (or 6 cm below male nipple). Bovie through latissimus and posterior aspect of serratus until down to rib. Place retractor under scapula, and lift to allow hand underneath to count ribs (cephalad-most palpable rib is the 2nd rib). Bovie along attachment of muscle to top of 6th rib for extent of incision to open pleural space. Place rib retractor (Finochietto) spread ribs. 2 chest tubes should be placed; one w/ a tip at the apex, and another inferior and posterior to the first.
        ii. *Closing*: approximate w/ 6–7 interrupted 2-0 Vicryl sutures around ribs w/ assistance of rib approximator. Next sew fascia together in 2 layers w/ 1-0 PDS. Approximate dermis w/ running 3-0 Vicryl, then staple skin.
    b. *Right upper lobectomy* [Johnson, www.vesalius.com]
        i. *Indications*: peripheral lobar carcinoma w/out hilar LN metastasis.
        ii. *Incidental*: on the right side, pulmonary vein is anterior to pulmonary artery, which is anterior to bronchus.

- Retract lung posteriorly, and open anterosuperior portion of hilar pleura caudal to azygous vein. Dissect out and ligate/divide truncus arterior branch of right pulmonary artery (gives off apical and anterior segmental arteries).
  - *Note*: on the right, the main pulmonary artery remains anterior to the upper lobe bronchus instead of passing posterior to it as on the left.
- Again retract posteriorly, and ligate/divide right superior pulmonary veins, taking care to preserve middle lobe vessels. (Posterior segmental vein may be better appreciated w/ anterior retraction of lung as in step below.)
- Retract lung anteriorly, then divide/open oblique fissure and ligate/divide posterior segmental artery. (Some prefer to switch order of this step w/ the step [bullet point] above.)
- Free up the upper lobe bronchus. (*Note*: there are no major vessels immediately posterior to it as on the left side.) Dissect distally until able to place the proximal bronchus clamp just distal to trifurcation. Suture the 3 segmental bronchi (not the upper lobe bronchus). Usu., it is possible (and recommended) to place a pleural flap over the bronchial stump, often using the relatively mobile pleura cephalad to the hilum, and passing anchoring sutures underneath the azygous vein, ligating that vein in the process.

V. HERNIA/AMPUTATIONS/LYMPHADENECTOMY/PAROTID

A. Herniorrhaphy, inguinal

1. *General notes*
   a. *Three nerves at risk from superior to inferior*: iliohypogastric, ilioinguinal, genital branch of genitofemoral nerve.
   b. May be done under general anesthesia, or w/ local.
      i. Ponka's 7-step approach for local anesthetic [Ponka JL, Seven steps to local anesthesia for repair of inguino-femoral hernia. *Surg Gynecol Obstetr.* July 1963;117:115–20] using 1% lidocaine w/ epinephrine and 25-g needle.
      - 2.5 cm cephalad and just *lateral* to ASIS, inject enough into epidermis to raise a wheal.
      - 5 cc superiorly, horizontally, and inferiorly above and just *lateral* to ASIS and deep to external oblique (find by passing needle just beyond drop in resistance). This will anesthetize ilioinguinal and iliohypogastric nerves.
      - Inject superomedially toward umbilicus to anesthetize 11th thoracic nerve intradermally. Inject toward and inferior to (several cm) ASIS intradermally. Inject along path of proposed incision, across midline, intradermally. [Make skin incision, dissect down to external oblique.]
      - Inject 2 mL every 2 cm along external oblique (just above ligament as well as just above planned incision). (Open external oblique fascia, do not apply undue traction on any structure.)
      - Inject into cord at level of internal ring.
      - Use 20-g needle and inject 5 cc into iliopectineal eminence (if performing McVay's) and pubic tubercle.
      - Anesthetize peritoneum w/ 5 cc of anesthetic.
2. *Anterior approach*
   a. *Exposure*:
      i. Make oblique incision 2 finger breadths cephalad and parallel to inguinal ligament beginning halfway from ASIS to pubis, and ending at level of pubis. Alternately, make equilateral triangle from mid-pubis to edge and apex equal length cephalad then connect w/ a more horizontal, Langer's line to a point slightly more inferior and medial than described above.
      ii. Place self-retaining retractor after get to level of external oblique fascia.
      iii. Locate external ring just cephalad and lateral to pubis. Make superficial stab incision in external oblique fascia (w/ blade up) at lateral extent of incision in line w/ fibers going to external ring. W/ tips up and closed, run Metzenbaum scissors under external oblique fascia to external ring, withdraw, and then w/ jaws locked in semi-open position and lifting up, divide fascia down through ring by gently pushing scissors. Repeat 180° for a few cm.

iv. Grasp each edge of divided external oblique fascia w/ hemostat and pull gently apart to reveal cord underneath. Attempt to identify the ilioinguinal nerve, which is usu. just under the cephalad leaf of divided fascia. Once found, remove hemostat from closest edge of fascia, and retract nerve out of harm's way over fascial edge, then replace hemostat. If interferes w/ dissection, division of nerve is acceptable. Separate upper leaf from underlying muscle/fascia superiorly 3 cm, inferiorly down to shelving edge, and medially 2 cm beyond lateral pubis pubic tubercle.

v. W/ fingers, Kuttner dissector, a/o moist Raytec sponge, isolate and lift up the spermatic cord at the level of the pubic tubercle, then pass Penrose drain around it. Clamp Penrose outstretched so as to expose cord fully.

vi. Divide appropriate amount of cremasteric fibers (Bovie, pulling w/ DeBakey forceps, etc.) longitudinally at the level of the internal ring, to expose indirect sac, which if present, is usu. along the anteromedial aspect of the cord. Begin dissection medially if possible.

vii. Open sac at its apex and reduce the contents. If sac spans entire canal, divide sac, leaving distal remnant open; do not dissect beyond pubic tubercle. Some recommend "fillet" of the distal sac to reduce chances of hydrocele. Close proximal w/ purse-string at base w/ 2-0 silk, then return to peritoneal cavity. If direct sac is found, reduce into peritoneal cavity, and superficially imbricate transversalis fascia over it to keep out of way for subsequent definitive repair. (*Note*: increasingly, some authorities note that simply returning sac into abdomen w/out division does not lead to increased recurrence, and causes less pain.) Evaluate femoral ring through Bogros' space through an opening in canal floor.

viii. Repair hernia w/ method of choice. *If performing Lichtenstein, be sure to skeletonize the floor and pubis w/ good view of shelving edge and pubis (trim out cremasteric and fat) before moving on.*

ix. After completing repair, close external oblique fascia w/ running 3-0 Vicryl. Approximate Scarpa's fascia w/ interrupted sutures of the same, and finally close skin w/ running 4-0 Monocryl (preferred) or Vicryl.

3. *Lichtenstein*

a. *Indications*: standard open approach for inguinal hernia.

b. *Instruments*: #10 blade; #15 blade; Metzenbaum scissors; Weitlaner retractors; small and medium Richardson retractors; 1/2-inch Penrose drain; DeBakey forceps; 2-0 Prolene on SH × 2; 8 × 16 cm polypropylene mesh; 3-0 Vicryl × 1; 4-0 Vicryl × 1; Adson forceps w/ teeth.

i. 8 × 16 cm polypropylene mesh is cut to conform to shape of medial end of canal and narrowed to dimensions of canal (at same time, measure length of slit needed). Create slit in lateral half of mesh dividing mesh into narrow (inferior) 1/3 and wider (superior) 2/3 tails. Position cord between the 2 tails.

ii. Suture rounded corner to fascia sheath over inferior pubic bone, overlapping the rectus sheath by 2 cm (do not suture to periosteum). Run suture laterally w/ lower edge of mesh to shelving edge of inguinal ligament until lateral to internal ring (occasionally pull up shelving edge to make sure it's not just rolled over external oblique or superficial inguinal ligament). *Note*: if femoral hernia present, suture mesh to Cooper's ligament, up to lateral aspect of femoral vein, then transition to inguinal ligament. Similarly, anchor suture above cord, and run along transversus abdominus/conjoined tendon until at level of internal ring. Periodically pull on mesh to flatten it out so that excess redundancy does not exist (some slight wrinkling OK). Alternately, use double-armed 2-0 Prolene at pubis, then run one arm inferiolaterally, the other superolaterally. Some surgeons prefer interrupted 2-0 Ethibond instead.

iii. *Retraction is key while suturing in the mesh*: best results obtained w/ small or medium Richardson retractor toed held from medial part of wound, w/ lip under the cord, lifting it up to expose pubis underneath. After finished medially, follow around edges of wound. Periodically identify the edges of the external oblique—if confused, trace back laterally to where the fascial incision begins.

c. Take upper/wider tail, and cross over the lower tail (both inferior edges now touching), and recreate internal ring by suturing w/ 2-0 Prolene the tails just lateral to the cord, or simultaneously recreate the shutter valve mechanism of the anatomic transversalis sling by suturing the inferior edges of both pieces of mesh to inguinal ligament just lateral to cord.

d. Trim excess lateral mesh, leaving 5 cm lateral to internal ring and tucked flat beneath external oblique aponeurosis. Close external oblique aponeurosis w/ absorbable suture (3-0 Vicryl), followed by Scarpa's (3-0 Vicryl) and skin (4-0 Monocryl/Steri-Strips/Telfa/Tegaderm/staples, etc.).

4. *McVay (Cooper's ligament repair)*
   a. *Indications*: an alternative open repair typically reserved for hernia repair if mesh or prosthetic is unavailable or contraindicated (e.g., contaminated field).
   b. *Instruments*: #10 blade; #15 blade; Metzenbaum scissors; Weitlaner retractors; small and medium Richardson retractors; 1/2-inch Penrose drain; DeBakey forceps; 2-0 Ethibond on SH, CT1 × 10; 3-0 Vicryl × 1; 4-0 Vicryl × 1; Adson forceps w/ teeth.
      i. Completely incise posterior wall of inguinal canal (transversalis fascia) including posterior ring. Retract spermatic cord superiorly w/ Deaver retractor, and clear off Cooper's and lacunar ligaments w/ Kuttner. Often, a thin malleable will be invaluable. Cooper's appears as fascia overlying convex pubic ramus, then runs under more lateral lacunar ligament, which arches superficially to create anterior femoral canal.
      ii. Beginning lateral to femoral vessels, identify femoral sheath (ant. fem. fascia), as well as femoral artery and vein. Dissect out fat and LNs from femoral canal. Divide, ligate crossing tributaries from obturator vessels rarely necessary.
      iii. Open spermatic cord and divide cremasteric fibers at internal ring. Remove fat from cord. Divide external spermatic artery from the inferior epigastric to facilitate moving cord laterally during repair.
      iv. Mobilize transversus abdominus arch (conjoined tendon), then make relaxing incision at line of fusion between external oblique aponeurosis and anterior rectus sheath, beginning at pubic tubercle and going superiorly 9 cm. A fair amount of blunt dissection cephalad to the pubis is necessary to visualize this line. Place pt in Trendelenburg.
      v. Open/explore/close indirect sac if present. Direct sacs may be inverted or excised.
      vi. Invert preperitoneal tissue w/ running 1-0 chromic suture to keep tissue away from repair.
      vii. Beginning at pubic tubercle and ending at medial edge of femoral vein, suture together transversus abdominus arch and Cooper's ligament w/ interrupted sutures (0 or 2-0 Ethibond). Do not tie any of the sutures until steps vii–ix are complete.
      viii. Close femoral canal w/ transition suture from (posterior to anterior) Cooper to medial 1/3 of Lacunar (obliterates excess space in femoral canal) to transversus.
      ix. Approximate the lateral inguinal ligament to transversus abdominus arch until at layer of internal ring, leaving new ring large enough to accept Kelly clamp tip.
      x. Relaxing incision margins may be secured w/ interrupted sutures or Marlex mesh and running 1-0 Prolene suture or left alone.
      xi. Marlex or other mesh may be overlaid as reinforcement.
      xii. Close external oblique, Scarpa's, and skin as described for Lichtenstein repair.

B. Ventral herniorrhaphy

1. *Laparoscopic*
   a. *Setup*: pt supine w/ arms out. Pneumoperitoneum w/ Veress needle in left subcostal position unless prior LUQ surgery (i.e., splenectomy, left colectomy)—RUQ access would then be preferred. Insufflate up to 15 mm Hg of CO_2.
   b. 5-mm angled laparoscope first introduced. Place 2 additional 5-mm ports ipsilateral to laparoscope, fairly far lateral.
   c. Adhesiolysis (sharp a/o blunt—avoid electrocautery) should begin in upper abdomen. Handle bowel w/ soft-jawed instrument.
   d. Bring sac content closer to operator by pressing down on hernia sac from outside.
   e. Divide hernia sac or abdominal wall fascia if encounter excessively dense adhesions w/ bowel.
   f. Inspect bowel for injury after dissection.
   g. *Mesh*:
      i. Gore-Tex dual Adhesiolysis sided mesh advantageous—durable yet minimal adhesive risk to bowel.
   h. Determine appropriate size by passing long spinal needle to define hernia defect edges (mark externally). After marking, deflate abdomen before measuring dimensions; add 2–3 cm to perimeter for overlay.
   i. Cut and orient mesh.

j. Place anchoring sutures at 4 corners, and cut sutures in staggered fashion.
k. Roll mesh (ventral surface inside) from both ends and squeeze to compress.
l. Reinsufflate abdomen and create 2 new 5-mm Adhesiolysis ports on contralateral abdomen.
m. Introduce lubricated mesh through LUQ port site using grasper from contralateral side.
n. Unfold mesh w/ right angle instrument.
o. Pass anchoring sutures through abdominal wall at skin marks (inject local anesthetic at each site)—cut skin w/ #11 blade and then use Gore-Tex suture passer. Inside abdomen, suture then repassed through same skin incision, but different fascial site.
p. Securely tie 4 anchoring sutures.
q. Tack or staple mesh to abdominal wall every 1 cm. Place additional anchoring sutures every 3–4 cm.

C. Amputation

1. Below knee amputation
   a. *Indications*: guillotine amputation should be performed for acutely infected/gangrenous distal lower extremity, followed by 4–5 d of IV abx to clear residual bacteria in skin/lymphatics. "Formal" or "revision" BKA should then be performed. In trauma pts w/ mangled foot, BKA may be performed as a single-stage operation.
   b. *Incidental*: 80% rate of healing if Doppler signal in popliteal artery.
      i. Anterior incision 11 cm below tibial tubercle (so that can transect tibia at 10 cm w/ 1 cm distal overlying skin), carry around anterior 2/3 diameter of calf.
      ii. Bovie through anterior compartment, divide neurovascular structures (see section c. on anatomy below). Divide fibula either at same level or 1 cm proximal to anticipated level of tibial transaction w/ Gigli or power saw. Divide tibia w/ Gigli or power saw, creating anterior bevel. Divide remaining neurovascular structures.
      iii. Posterior incision parallel to long axis. Can either carry all the way to end of wound, or make the length equal to the diameter of the calf at the level of proximal skin incision.
      iv. Regardless of length, prepare posterior myocutaneous flap by bluntly dissecting superficial from deep posterior muscles, then bring up flap and trim to appropriate length. Alternately, can use "cake knife" to create tapered flap w/ fascia all the way to end. No need to fashion bulky muscular "pad" to lie over stump.
   c. *Anatomy*:
      i. *Anterior compartment contains*: anterior tibial artery/vein and deep peroneal nerve along posterior fascia.
      ii. *Deep posterior compartment*: contains posterior tibial artery/vein and tibial nerve along posterior fascia and peroneal artery/vein along medial aspect of fibula.
      iii. *Lateral compartment*: no neurovascular structures.
      iv. *Superficial posterior compartment*: no neurovascular structures, contains gastrocnemius, soleus complex.

D. Lymphadenectomy

1. *Axillary lymphadenectomy*
   a. *Indications*: (+) SLNBx or palpable LAD in breast CA or melanoma.
   b. *Incidental*: main risks include injury to lateral pectoral (motor pectoral), long thoracic (motor serratus anterior), thoracodorsal nerve (motor latissimus dorsi), brachial plexus. Intercostal brachial nerves (purely sensory to medial arm) almost invariably sacrificed.
      i. Incision roughly parallels axillary vein, beginning at lateral aspect of pectoral major and extending to latissimus. Alternately, a shorter, gentle convex-down curvilinear incision along the contour of the hair-bearing skin.
      ii. Dissect superior skin flap up to pectoralis major, fat overlying axillary vein, and latissimus. Dissect inferior skin flap down ~ 8 cm.
      iii. Incise fascia over lateral pectoral fascia, retract pectoralis superomedially to expose coracobrachial muscle. Dissect fat/fascia off inferior surface of muscle. If level III node harvest is indicated, divide pectoralis minor muscle at its insertion.

- *Note*: take care not to injure the medial pectoral nerve (innervates pectoralis major) as it passes medial to minor pectoral muscle.

iv. Incise corococoracoid ligament cephalad to axillary vein, then gently bring down fat to expose axillary vein. Electrocautery in this area risks injury to brachial plexus.

v. Sharply divide adventia over axillary vein, then ligate and divide any inferior branches of the vein. The subscapular vein posteriorly should be preserved.

vi. Vertically incise clavipectoral fascia caudal to axillary vein for ~ 5 cm. Sweep down lymphatics and fat, dividing intercostobrachial nerve as it enters the specimen medially.

vii. Use a Kuttner, sponge stick, or Raytec sponge to sweep fatty tissue down from subscapular space. Identify and preserve the long thoracic nerve as it runs along the thorax as well as the thoracodorsal nerve that (along w/ thoracodorsal vessels) runs parallel and lateral to long thoracic nerve.

viii. Divide any remaining attachments of specimen to latissimus and chest wall. Orient specimen for pathology.

ix. Drain space w/ closed drain via separate puncture wound.

2. *Inguinal and pelvic lymphadenectomy*

a. *Indications*: most frequently melanoma (therapeutic LN dissection for clinically or microscopically [+] LN). Histologically positive Cloquet's node (read below) has historically been used as an indication for pelvic LN dissection, but this has been questioned by recent articles [i.e., Strobbe LJA, et al., *Ann Surg Onc*. 2001;8(3):209–14.]. Some authors now advocate preoperative CT of the pelvis, using imaged pelvic lymphadenopathy as an indication for pelvic dissection. Others assert that palpable inguinal LN metastasis is an acceptable indication. Unlike pts w/ breast cancer, those w/ melanoma who undergo regional lymph node dissection may obtain benefit of prolonged survival.

b. *Incidental*: preop, have pt fitted for Jobst stocking, which should then available in OR.

i. *Inguinal*:

- *Anatomy*:
    - *Superficial inguinal*: defined by "femoral triangle" bounded superiorly by inguinal ligament, medially by adductor longus, and laterally by sartorius. LNs located beneath Camper's fascia above, and cribriform fascia (covers femoral vessels) below.
    - *Deep inguinal*: 3–5 nodes beneath cribriform fascia (read above), medial to femoral vein. The most cephalad of these nodes is usu. under the inguinal ligament and termed Cloquet's node.
- *Incision*: formerly, large vertically oriented flaps were advocated, but assoc. w/ risk of flap necrosis. An oblique, sigmoid incision oriented ~ 1 cm below and along inguinal crease is adequate to expose the boundaries of the femoral triangle. Laterally, begin 2 cm cephalad and just medial to ASIS and end medially 5 cm below medial extent of inguinal ligament. Incision should extend deep enough to reach fascia of abdominal wall.
- *Lymphadenectomy*:
    - Sharply remove fat over adductor longus immediately inferior to inguinal ligament, beginning a finger breadth lateral to pubis, continuing inferiorly to the point where sartorius crosses this muscle. Divide small venous branches as necessary.
    - Divide sartorius fascia, and then work superiorly to remove underlying fat medial to and overlying the sartorius.
    - Dissect and remove remaining lymphatics and fat from femoral triangle, ligating saphenous vein at its confluence w/ the femoral vein. Cloquet's node is generally in femoral canal, underneath inguinal ligament, just medial to femoral vein.
- *Closure*:
    - Divide origin of the sartorius w/ electrocautery, free the proximal 7 cm of the muscle, then swing it medially so that it directly overlies the femoral vessels. Suture end of sartorius to inguinal ligament w/ permanent suture (i.e., 3-0 braided polyester).
    - Place 1–2 bulb-suction drains in wound through stab incisions. Close skin as for similar cases.
    - Place elastic stocking on involved lower extremity after dressing wound.

ii. *Pelvic*:
- *Anatomy*: defined inferiorly by fascia over obturator foramen, and superiorly by bifurcation of common iliac artery (forms a triangle).
- *Incision*: if not already in the area from an inguinal lymphadenectomy, make an incision just lateral to that used for inguinal hernia repair—specifically, ~ 3 cm above inguinal ligament from external ring to ASIS.
- Divide through abdominal wall musculature (and deep inferior epigastric vessels) down to peritoneum. Sweep and retract peritoneum (and ureter) cephalad.
- Remove lymph nodes and adipose tissue overlying external iliac artery and vein (artery will be lateral to and superficial to vein) beginning at inguinal ligament and working cephalad.
- Close any femoral canal defect by suturing inguinal ligament down to Cooper's ligament. Close abdominal wall as for other cases. No drains indicated.

E. **Mastectomy** (can be simple or skin sparing w/ immediate reconstruction)

1. *Indications*: breast cancer in a woman not desiring breast conservation tx, inflammatory breast cancer, tumors involving the chest wall or skin, tumors > 5 cm.
2 *Anatomy*:
   a. The breast tissue extends to the clavicle superiorly, the sternal edge medially, the 2–3 cm below the inframammary fold inferiorly, and the latissimus laterally.
3. *Procedure*:
   a. Prepping usu. includes the entire arm, esp. if completion axillary dissection is anticipated. Pt positioned at the margin of the table.
   b. Mastectomy will often be done w/ a sentinel lymph node biopsy. Skin incision is elliptical and includes the nipple and areola. The orientation and size depend upon the location of the tumor and size of the breast. The lateral corner of the standard incision can be placed to allow the sentinel lymph node biopsy to be done via 1 incision. Try to include the biopsy site if possible, but this is not mandatory.
   c. Sentinel node assessment is done first (see separate description). Completion axillary dissection can be done immediately if the sentinel node is positive.
   d. Skin flaps are then created. Traction on the edges is often achieved w/ Layhey or Allis clamps. The plane between the breast and subcutaneous tissue is usu. developed w/ cautery, but sharp dissection is also used by some surgeons.
   e. The breast is removed from the chest wall w/ the pectoralis fascia included in the specimen. Perforator vessels from the pectoralis to the breast often require ties. Dissection usu. proceeds from superior to medial to inferior w/ the lateral aspect taken last. If axillary dissection is necessary, this can be done so that the breast and axillary contents are removed together.
   f. The specimen is carefully marked or inked for orientation and margin determination.
   g. A 19 French round drain is placed via a separate stab incision and trimmed and positioned under the inferior flap and medially. A 2nd drain would be placed in the axillary bed if a dissection is done.
   h. The skin is closed w/ deep dermal interrupted absorbable sutures followed by a running subcuticular stitch.

F. **Modified radical mastectomy**

1. *Indications*: mastectomy w/ axillary dissection (see separate descriptions).
   a. [Excellent technique using infiltration and creation of skin flaps w/ scissors described in detail by: Shower, et al., *J Surg Onc*. 2003;83:191–3.]

G. **Sentinel lymph node biopsy** (breast)

1. *Indications*: assessing the regional lymph node(s), which receive lymphatic drainage directly from a cancer; currently used for melanomas and breast cancer primarily. Usu. 1–4 nodes are removed.
2. *Instruments*: gamma probe, blue dye (either methylene blue or Lymphazurin).
3. *Incidentals*: lines of Sappey; horizontal (just above umbilicus) and vertical (midline) lines; traditional teaching was that lymphatic drainage would not cross these lines (i.e., a lesion above the umbilical line on the right side would drain to the right axilla; one below would drain to the right groin). In reality, lymphatic drainage is highly variable.

4. *Procedure*: radiocolloid injection done 30 min to 3–4 h beforehand. Lymphoscintigraphy is optional, esp. if a handheld gamma probe will be used intraop.
   a. Injection of blue dye in the operating room in the interstitial space, usu. 5 mL in 1-mL increments. Peritumoral or periareolar injections are advocated. Breast massage for 5 min afterward helps propagate the dye.
   b. Gamma probe used to identify the area of highest counts. In the axilla for breast cancer, this is usu. at the junction of the breast and axilla at the pectoralis edge.
   c. The skin is incised. Subcutaneous blue lymphatics are sometimes noted. Dissection should continue through the clavipectoral fascia. Blue lymphatics can again sometimes be identified.
   d. Gentle dissection should be used to identify a node. Hopefully the node is blue and hot. *In situ* counts should be obtained. The node is isolated from the surrounding tissues, taking care to ligate any lymphatics or vessels leading to it. This can be done w/ clips or ties.
   e. Ex vivo counts should be checked. The node is sent to pathology for immediate frozen or touch prep analysis.
   f. Reassessment of the area to check for additional hot, blue, or palpable nodes. The residual radioactivity should be less than 10% of the ex vivo count. Values higher than that require searching for additional nodes.
   g. Attention is then turned to the cancer excision while the pathologist does the rapid assessment. Findings of cancer in the sentinel nodes mandate completion lymphadenectomy.
   h. The clavipectoral fascia is reapproximated. The wound skin is closed w/ a deep dermal interrupted layer followed by a running subcuticular for the skin.

H. Parotidectomy

1. *Indications*: parotid mass is sufficient indication (FNA, imaging rarely change management; exception is if suspect lymphoma or in pt w/ AIDS). Facial melanoma requiring lymphadectomy may mean parotidectomy as well.
2. *Incidentals*: early in the dissection, one must identify, and, when possible, preserve branches of the facial nerve. Aside from facial nerve injury, potential complications include injury to Stensen's duct (requires repair over cannula) and Frey's syndrome (gustatory sweating) due to aberrant postoperative innervation of cholinergic sweat glands by auriculotemporal nerve.
   a. Begin w/ a Y-shaped incision w/ one limb along anterior ear/tragus, another limb along posterior 1/2 of ear (over mastoid), then joining inferior to lobule and continuing w/ gentle anterior curve anterior to SCM.
   b. Divide platysma, apply skin rakes, and develop anterior skin flap until parotid is seen (may divide superficial fibers over parotid w/ impunity). Dissect cephalad until zygomatic process is reached.
   c. Dissect flap posteriorly to expose EAC cartilage, mastoid, and 2 cm of SCM.
   d. *Identify, preserve the great auricular nerve*: it passes over SCM 3–4 cm inferior to mastoid. Divide branch of this nerve that enters parotid. (External jugular vein is usu. just anterior to this and may be divided/ligated as well.)
   e. *Identify, preserve the facial nerve*:
      i. Tympanomastoid fissure is the recess between the cartilaginous EAC and mastoid process. Sharply divide over tonsil clamp the fascia, which extends from here to the parotid.
      ii. Main trunk of facial nerve is roughly 1 cm anterior to and 1 cm deep to tympanomastoid fissure.
      iii. Bluntly dissect to retract posterior parotid from the mastoid and free the main trunk of the facial nerve. Posterior belly of digastric muscle will be visualized just inferiorly, deep/medial to SCM.
   f. W/ a tonsil clamp or similar instrument, lift up fibrous tissue overlying facial nerve (work proximal to distal) and sharply divide until each of the branches has been cleared of overlying parotid tissue.
   g. Identify Stensen's duct at the anterior margin of the parotid, then ligate and divide it.
   h. Remove the superficial lobe of the parotid.
   i. *If excision of deep lobe indicated*:
      i. Dissect deep lobe free from overlying branches of facial nerve.

ii. Identify the marginal mandibular and the posterior facial vein, which usu. runs inferior to it. Ligate and divide the latter.
iii. Ligate and divide the *superficial temporal artery* and vein just cephalad to the main trunk of the facial nerve.
iv. Retract cephalad the lower aspect of the gland, then ligate and divide the *external carotid artery* as it emerges inferior to the main trunk of the facial nerve.
v. Ligate and divide *internal maxillary* and *transverse facial arteries* at anterior aspect of the deep parotid.
vi. Remove the deep lobe of the parotid.

j. Place small closed-suction drain into the wound bed via separate stab wound posterior to incision.
k. Close platysma, subcutaneous tissue, and skin in separate layers.

VI. TRAUMA/CRITICAL CARE

A. Burn surgery (acute)

1. *Excision*:
   a. Traditionally recommended to not excise more than 20% BSA at a time, but this has been challenged. First surgery should be w/in 72 h of injury.
   b. *Preparation*: to minimize bleeding, tourniquet or clysis (solution of 1 L LR w/ 30 mg neosynephrine) should be utilized.
   c. *Tangential* (w/ Humby or Weck blade): usual means of excising tissue. Excise down to healthy yellow fat w/ no thrombosed vessels (preferable), or at least to white (not purple/hemorrhagic) dermis.
   d. *Fascial* (w/ Bovie): for deep/4th-degree burns. Cut down to fascia. Minimizes bleeding, but leaves considerable cosmetic defect.
   e. *Dressing*: consider use of biologic (allograft, xenograft) or synthetic (Alloderm, Biobrane, TransCyte).

B. Celiotomy, trauma exploratory

1. *Insights*: be systematic in approach, and know when to employ damage control techniques. Remain in conversation w/ anesthesiologist about pt's physiology.
   a. Vertical midline incision, ideally "w/ 3 passes of scalpel"—linea alba usu. thinnest just above umbilicus. Can use scissors to continue once have hand inside peritoneal cavity.
   b. If blunt mechanism, pack off all quadrants first.
   c. If penetrating, direct attention to path of injury.
   d. *Kocher maneuver*: incise peritoneum lateral to duodenum C-loop, then lift up pancreatic head.
   e. *Cattel-Braasch maneuver*: perform Kocher, then continue by mobilizing right colon along white line of Toldt, and then continue dividing peritoneum from cecum toward ligament of Treitz. Provides excellent exposure for inframesocolic hemorrhage (infrarenal IVC and aorta, both kidneys).
   f. *Mattox maneuver*: medial rotation of left colon, followed by extension of cephalad, lateral to spleen, rotating spleen +/– kidney, then dividing left crus of diaphragm, affording exposure of aorta potentially from T-6 to supraceliac region. Excellent exposure for supramesocolic hemorrhage.
      i. Alternate means to rapidly gain access to supraceliac aorta is by making hole in lesser omentum and applying direct pressure.

C. Escharotomy

1. *Indication*: to release circumferentially constricting eschars from burns, which compromise circulation (in extremities or respiration [chest]).
2. *Instruments*: scalpel or electrocautery (latter useful as significant bleeding may occur).
3. *Incidentals*: as involved regions typically have full-thickness injury, anesthesia is generally unnecessary.
   a. *Upper extremities*:
      i. *Arms/forearms*: along medial and lateral aspects, staying anterior to epicondyles at elbow.
      ii. *Hands*:
         - *Fascial escharotomy*:
            - Thenar and hypothenar eminences.
            - Radial aspect of each finger, staying dorsal to neurovascular bundle (located just volar to mid-axis).

- Ulnar aspect of thumb, dorsal to neurovascular bundle (located just volar to mid-axis).
- Over each of the 3 interosseous spaces of the dorsal hand.

- *Tangential escharectomy*: involved tissue may be excised under tourniquet control for hemostasis.

b. *Lower extremities*:
   i. *Thigh/calf*: along medial and lateral aspects, staying anterior to malleoli at ankle.
   ii. *Foot*: medial and lateral aspects along long axis (separate incision from above).

c. *Chest*: along mid-axillary line bilaterally (from upper arm to distal flank), connecting to incision arching along subcostal line.

D. Fasciotomy

1. *Indications*: extremity compartment syndrome, manifested by the classic "P" mnemonic: **p**ain, **p**aralysis, **p**aresthesias, **p**oikilothermia (coolness), **p**allor, **p**ulselessness. Pain (particularly w/ passive extension) out of proportion to anticipated level w/ a suitable mechanism or risk factor is the only finding that is not a very late finding—one should not wait for the other signs to manifest before taking action. Objective measurements that buttress the case for fasciotomy include compartment pressure ≥ 30, a narrowed difference between the diastolic pressure and the compartment pressure (hypotensive pts at higher risk), or a trend of increasing compartment pressure. Note that compartment pressures can vary significantly in a given compartment in relation to site of maximal injury (i.e., fracture).
2. *Risk factors and markers*: fractures (esp. tib/fib, calcaneal, humeral), crush injuries, circumferential burns, massive resuscitation, hypotension, myoglobinuria (esp. w/ sediment), extremity ischemia > 4 h.

a. *Lower extremity*:
   i. *Anatomy*
      - *4 compartments* (calf):
        - Anterior
        - Lateral
        - Superficial posterior
        - Deep posterior
   ii. *Technique* (2 incisions, each ~ 15–20 cm, can access all 4 compartments)
      - Medial incision 2 finger breadths posteror to tibia down to, through fascia (sup post/deep post).
      - Lateral incision 1 finger breadth anterior to fibula down to, through fascia, avoid injury to peroneal nerve (ant/lat).

b. *Upper extremity*:
   i. *Anatomy*
      - *3 compartments* (forearm):
        - *Anterior forearm* (flexor compartment):
          - *Superficial*: pronator teres, pronator quadratus, palmaris longus, FDS, FCU, FCR; *Deep*: FPL, FDP.
        - *Posterior forearm* (extensor compartment): abductor pollicis longus, EPB, EPL, EIP, EDQ, ECU.
        - *Mobile wad*: brachioradialis, ECRB, ECRL.
   ii. *Forearm technique*
      - "Classic" incision is curvilinear from medial elbow over to radial forearm (for mobile wad), then back ulnar, before curving radialward again to continue as carpal tunnel release.
      - *Alternatively, 3 lesser incisions can be made*: 1 longitudinal over posterior extensors, a 2nd longitudinal along ulnar border of anterior surface (can retract FCU anteriorly to expose ulnar and median nerves and directly visualize deep group), and a 3rd for the carpal tunnel release.

iii. *Hand technique*
   - 10 compartments (4 dorsal interossei, 3 volar interossei, adductor pollicis, thenar, hypothenar).
   - Incise over 2nd and 4th metacarpals then bluntly dissect along each w/ hemostat. Repeat over thenar and hypothenar eminences.

iv. *Fingers*: exceedingly rarely indicated. If performed, longitudinal incisions just dorsal to midaxial line to avoid injury to digital nerve and artery.

E. Liver

1. *Total vascular isolation*: particularly useful for retrohepatic hemorrhage.
   a. Begin w/ Pringle maneuver (clamp the hepatoduodenal ligament, which contains hepatic artery and portal vein, w/ avascular clamp, finger, or Rommel tourniquet). Usu. stops bleeding if not retrohepatic.
   b. Gain access to infrahepatic, suprarenal IVC via Kocher maneuver.
   c. Gain access to supradiaphragmatic IVC via median sternotomy, followed by opening pericardium . . .
   d. *Atriocaval shunt*: expose intrapericardial and suprarenal IVC, encircle both w/ Rommel tourniquet, incise right atrial appendage, and span venous defect w/ 34 Fr chest tube or #8 ETT. Pursestring appendage, tighten tourniquets.
2. *Intraparenchymal adjuncts*:
   a. Mobilize and compress.
   b. Pack.
   c. Surgicel.
   d. Bovie a/o argon beam coagulation.
   e. Hepatorrhaphy w/ chromic suture.
   f. Tamponade tract w/ Foley catheter w/ Penrose drain tied over it and distended w/ saline.
   g. Finger/Pean clamp fracture w/ clamping and ligation of vessels.

F. Pericardial window

1. *Indication*: pericardial fluid visualized on U/S or based on clinical suspicion in unstable pt.
   a. Midline incision 2 cm cephalad to xiphoid continued 3–5 cm below xiphoid.
   b. Retract xiphoid w/ Army-Navy, bluntly dissect tissue down off left inferior rib margin next to xiphoid.
   c. Grasp pericardium w/ 2 Allis clamps, and incise.
   d. If nonclotting blood returns, convert to median sternotomy.

G. Spleen

1. *Splenectomy*
   a. *Indications*: see Chapter 18.
   b. *Instruments*: Balfour, Metzenbaum, laparotomy pads.
      i. Pt supine, rotated 10–15° to pt's right. Surgeon on pt's right. Headlamp, NGT recommended.
      ii. Midline incision from xiphoid to ~ 4 cm below umbilicus.
      iii. Unless pt is massively hemorrhaging, begin to mobilize spleen by first dividing splenocolic ligament (usu. avascular), aided by gentle downward traction on the colon.
         - If do encounter massive hemorrhage, can access splenic vessels through lesser sac, and manually compress.
      iv. Next, gentle medial retraction exposes splenorenal ligament (avascular). Divide from caudad to cephalad, continuing on to divide splenophrenic ligament (judicious downward traction facilitates dissection of latter).
      v. Insinuate fingers of left hand over spleen into plane below pancreatic tail, but anterior to Gerota's fascia—mobilize medially/anteriorly w/ blunt/finger dissection.
      vi. Once spleen is mobilized somewhat, pack posteriorly w/ laparotomy pads before dividing gastrosplenic ligament.
      vii. Gently retract spleen downward and stomach medially to expose gastrosplenic ligament. Divide short gastric vessels in continuity using Mixter clamp and 2-0 silk.
      viii. Irrigate off or gently pick off clot to assess damage.
      ix. If decide to perform splenectomy, isolate splenic vessels, doubly ligate in continuity (or stick tie) and divide.

2. *Splenorrhaphy*
    a. *Instruments*: JP drain (if pancreatic tail injury).
        i. Expose the spleen as described above in "splenectomy."
        ii. *Salvage options*:
            - *Grade I*: tamponade w/ lap pad, topical hemostatic agents *(small, nonexpanding hematoma or superficial, nonbleeding laceration)*.
            - *Grade II*: achieve hemostasis w/ electrocautery, sutures (running closure of capsure, tie off vessel ends, etc.), or clips. Hemostatic agent packing may also help *(10–50% SA, nonexpanding hematoma or actively bleeding parenchymal laceration)*.
            - *Grade III*: may incise over large subcapsular hematomas, evacuate clot, and methods above *(expanding or ruptured subcapsular hematoma or deep parenchymal laceration w/out splenic devascularization)*.
            - *Grade IV*: splenic resection, deep sutures, debridement by finger fracture; retracted vessel bleeding gets horizontal mattress sutures + hemostatic agent, possibly omental patching; deep stellate lacs → try to wrap in mesh; horizontal mattress suturing w/ pledgets useful for hemostasis of a resected/avulsed end *(ruptured intraparenchymal hematoma or laceration through polar trabecular arteries w/ avascular segment)*.
            - *Grade V*: splenectomy *(near total maceration or severe hilar injury w/ avulsion of splenic artery)*.

H. Tracheostomy

1. Transverse incision below cricoid cartilage approx. 2 finger breadths above sternal notch.
2. Afterward make longitudinal incisions in midline.
3. Divide thyroid isthmus if necessary.
4. Trachea hook helps retract cephalad if trachea is deep—place on base of thyroid or cricoid cartilage.
5. Transverse incision between 2nd and 3rd tracheal rings; place lateral "stay" sutures.
6. If pt already intubated, gradually back out ETT and insert tracheostomy tube when ETT tube cephalad to tracheostomy. Use of tracheal spreader or right-angle clamps can help guide tube.
7. Most feared delayed complication is tracheoinnominate fistula.
    a. Can attempt to place larger balloon to tamponade.
    b. Can perform Utley maneuver, applying pressure to artery manually, followed by median sternotomy and ligation.

I. Thoracotomy

1. *Emergency department*
    a. Supine position.
    b. Incise from xiphoid to latissimus along left 4th intercostals spac down to intercostal muscles.
    c. Cut through intercostals along top of rib w/ heavy curved Mayo scissors.
    d. Retract lung inferiorly, lift up pericardium w/ toothed forceps and incise anterior to phrenic nerve.
    e. *Additional maneuvers of potential utility*: 2-hand cardiac massage, Satinsky clamp across descending aorta (retract lung anteriorly for this), clamp pulmonary hilum for hemorrhage, clamp across tracheobronchial injury.

VII. PEDIATRIC

A. Congenital diaphragmatic hernia

1. Subcostal transverse incision.
2. Pull herniated contents back into peritoneal cavity.
3. Primarily close defect if possible w/ interrupted permanent sutures. If unable to close primarily, repair w/ patch.

B. Ladd's procedure

1. Midline vertical incision.
2. Devolve bowel if twisted.

3. Divide Ladd's bands over duodenum (extend from hepatic flexure to right upper abdominal wall) to free right colon.
4. Place cecum in LUQ, +/– suture to splenic flexure of colon.
5. Remove appendix.

C. Pyloromyotomy

1. Ensure pt is adequately resuscitated (normal potassium, bicarb < 30).
2. Make transverse incision in RUQ w/ 15 blade, then Bovie down to anterior abdominal wall. Lift up abdominal musculature, and w/ Bovie, make longitudinal incision about the same length as the skin incision. Open into peritoneal cavity w/ hemostat.
3. Grasp the enlarged pylorus and pull into wound.
4. Lightly incise the serosa of pylorus in longitudinal fashion w/ 15 blade from just proximal to pylorus to just proximal to vein of Mayo. Gently distract underlying muscle fibers w/ Benson spreaders until down to mucosa for length of incision.
5. Return pylorus to peritoneal cavity and close abdomen.

D. Tracheoesophageal fistula (technique for esophageal atresia and distal TE-fistula)

1. After intubation, place 18 Fr red rubber catheter in esophageal pouch to aid in location.
2. Place in lateral position for right thoracotomy.
3. Incise through 4th intercostals space to achieve an extrapleural approach.
4. Perform pleural dissection sharply to cephalad lung apex, caudad several rib spaces, and posteriorly to spine.
5. Divide IC veins and retract azygous vein anteriorly. Identify the vagus nerve.
6. Place umbilical tape around distal esophagus and dissect to location of fistula; divide fistula, and close trachea w/ 5-0 permanent suture.
7. Mobilize esophageal ends, and perform end-to-end, single-layer anastomosis.
8. Place retropleural chest tube away from anastomosis.
9. Close in layers as for thoracotomy.

VIII. OB/GYN

A. Total abdominal hysterectomy

1. *Indication*: most often for the general surgeon, uterine involvement in intraabdominal malignancies. Gynecologic indications include myomata, endometriosis, endometrial carcinoma, or prolapse.
2. *Instruments*: Balfour retractor, tenaculum, Kocher or Ochsner clamps, Allis or Teale clamps.
   a. Place Foley catheter and prep abdomen, perineum, and vagina.
   b. Lower midline or Pfannenstiel's incision (latter not indicated if large uterus or exploration of abdomen anticipated) is used on the skin, then fascia is divided inferiorly down to symphysis.
   c. After entering the abdomen, pack small bowel cephalad using moist laparotomy pads and place self-retaining retractor.
   d. If possible, grasp uterus w/ tenaculum and pull cephalad. Grasp peritoneum over cervicovesical fold and divide transversely w/ scissors, exposing distal uterus beneath.
   e. Run nondominant index finger underneath ovarian vessels and fallopian tube, then up through posterior leaf of broad ligament to emerge in space created by peritoneal division in step d. At this point, the tube and ovarian vessels are encircled by the finger.
   f. Clamp adjacent infundibulopelvic (supports ovary and contains ovarian vessels) and round (supports uterus) ligaments w/ Kocher or Ochsner clamps bilaterally flush w/ the uterine edge, then divide and suture ligate them w/ 2-0 suture.
   g. Under the divided peritoneum, bluntly dissect anteriorly and displace bladder caudad, facilitating palpation of cervix anteriorly and posteriorly. Dissect rectum off of posterior vaginal wall if adherent.
   h. Apply Kocher or Oscher clamps to both sides of distal uterus/proximal cervix, incorporating a small amount of cervical tissue in order to ensure complete occlusion of uterine vessels. Clamps are angled 45° caudad to avoid injury to ureters. Divide uterine vessels between clamps and doubly ligate.

i. Apply Allis or Teale forceps to paracervical tissue between cervix and stumps of uterine vessels. Rotate uterus anteriorly and divide posterior peritoneum and wall of vagina w/ scissors adjacent to the cervix. Continue incision anteriorly until specimen is free.

j. Approximate anterior and posterior vaginal walls w/ forceps used in step i., then sew together after first placing 2-0 absorbable, figure-of-eight stitches at the lateral corners of the vaginal vault.

k. Return intestines to pelvis, then close peritoneum, fascia, and skin.

B. Caesarean section

1. *Indications*: imminent fetal demise during labor, 42-wk intrauterine pregnancy, failed induction.
2. *Instruments*: #10 scalpel, Kocher clamp, Metzenbaum and Mayo scissors, bladder blade retractor.
3. *Positioning*: pt supine, tilted slightly to left.
4. *Incision*: Pfannenstiel skin incision w/ knife, continue down to fascia w/ Bovie.
   a. Incise fascia in midline, then extend laterally w/ Mayo scissors.
5. *Dissection*: grasp superior fascia w/ Kocher clamps, and bluntly dissect away from underlying muscles.
   a. Repeat w/ inferior fascia and abdominal muscles.
   b. Incise peritoneum vertically to expose bladder, then insert bladder blade retractor.
   c. Identify vesicouterine peritoneum, grasp, and divide w/ Metzenbaum scissors.
   d. Extend incision laterally and create bladder flap w/ finger.
6. *Delivery*: reinsert bladder blade and incise lower uterine segment transversely w/ scalpel.
   a. Extend incision laterally w/ heavy scissors.
   b. Remove bladder blade and deliver infant head.
   c. Suction nose and mouth, cut and clamp cord, hand infant off.
7. *Closure*: remove placenta, exteriorize uterus and clear of debris.
   a. Repair uterus w/ 2 layers of running, locked 1-0 chromic gut suture.
   b. Repair bladder flap w/ running 3-0 Vicryl, then return uterus to abdomen.
   c. Do not repair peritoneum.
   d. Close fascia w/ #1 PDS placed in running fashion.
   e. Close skin using surgeon's preference.

IX. VASCULAR EXPOSURES AND OPERATIONS

A. General principles

1. *Anastomosis, vascular*
   a. Systemically heparinize when able.
   b. Obtain proximal and distal control.
   c. Heparin flush periodically.
2. *AV fistulas*
   a. Use veins w/ internal diameter of at least 3 mm.
3. *Exposures below indebted to following sources*:
   a. Valentine RJ, Wind GG, *Anatomic Exposures in Vascular Surgery*, 2nd ed. Philadelphia: Lippincott Williams & Wilkins; 2003.
   b. Ouriel K, Rutherford RB, *Atlas of Vascular Surgery*. Philadelphia: WB Saunders Co.; 1998.
   c. Thal ER, Weigelt JA, Carrico CJ, *Operative Trauma Management*. New York: McGraw-Hill Professional; 2001.

B. Regional exposures

1. *Neck*
   a. *Carotid*
      i. *Zone I*: prepare for median sternotomy.
      ii. *Zone II*: incise along anterior border of SCM w/ head rotated away, curving slightly posterior once near marginal mandibular nerve (toward the mastoid process below the earlobe-leave earlobe prepped in for landmarking). Continue through platysma and deep

cervical fascia. Ligate branch of superior thyroid artery as necessary. Preserve CN XI as it enters the SCM in superior part of exposure. Vascular sheath is then identified, and then divide the facial vein to facilitate retracting IJ vein posteriorly along w/ SCM. Carotid artery is then visualized. The facial vein provides a good general landmark for the carotid bifurcation.

iii. *Zone III*: difficult to expose, and many maneuvers have been described. Consider nasotracheal intubation in order to sublux ipsilateral mandibular condyle (fix w/ transnasal or transoral wire). Incise as for zone II, and extend superiorly and posteriorly behind earlobe. One may divide posterior belly of digastric to visualize last 2 cm of internal carotid before it dives into skull base. Further exposure requires resection of styloid (and, along w/ it, stylohyoid ligament, stylopharyngeus, and styloglossus muscles). Of note, exposure of the distal ICA puts the glossopharyngeal nerve at great risk.

b. *Vertebral artery*

i. *V1* (subclavian origin to C6):

- *Supraclavicular approach* (usu. elective cases): w/ head turned away, incise 1 cm above and parallel to clavicle from clavicular head for ~ 8 cm. Continue through platysma and superficial fascia, then divide EJ vein at lateral SCM. Divide the clavicular head of the SCM and retract the clavicular head medially, exposing the carotid sheath. The carotid sheath should be opened and the carotid and IJ mobilized to facilitate medial retraction w/ the SCM. W/ medial retraction, the scalene fat pad can be mobilized medially exposing the anterior scalene (take care to preserve the phrenic nerve). The vertebral artery should be at the medial border of the anterior scalene muscle. The nerve can be followed superiorly w/ this dissection until it becomes intraosseous.
- *Anterior cervical approach* (usu. emergency cases): w/ head turned away, incise along full length of anterior SCM, through platysma and overlying fascia down to SCM, which is retracted laterally. Divide superior belly of omohyoid. Carefully dissect and then retract medially the carotid sheath/contents. Scalene fat pad is mobilized on medial aspect then retracted laterally as well. Anterior scalene should now be visible w/ phrenic nerve overlying it ventrally. Next, ligate and divide the inferior thyroid artery along the medial border of the anterior scalene. The vertebral artery should be apparent after laterally retracting the anterior scalene.

ii. *V2* (intraosseous: transverse processes of C6–C2): this segment is generally treated by endoluminal means, but exposure is possible w/ resection of the anterior aspect of the canal using bone rongeurs.

iii. *V3* (transverse process C2 to base of skull): rarely needed w/ advent of endoluminal. Incision similar to anterior surgical approach w/ the superior curvilinear portion of the incision extending further posterior and behind the mastoid process. SCM can be completely divided below the mastoid to facilitate the exposure, but great care should be taken not to injure the spinal accessory nerve that will be in the field at that level. The prevertebral fascia can then be opened parallel to the spinal accessory nerve. The nerve should then be carefully retracted anteriorly and the levator scapulae and splenius cervicis muscles divided as close to their insertion on the transverse process of C1 as possible. Excision of these muscles over the C1/C2 interspace will expose that portion of the vertebral artery for a short distance.

iv. *V4* (intracranial: atlantooccipital membrane to basilar artery): rarely needed exposure w/ advent of endoluminal therapies, can be obtained w/ the pt in the prone position and the head turned away. A curvilinear incision is made starting at the occipital protuberance toward the mastoid process and then inferiorly along the posterior border of the SCM. The deep fascia/muscle fibers of the underlying muscles (trapezius, splenius capitis, semispinalis capitis, and longissimus capitis) should be divided. The occipital nerve may be seen and can be divided as necessary to facilitate exposure. The SCM should be divided near its insertion on the mastoid process and the IJ and spinal accessory nerve exposed in the lateral portion of the wound. The transverse process of C1 should be apparent w/ palpation and the condyloid emissary vein can be divided. The rectus capitis can be divided transversely in the medial portion of the wound, which will expose the vertebral artery. The artery will be surrounded by a dense venous plexus at this level, which will require meticulous division for mobilization of the artery.

2. *Thorax*

a. *Subclavian*: for proximal left subclavian, a left anterolateral or posterolateral thoracotomy is used. For proximal right subclavian, a median sternotomy w/ supraclavicular extension may be useful. For more distal exposure on either side, a supraclavicular incision +/– mid-clavicular resection is optimal.

b. *Heart*: median sternotomy, unless unstable, then left anterolateral thoracotomy is faster, and a "clamshell" thoracotomy can be performed for further exposure (extension of the thoracotomy across the sternum using a Lebsche knife, Gigli saw, or other suitable instrument). The internal mammary arteries will require ligation w/ this exposure.

c. *Thoracic aorta*: left anterolateral (emergent) or posterolateral thoracotomy (ideal).

3. *Upper extremity*

a. *Brachial artery* (#10 blade, Weitlaner/Gelpi retractors, small and medium vessel loops, 3-0/4-0 silk ties, right angle clamps, thin malleable retractors).

b. *Arm*

i. Axillary artery becomes brachial artery lateral to the teres major muscle. Proximally, a deep brachial artery branch comes off to anastomose around the elbow w/ the recurrent radial artery. The brachial artery rarely branches into duplicate arteries high in the arm.

ii. Pt in supine position w/ arm abducted 90° on board. Keep hand/forearm in stockinette.

iii. Incise 5–8 cm along medial groove in arm between biceps and triceps w/ extension across the proximal forearm in a "lazy S" fashion. Basilic vein may be encountered in distal 1/2 of arm, and should be retracted posteriorly (ligate crossing branches).

iv. Incise deep fascia along medial/posterior biceps, which is retracted anteriorly (watch for basilic v. medial/posterior to this and retract *posteriorly* if necessary). Median nerve is most superficial structure in brachial sheath, and should be retracted *anteriorly*.

v. Brachial artery will be deep to median nerve, w/ 2 brachial veins running parallel and ulnar nerve posteriorly. Ligate crossing veins as necessary. Occasionally, brachial artery will bifurcate high in the arm w/ double arteries running through the usual location.

c. *Antecubital fossa*

i. Brachial artery bifurcates at radial tuberosity, distal to elbow joint, w/ radial artery continuing in-line, and ulnar artery branching almost perpendicularly.

ii. 4 cm transverse/oblique skin incision 1 cm distal to mid-antecubital fossa if narrow segment needed ("Lazy S"). For wider exposure, a sigmoid incision running from distal medial border to biceps, curving radial/lateral across flexor crease, then turning longitudinal again for ~ 4 cm lateral to mid-volar forearm.

iii. Dissecting through skin, look for basilic vein and retract medially along w/ medial antebrachial cutaneous nerve.

iv. Divide bicipital aponeurosis to expose brachial artery, flanked by 2 deep veins and their branches.

d. *Forearm branches* (radial and ulnar arteries)

i. *Radial artery* (supplies deep arch in hand)

- Pt supine, arm abducted 90°, 5-cm longitudinal incision made over area of interest; follow line from midpoint of antecubital crease to styloid process of radius (corresponds w/ groove on medial brachioradialis).
- Divide/ligate subcutaneous veins, deepen wound, incise antebrachial fascia along medial border of brachioradialis.
- *Proximal/middle 1/3 of forearm*: radial artery underneath medial fibers of brachioradialis —retract this muscle laterally and (FCR distally, pron. teres proximally) medially apart for access. Watch for/preserve superficial radial nerve along lateral aspect of radial artery in middle 1/3 of forearm. Separate paired veins as necessary.
- *Distal 1/3 of forearm*: radial artery lies beneath antebrachial fascia between tendons of brachoradialis and flexor carpi radialis. (Radial and ulnar arteries lie just radial to their respective flexor tendons, FCR and FCU.) Separate paired veins as necessary.

ii. *Ulnar artery* (supplies superficial arch in hand)

- Pt supine, arm supinated, hand slightly flexed.
- *Proximal 1/3 forearm*: incise 9 cm beginning 4 finger breadths distal medial epicondyle of humerus, along line from medial epicondyle to pisiform. Ligate superficial veins, incise

antebrachial fascia entire length of exposure. Ulnar artery will be in plane between FCU and FDS muscles (often bound in fascia to FDP); retract FDS radially/laterally to expose. *Note*: proximally, ulnar artery gives off common interosseous artery.

- *Middle 1/3 of forearm*: ulnar artery deep to FCU; retract muscle medially/ulnarly to expose. Watch for/preserve ulnar nerve just medial/ulnar to artery bound to FDP fascia.
- *Distal 1/3 of forearm*: make longitudinal incision just radial/lateral to FCU tendon; artery just beneath antebrachial fascia. Watch for/preserve palmar branch of ulnar nerve superficial to antebrachial fascia here.

4. *Abdomen*
   a. *Aorta*: transabdominal access to the aorta can be achieved by the following:
      i. Midline vertical incision is fast and generally preferred, although transverse abdominal is used by some to diminish pulmonary compromise.
         - Bring up transverse colon and greater omentum, rest them on lower ribs. Small bowel then brought to right, then packed off in abdomen or eviscerated.
         - Make longitudinal incison along base of mesentery along right side of aorta halfway between aorta and IVC to avoid excessive tissue. Duodenum lies over upper infrarenal aorta, and will require mobilization from its retroperitoneal attachments to exposure the aorta at the elvel of the renal vein.
         - Lymphatic-rich tissue surrounding left renal vein should be divided in continuity. IMV may need to be divided before joining the splenic vein as it courses from left to right superiorly. Be wary of potential retroaortic left renal vein (this should be identified on the preoperative CT when possible).
         - After identifying left renal vein, move caudad by dividing the retroperitoneal tissue overlying the aorta down to the iliac arteries. In young males, attempt to avoid dividing tissue from distal aorta to over left common iliac artery to avoid retrograde ejaculation from injured sympathetic fibers. The IMA will be encountered in the mid-abdomen and should be controlled or divided when appropriate.
      ii. *Supraceliac*:
         - Left medial visceral rotation (Mattox maneuver), divide lesser omentum, retract esophagus to left. An NGT should be placed prior to this to facilitate identification of the esophagus.
         - Retract stomach and transverse colon away from each other, divide lesser omentum.
      iii. *Infraceliac*:
         - Right medial visceral rotation (Cattell-Braasch maneuver). The IVC, right kidney and renal vein will be overlying the aorta from the right side and will require mobilization for exposure of the aorta/right renal vein.
   b. *IVC*:
      i. *Suprahepatic*: requires mobilization of the liver for caudad retraction to see the IVC at the top of the liver entering the chest through the diaphragm. The falciform ligament as well as the right and left triangular ligaments must be divided for full mobilization. Care should be taken not to injure the left hepatic vein when freeing the left hepatic ligament as this will be the first structure encountered when lysing that ligament.
      ii. *Infrahepatic*: perform a Cattell-Braasch maneuver (hepatic flexure mobilization and Kocher maneuver) to expose the infrahepatic IVC as well as the right kidney w/ its associated vein and artery.
   c. *Iliacs*: the iliac arteries can be exposed through a transabdominal incision (midline celiotomy vs transverse abdominal incision) or through retroperitoneal incisions. When exposing through a midline incision, the small bowel is reflected toward the right and the retroperitoneal tissue overlying the aorta and the iliac arteries should be divided to expose the vessels. The ureters cross anterior to the iliac arteries at the pelvic brim. These should be identified, mobilized, and carefully protected during the procedure. The periadventitial tissue overlying the aortic bifurcation and left CIA should be preserved in men when possible as division of this can lead to ejaculatory dysfunction. Circumferential dissection of the iliac arteries can lead to iliac vein injury, and should be avoided unless specifically needed for exposure of the iliac veins or iliac artery reconstruction. If the CIA is not adequately exposed, the sigmoid colon can be mobilized from its retroperitoneal attachments and reflected medially to expose more of the left iliac

arteries as necessary. Retroperitoneal incisions can be performed w/ an oblique incision in the right or left lower quadrant or a paramedian incision w/ division of the anterior rectus sheath and medial retraction of the rectus muscle and abdominal contents for exposure of the retroperitoneal plane. When using an oblique or transverse incision, the retroperitoneal plane is best entered laterally as the peritoneum tends to be adherent to the transversalis fascia toward the midline. The abdominal contents and the ureter should be reflected medially off of the vessels.

5. *Lower extremity*
   a. *Popliteal artery* (#10 blade, Weitlaner retractor, small and medium vessel loops, 3-0/4-0 silk ties, right-angle clamps).
   b. *Medial suprageniculate*
      i. *Indication*: preferred for distal anastomosis of fem-pop bypass *if* no distal dz (rarely occurs).
         - Pt supine, leg externally rotated, knee flexed 30°.
         - Incise distal 1/3 of medial thigh along anterior border of sartorius, then incise fascia over sartorius before retracting the muscle posteriorly. Popliteal artery may be seen by retracting vastus medialis anteriorly. Distally, some division of fascial bridge between the anterior adductor and posterior semimembranosus may help expose artery as well. Proximally, division of part of adductor magnus tendon may be needed for exposure as artery passes deep to it.
         - Attempt to preserve highest geniculate artery and saphenous branch of femoral nerve.
         - Artery will be encased in fibrous sheath, and medial to vein(s), which may have communicating branches requiring division.
   c. *Medial infrageniculate*
      i. *Indication*: most common site actually used for fem-pop bypass.
         - Pt supine, leg externally rotated, knee flexed 30°.
         - Incise longitudinally 1 cm posterior to posterior tibial border, 1/3 down the calf beginning at posterior aspect of medial tibial condyle, w/ precautions to preserve greater saphenous vein, usu. by posterior retraction (can ligate branches as needed).
         - Incise crural fascia 1 cm posterior to tibia, extending proximally to semitendinosus m. (distal—most of the 3 muscles that insert onto the pes anserinus: semitendinosus, gracilis, sartorius, semimembranosus).
         - Posteriorly retract medial gastrocnemius to expose neurovascular sheath—divide soleus off tibia if need to (if need more proximal exposure, can divide the 3 pes anserinus muscles, but must reapproximate at end of case; for distal exposure, divide tibial attachments of soleus).
         - Open neurovascular sheath, encountering popliteal vein first, often paired. Divide communicating veins to get access to artery, which may be elevated w/ vessel tapes. Preserve the posteromedial tibial nerve.
   d. *Posterior*
      i. *Indication*: disadvantage—need to be prone; difficult to get proximal extension.
         - Useful for reoperative cases as well as popliteal entrapment syndrome, cystic adventitial dz, traumatic intimal flaps from posterior dislocation, and local aneurysms.
         - Pt prone, knee slightly flexed.
         - Sigmoid incision (longitudinal, begin medially, then transverse across fossa, then longitudinal and lateral) is made, ligating and dividing the short/lesser saphenous vein, which runs longitudinally in the subcutaneous fossa.
         - Incise deep fascia vertically, and laterally retract the medial sural nerve revealing the underlying vertical tibial nerve. The peroneal nerve is more lateral and oblique. Laterally retract the latter 2 nerves to better expose the vessels. Retracting the gastrocnemius heads (possibly w/ vertical releasing incision) will better show distal aspect of vessels.
         - The popliteal vein will be anteromedial to the tibial nerve and the popliteal artery will be anteromedial to the vein. *Note*: the divided short saphenous vein will lead to the popliteal vein.

C. Regional operations

1. *Neck*
   a. *Carotid TEA*
      i. *Indications*: symptomatic carotid stenosis of ≥ 50%. Asymptomatic dz ≥ 60% (more controversial).
      ii. *Instruments*: #10 blade, Weitlaner, Rummel tourniquet, Dacron patch, umbilical tapes, Argyle shunt, 6-0 Prolene, vascular needle drivers.
      iii. *Incidental*: carotid TEA can be performed through a longitudinal arteriotomy or using an eversion endarterectomy technique. The eversion technique is faster as does not require a patch angioplasty, but is difficult to perform if shunting is desired or needed. The technique described below is through a longitudinal arteriotomy.
         - Place pt supine w/ head extended and rotated to opposite side. Incise along upper $^2/_3$ of anterior border of SCM, curving posteriorly if above level of ear lobe to avoid injury to marginal mandibular nerve.
         - Bovie through platysma, then divide, ligate facial vein to expose carotid sheath—apex of ansa cervicalis (ansa hypoglossi) often found at this point, and may be divided w/ relative impunity if necessary.
         - The facial vein is generally a good landmark for the location of the carotid bifurcation. This vein will require division for adequate exposure of the carotid artery.
         - Open sheath over common carotid artery, then encircle inferiorly w/ umbilical tape (+/– and Rummel tourniquet) or vessel loop. Next approach external carotid artery, encircling first branch (superior thyroid artery) followed by separate umbilical tape (w/ Rummel) or loop around external carotid. Place a loop around the distal internal carotid in a palpably soft segment.
         - If higher exposure is required, the digastric muscle can be divided and the hypoglossal nerve mobilized. The hypoglossal nerve is fixed in place by the SCM branch of the ECA. If this small artery is divided, the hypoglossal nerve can be more easily mobilized. For higher exposure toward the skull base, the stylohyoid tendon can be divided and the stylohyoid process can be removed using a bone Rongeur. This places the glossopharyngeal nerve at great risk and should be done w/ care. If lower exposure is necessary, the omohyoid muscle can be divided. Further proximal exposure requires median sternotomy.
         - Heparinize pt (5000 U IV), then occlude internal carotid, external carotid, and common carotid (in order).
         - Anterolateral arteriotomy from CCA across ICA lesion then made. Decision for shunt (*several choices*: Argyle, Pruitt-Inahara, Javid, etc.) can be done nonselectively, or based on stump pressure (want at least 50 mm Hg in CCA after occlusion of all but ICA), EEG findings if neuro-monitoring utilized, or mental status changes if done under awake anesthesia.
         - Endarterectomy performed, including high-pressure injection of heparinized saline at edges to identify shelves/flaps.
         - Randomized controlled trials as well as large series have demonstrated a benefit to patching (decreased restenosis), and this should be done in essentially all pts. Can use vein (saphenous vein from ankle in men, from groin in females due to risk of patch blowout), Dacron, PTFE, bovine pericardium. No differences have been found in terms of stroke, restenosis w/ different patch types.
         - *Unclamp in the following order*: ECA, CCA (allow several cardiac cycles to pass to clear the endarterectomy site), ICA.
         - Many surgeons obtain postop Duplex scan, then awaken pt in operating room to check for gross neuro deficits before extubation.
2. *Upper extremity*
   a. *Axillobifemoral bypass*
      i. *Indications*: most commonly indicated for inflow dz of lower extremities complicated by contaminated peritoneal cavity (i.e., after removal of infected aortic graft), or a pt who is physiologically not able to tolerate an open abdominal operation for tx of aorto-iliac occlusive dz.

ii. *Instruments*: large vascular instruments w/ variety of medium/small vascular clamps, self-retaining retractors (e.g., Weitlaner, Gelpi).

- Pt supine w/ target upper extremity abducted (note, right innominate/subclavian artery usu. less burdened w/ plaque than proximal left subclavian artery).
- Make vertical incisions over both common femoral arteries, which will be revisited later in the case.
- Incise 2 cm beneath and parallel to clavicle from sternoclavicular joint to coracoid process. Split pectoralis major fibers then divide clavipectoral fascia to expose subclavian vein.
- Mobilize subclavian vein, then retract caudad to expose subclavian artery. Divide and ligate highest thoracic artery coming off inferior, proximal portion of exposed artery.
- Pass tunneling instrument (prior to heparinization) from exposed artery underneath pectoralis muscles then along midaxillary line, anterior to ASIS, then medially to pass superficial to inguinal ligament into groin incision. Attach ringed graft (8- to 10-mm diameter, depending on subclavian diameter) to tunneling device and pass it.
- *Proximal anastomosis*:
  - Clamp subclavian artery proximally and distally, then create longitudinal arteriotomy exactly the diameter of selected graft.
  - Fashion anastomosis w/ running 5-0 or 6-0 monofilament nonabsorbable suture, w/ graft passing posterior/deep to subclavian vein as the latter is retracted caudad for exposure.
  - Place rubbershod clamp on graft close to the level of the anastomosis, then restore perfusion to upper extremity by releasing arterial clamps.
  - Make sure to leave enough slack in the bypass to prevent avulsion once the pt begins using the arm.
- *Distal (ipsilateral) anastomosis*:
  - Clamp common femoral, superficial femoral, and profunda femoral arteries. Create longitudinal arteriotomy on common femoral artery. Endarterectomy a/o extension of incision onto SFA or PFA is/are performed as appropriate.
  - Fashion anastomosis w/ running 5-0 monofilament nonabsorbable suture.
  - Before releasing arterial clamps, excise an ellipse of graft from the hood over the distal anastomosis, and fashion an end-to-side anastomosis w/ a 2nd segment of graft, which will perfuse the contralateral lower extremity.
  - Release clamps from subclavian anastomosis and CFA, then flush blood through crossover limb. Reapply these clamps, then release SFA, PFA clamps to flush again w/ backbleeding. Finally, clamp crossover limb, and remove all other clamps to restore perfusion to lower extremity.
- *Distal (crossover) anastomosis*:
  - Pass crossover limb to contralateral side via a subcutaneous, suprapubic tunnel made w/ finger dissection or a tunneling device (care should be taken to prevent passage through the fascia and into the bladder; some surgeons prefer a subcutaneous tunnel, while others prefer a subfascial tunnel for passage of a fem-fem graft).
  - Clamp CFA, SFA, and PFA on the new side, then create longitudinal arteriotomy as described above. Fashion anastomosis as described above, flushing just before completion.
- If done for an infected aortic graft, the graft excision can be done immediately after the Ax-femoral bypass or on the following day, depending on the stability of the pt.

b. *Vascular access*

i. *Native*:

- *Radiocephalic (Brescia-Cimino) fistula*: evaluate vein w/ tourniquet below elbow—want at least 3-mm diameter. Incise 2–3 cm longitudinally midway between vein and radial artery (distal radius). Dissect both vessels, place loops, ligate vein, swing down to form end-to-side anastomosis w/ 6-0 Prolene. Avoid injury to median nerve and FCR tendon. Verify flow w/ Doppler more proximal in arm.

- *Brachiocephalic fistula*: make transverse incision proximal to antecubital crease. Dissect cephalic vein in upper arm, and distally ligate. Divide bicipital aponeurosis to mobilize brachial artery. Fashion end-to-side anastomosis proximal to crease. Avoid injury to median nerve.
- *Basilic vein transposition*: incise over brachial artery. Divide brachial fascia, and dissect basilic vein from axilla to antecubital fossa, ligating branches. Transpose to superficial location (more anterior/lateral) via tunneling. Some surgeons will perform this operation in 2 stages w/ the brachiobasilic anastomosis done at the first procedure and the transposition done at a later time after maturation of the fistula.

ii. *Prosthetic grafts*:

- *Forearm loop*: incise distal to antecubital crease. Tunnel graft w/ counterincisions along volar surface of forearm. Use brachial artery and cephalic, brachial, or basilic vein (want at least 4 mm).
- *Upper arm loop*: make longitudinal incision in distal upper arm and dissect out brachial artery. Next, make more proximal incision for appropriate vein (cephalic, brachial, axillary, or basilic). Can also be done w/ autogenous femoral vein/saphenous vein or cryopreserved femoral artery/vein.

3. *Abdomen*

a. *Abdominal aortic aneurysm* (ruptured)

i. *Indications*: abdominal pain in pt w/ known AAA.

ii. *Instruments*: general abdominal instruments, large vascular instruments/clamps, self-retaining retractor (Omnitract, Bookwalter, Thompson-Farley, Iron Intern, etc.).

- Make vertical midline incision from xiphoid to pubis.
- *Location and size of hematoma dictates where to gain proximal control*:
  - *Below renal vessels*:
    - Incise peritoneum over the hematoma to the left of duodenum.
    - Use finger through hematoma to guide straight or curved vascular clamp to obtain initial control through the hematoma.
    - If this maneuver is unsuccessful, consider passing a Foley or other inflatable balloon catheter retrograde through an incision in the visualized anterior aneurysm wall below the vessels.
  - *At diaphragm*:
    - Divide gastrohepatic omentum.
    - Retract lesser curvature of stomach inferiorly and to the left.
    - Aorta passes through crura posterior and to the right of the esophagus; occlude w/ vascular clamp or compression w/ sponge stick.
    - Incise peritoneum overlying aneurysm, then bluntly dissect w/in hematoma to gain access to and control of infrarenal aorta before releasing control at level of diaphragm.
- Distal control is achieved by dividing peritoneum overlying iliac arteries and clamping, taking care to avoid injury to the ureters as they cross over the iliac arteries and the veins that run underneath the arteries.
  - Again, if hematoma obscures ability to visualize iliacs, intraluminal balloon tamponade from w/in the aneurysm may be used to occlude the iliacs arteries.
- After clamping, consider regional heparinization via injection into iliac arteries.
- Remove mural thrombus and suture ligate lumbar vessels to prevent backbleeding. Suture ligate IMA unless reimplantation is planned. If occluded or brisk pulsatile backbleeding, suture ligation OK; if weak backbleeding indicating poor collateral flow is seen, reimplantation should be considered.
- Suture woven (not knitted—too permeable) Dacron graft w/ 3-0 Prolene suture (tube graft usu. appropriate, unless iliac involvement requires aortoiliac or aortofemoral bypass) (see aortobifemoral description below).
- Before finishing distal anastomosis, release occlusion of iliacs to assess patency from backbleeding.

    - If no backbleeding, pass embolectomy catheter to remove thrombus.
  - Close aneurysm wall, then peritoneum, over graft w/ sutures.

b. *Mesenteric artery embolectomy*

   i. *Indications*: acute mesenteric ischemia from embolus of thrombosis of SMA.

   ii. *Instruments*: general abdominal instruments plus large vascular instruments and a self-retaining retractor (Omnitract, Bookwalter, Thompson-Farley, Iron Intern, etc.).

   iii. *Insights*: prompt clinical dx confirmed w/ arteriography is critical.

   - Enter abdomen through generous vertical midline incision, then explore peritoneal contents.
   - Lift transverse colon and omentum cephalad, then retract small bowel and mesentery cephalad and to the pt's right. Locate SMA at root of mesentery and transverse mesocolon before it passes under duodenum and pancreas (often finding the middle colic artery and following it down to the SMA can be helpful).
   - Incise mesentery overlying SMA, dissect out target section of artery, then pass proximal and distal vessel loops.
   - Systemically heparinize the pt, then create a transverse or longitudinal arteriotomy (transverse arteriotomy only if the vessel feels normal in quality; if diseased, a longitudinal arteriotomy will be useful if a patch angioplasty or subsequent bypass needed), through which a balloon catheter is advanced, inflated and then w/drawn (proximally, then distally).
   - If successful, close w/ nonabsorbable monofilament suture or vein/bovine pericardial patch.

c. *Mesenteric artery bypass*

   i. *Indications*: mesenteric ischemia due to proximal celiac a/o SMA occlusive lesion not amenable to embolectomy.

   ii. *Instruments*: abdominal instruments and large/medium vascular clamps and instruments; self-retaining abdominal retractor system (Omnitract, Bookwalter, Thompson-Farley, Iron Intern, etc.).

   iii. *Insights*: conduit may be synthetic (ribbed Dacron resistant to compression) unless significant bowel ischemia/necrosis or spillage of succus—contamination risk mandates use of vein (saphenous or femoral vein; can also use cryopreserved femoral vein/artery). Priority should be given to fashioning end-to-side anastomosis between SMA and aorta. Celiac may be also considered after restoring SMA.

   - Expose SMA as described for mesenteric artery embolectomy. Create longitudinal arteriotomy on SMA if not already accomplished.
   - Fashion end-to-side graft to arteriotomy w/ reversed saphenous vein or prosthetic graft using 6-0 running nonabsorbable monofilament suture. Anastomose graft distally to segment of infrarenal aorta/iliac artery that is accessible w/out kinking the graft (evaluate how graft will lie *after* returning bowel to usual location).
   - Celiac axis may be also be revascularized in retrograde fashion w/ graft between infrarenal aorta/iliac artery and common hepatic artery. Mobilization of duodenal c-loop and pancreatic head w/ Kocher maneuver facilitates passage of graft behind c-loop, which minimizes kinking.
   - *Alternately, antegrade anastomosis to both celiac and SMA may be accomplished in the following fashion* (less potential kinking, but dissection is more difficult):
     - Divide gastrohepatic omentum to enter lesser sac, then mobilize and retract left lobe of liver.
     - Retract esophagus (after placing OGT) laterally, identify right diaphragmatic crus, then divide crus until down to celiac plexus overlying aorta.
     - Systemically heparinize then occlude aorta w/ side-biting vascular clamp (i.e., c-clamp, Satinsky clamp, or Lemole clamp).
     - Perform end-to-side anastomosis between graft and aorta w/ running 3-0 Prolene. If use a single limb graft, implant celiac axis onto side of graft then anastomose end of graft into side of SMA. Alternately, a bifurcated (i.e., 12 × 6) graft can be anastomosed end-to-end into celiac and end-to-side into SMA.

4. *Lower extremity*
   a. *Aortobifemoral bypass*
      i. *Indications*: aortoiliac occlusive dz, aortoiliac aneurysm.
      ii. *Instruments*: self-retaining abdominal retractor, 3-0 Prolene, 5-0 Prolene, bifurcated Dacron graft, angled vascular clamps, Weitlaner retractors, rubber-shod hemostats, umbilical tape, vessel loops, rubber-shod straight vascular clamp, Satinsky clamp, Rummel tourniquets.
      iii. *Incidental*: an end-to-side proximal anastomosis is generally preferred, but an end-to-end anastomosis is preferred. When there is an aortic aneurysm requiring repair, bilateral CIA occlusion negating the benefit of leaving antegrade perfusion for the pelvis.
         - Make vertical or transverse incisions over the common femoral arteries to expose them from inguinal ligament down to their bifurcations. Gain individual control over SFA and profunda (divide and ligate branches of profunda vein as necessary for exposure). Divide posterior portion of inguinal ligament and transversus fascia as it crosses the femoral artery. Pass a finger anterior to the femoral/EIA into the retroperitoneum and gently clear the retroperitoneal tissues anterior to the EIA as far proximal as possible before proceeding w/ opening the abdomen.
         - Make a vertical midline or transverse abdominal incision, explore intraabdominal organs, and retract transverse colon superiorly before packing small bowel off to the right and sigmoid in LLQ.
         - Incise parietal peritoneum over aorta, and continue incision to ligament of Treitz. Divide between 4th portion of duodenum medially, and IMV laterally (may divide IMV if necessary), exposing left renal vein crossing over aorta just above and posterior.
         - Expose artery between renal vessels and IMA.
         - Using gentle blunt dissection w/ a finger, the retroperitoneal tunnel should be created prior to heparinization to prevent hemorrhage w/in the tunnel. An umbilical tape or ringed clamp can be left in the tunnel for passage of the graft after completion of the proximal anastomosis.
         - Systemically heparinize w/ 100 mg/kg, and cross-clamp infra-renal aorta just below renal arteries and further distal for distal control. If an end-to-side anastomosis is planned, perform a longitudinal arteriotomy for the proximal anastomosis. A local endarterectomy may be required if this portion of the aorta is diseased. If an end-to-side anastomosis is planned, transect section of infrarenal aorta between clamps. Oversew distal stump w/ running 3-0 Prolene in 1–2 rows. Perform local endarterectomy if necessary to get good tissue for closure.
         - Inspect proximal stump and remove loose plaque or thrombus. Suture prosthesis to infrarenal aorta in end-to-end fashion w/ running 3-0 Prolene using large bites. Begin posteriorly, and tie anteriorly.
         - Pinch graft closed w/ left hand, ensure distal ends are clamped, and slowly release proximal clamp to check adequacy of anastomosis. Reclamp, flush graft w/ heparinized saline.
         - Using a clamp, pass the graft limbs (under pressure to prevent kinking) through the tunnels created previously.
         - Vascular clamps are applied to CFA, SFA, and PFA, and longitudinal arteriotomy is made in CFA. Plaque or stenosis in either outflow vessel may require local endarterectomy a/o extension of incision.
         - Stretch Dacron graft and cut to length (can test by pinching limb and releasing proximal clamp to fill w/ blood). Cut obliquely for end-to-side anastomosis. Sew anastomosis w/ running 5-0 Prolene from heel to toe. Notify anesthesia when you are about 10 min from finishing anastomosis so they can prepare for revascularization physiology.
         - Briefly release distal clamps of right groin to allow backbleeding (removes air). Reclamp, then briefly release proximal aortic clamp, flushing blood through open left limb (evacuates debris).
         - Place vascular clamp on proximal left limb of graft. Reapply SFA and PFA clamps to further flush material retrograde up right; after several seconds, release the right clamps to reperfuse the right leg.

- Evacuate blood from left limb and rinse w/ heparinized saline. Apply clamps to left CFA, SFA, and PFA. Make left arteriotomy and anastomosis as on other side. Before completing anastomosis, flush left limb of graft by releasing proximal left clamp, then complete suture line (again, inform anesthesia of your progress). Remove distal clamps.

b. *Femoral-popliteal bypass*

i. *Insights*: this technique describes use of reversed saphenous vein for conduit; the use of *in situ* vein is acceptable, but less frequently used primarily due to surgeon preference and comfort level. Some dislike the *in situ* technique because of the superficial nature of the graft and the possibility of graft exposure w/ wound dehiscence. In trauma cases, vein should be taken from contralateral extremity unless that extremity injured equally or worse. If the vein is reversed, a valvulotome is not necessary. If nonreversed/transposed or *in situ*, a variety of valvulotomes may be utilized.

- Prep and drape both legs from groin to ankle w/ hips externally rotated and knees gently flexed.
- *Exposure of arterial targets*:
  - Make a longitudinal or transverse incision over common femoral artery (longitudinal preferred if a femoral endarterectomy/profundaplasty are needed), then a 2nd longitudinal incision over the medial knee extending from the medial femoral condyle, for ~ 10 cm.
  - Anterior muscle in the distal incision will be sartorius; just posterior will be gracilis, which is divided along w/ semitendonosus just posterior to gracilis and semimembranosus, which is deep/lateral to semitendonosus.
  - Divide the medial head of gastrocnemius and retract posteriorly to visualize the Infrageniculate popliteal artery anterior to it corresponding vein and tibial nerve. Encircle target arterial segment w/ vessel loops proximally and distally.
- *Harvesting/preparation of vein* (assuming harvesting from contralateral extremity):
  - Incise over saphenous vein and dissect distally from saphenofemoral junction until adequate length achieved.
  - Ligate and divide all side branches. Vein may be harvested via single long incision or multiple shorter ones.
  - Excise saphenous vein and flush w/ heparinized saline. Distend w/ saline to check for leaks, then soak in papaverine/heparinized saline solution.
  - Pass tunneling device from groin incision under sartorius until in popliteal incision. The vein can be tunneled now, or after the proximal anastomosis. Passing under pressure after the anastomosis helps prevent twisting of the graft. If passing prior to the anastomosis, the graft should be pressurized w/ vein solution, tied to the tunneling device, and passed while still distended.
- *Creation of proximal anastomosis*:
  - Clamp CFA, SFA, and PFA, then create longitudinal arteriotomy over CFA.
  - Spatulate vein and fashion end-to-side anastomosis w/ running 6-0 suture as above.
- *Creation of distal anastomosis*:
  - Systemically heparinize, then clamp (i.e., w/ Heifetz clamps) popliteal artery. Create longitudinal arteriotomy.
  - Cut end of vein longitudinally the same length as the arteriotomy. Fashion end-to-side anastomosis w/ 6-0 nonabsorbable monofilament suture.
- Remove femoral artery clamps followed by proximal popliteal clamp to wash debris into diseased segment. Finally release distal popliteal clamp and obtain a completion study (e.g., arteriogram or intraoperative duplex). Confirm distal signals and graft-dependent flow (clamp graft while listening to signals).

INDEX

NOTES

NOTES

NOTES